WorldCALL

Routledge Studies in Computer Assisted Language Learning

EDITED BY CAROL CHAPPELLE

WorldCALL

International Perspectives on
Computer-Assisted Language Learning

Edited by Mike Levy, Françoise Blin, Claire Bradin Siskin and Osamu Takeuchi

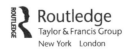

Routledge
Taylor & Francis Group
New York London

First published 2011
by Routledge
711 Third Avenue, New York, NY 10017

Simultaneously published in the UK
by Routledge
2 Park Square, Milton Park, Abingdon, Oxfordshire OX14 4RN

First issued in paperback 2014

Routledge is an imprint of the Taylor & Francis Group, an informa business

Library of Congress Cataloging in Publication Data
    WorldCALL: international perspectives on computer-assisted language learning / edited by Mike Levy...[et al.].
        p. cm. — (Routledge studies in computer assisted language learning; 5)
    Includes bibliographical references and index.
    1. Language and languages — Computer-assisted instruction. 2. Language and languages — Globalization. I. Levy, Mike, 1953–
    P53.85.W68 2011
    418.0078'5 — dc22
    2010031672

ISBN 978-0-415-88086-2 (hbk)
ISBN 978-1-138-81055-6 (pbk)
ISBN 978-0-203-83176-2 (ebk)

Contents

PART II:
Developing Language Skills through Technology

PART III:
Materials Design and Development

Figures

Tables

Preface

From its successful beginning in Melbourne (1998), and equally ambitious second conference in Banff (2003), WorldCALL has consistently attracted a broad spectrum of international CALL researchers, representing both highly developed and less well-served nations, and highly experienced and neophyte researchers alike. Those conferences represented collective aims of the founding organizations (EUROCALL, CALICO, ATELL, CCALL) and tended to reflect the early strength of CALL in Europe and the English-speaking world. LET (the Japan Association for Language Education and Technology), the hosts of WorldCALL III in Fukuoka in August 2008, were anxious to continue the same wide-ranging, global tradition whilst at the same time providing an attractive, accessible venue for the rapidly growing numbers of CALL colleagues in Asia-Pacific regions. In that, they were resoundingly successful, as the chapters printed here also testify. Entitled "CALL Bridges the World," the formal part of the conference consisted of 157 presentations. As well, continuing another tradition of WorldCALL, 13 scholarship winners from "underserved" CALL regions were able to hear and meet with some of the approximately 650 attendees from 33 countries.

The range of chapters in this volume is too broad (and deep) for me to introduce individually here, but a sense of their scope can be seen in the part headings, which gather chapters addressing innovation in technology and pedagogy, aids to skills development, materials design issues, and concerns in training learners, as well as an often-forgotten necessity—teacher education in using CALL. Our thanks to these authors, and all those who presented their work "live" in Fukuoka.

As Liaison Officer for LET, it was my honor to work with some extremely dedicated national and international colleagues. Principal among them, of course, was Professor Mike Levy, who was behind this third WorldCALL from the very beginning. Without his vision and commitment, nothing could have been accomplished. His firm editorial hand also guides this volume.

I cannot name all those who contributed to the success of the conference here, but I would like to acknowledge particularly the tireless LET

Organizing Committee members, and Françoise Blin and Claire Bradin Siskin, the co-chairs of the Program Committee, who did so much to encourage submissions and shape the formal part of the conference.

Akio Iwasaki
School of Language Communication
Tokyo International University

Introduction

WorldCALL: International Perspectives on Computer-Assisted Language Learning

With the third WorldCALL conference in Fukuoka, Japan, in August 2008, the WorldCALL concept has gathered further momentum and focus. From its infancy in 1998 at the inaugural WorldCALL conference in Melbourne, it has moved forward with confidence. At the most recent conference the worldwide representation, including the participation and significant contribution of the 13 scholarship holders, helped shape a long-term commitment to collaboration and the exchange of ideas at a face-to-face conference at the global level. Also essential to this process is recording the ongoing work of the conference participants. As such, this book represents the distillation of ideas initially presented at the conference. The first two conferences were represented by publications of key works presented, and this volume follows that tradition with the most recent contributions to this collective endeavor. With 20 chapters and 35 authors from 15 countries and all five continents, the book is both an expression of the diversity of CALL around the globe and an expression of a desire for collaboration and the exchange of ideas.

The five parts of the book on new technologies/new pedagogies, language skills, materials design and development, learner training, and teacher education represent a well-rounded yet still evolving collection of perspectives on the application of new technologies to language learning. Together the sections reflect the range, interests, and goals of modern-day CALL.

Part I, "New Technologies, New Pedagogies," covers a range of contemporary technologies in use in language learning together with their attendant pedagogies.

To begin, Hsien-Chin Liou (Chapter 1) investigates how blogging may be employed effectively in a collaborative approach to writing and multimodal literacy. The pedagogy emerges in the shape of the assignments and the task goals and also, importantly, in the ways in which language learners are required to collaborate with each other through co-writing, peer review, and self-reflection. In this chapter, students' perceptions of the process are carefully evaluated so that refinements may be made. In Chapter 2, Wai Meng Chan, Ing Ru Chen, and Martin Döpel consider podcasting, where again the pedagogical approach is paramount. In this regard, a detailed rationale for the pedagogical design of supplementary podcast lessons associated with a German course is described. Each podcast lesson requires a well-constructed blend of language content and pedagogical elements. The pedagogy is operationalized through the choice of elements in each podcast, sequencing that encourages engagement and careful pacing, and the integration of the podcasts week by week into the course as a whole. As with all chapters in this part, the innovation is followed by systematic evaluation with students.

Mobile learning is another important new development that is fast making inroads into mainstream CALL. Midori Kimura, Hiroyuki Obari, and Yoshiko Goda (Chapter 3) look at this topic with a particular emphasis on the options available and their relative merits for language learning. In particular, this chapter compares a mobile group of learners with a PC group, and the authors also consider how mobile technologies can effectively support and foster autonomous learning. Again, locating the optimal pedagogy is critical. This focus is also highlighted in the following chapter where a pedagogical innovation has become possible through the creative use of an established technology. Such is the case with e-mail tandem whereby learners with a different native language (L1) communicate via e-mail using their respective target languages (L2) while providing feedback on their partners' messages in their L1. Akihiko Sasaki and Osamu Takeuchi (Chapter 4) develop and extend the existing body of work on e-mail tandem by investigating metalinguistic awareness in this setting, and again the authors evaluate the results from a learner's perspective. In the final chapter in this part, Yuri Nishihori considers collaborative learning at a distance with multicultural classes located in different countries with an emphasis on learner awareness and cross-cultural understanding. In this study, connections are made through a variety of broadband network technologies, including video-conferencing, text-based discussion, and network-based display sharing systems. The pedagogical implications of each option are described, compared, and evaluated.

Part II of the book, "Developing Language Skills through Technology," considers the learning and teaching of pronunciation, writing, and grammar with specially designed programs and applications to address these goals. This part includes some of the more technical contributions to the volume, illustrating some of the programming and linguistic challenges being addressed in the CALL arena. The part begins with Ferit Kiliçkaya (Chapter 6) with a focus on pronunciation and brings with it a valuable overview of recent developments, especially in relation to text-to-speech software. The chapter then evaluates accent reduction and text-to-speech software as it might be applied in elementary language classes. In Chapter 7, Erifili Roubou looks at learners' patterns of revision in writing by making use of computer keystroke recording software to catalog and explore writing processes. The effects of the word processor on writing are examined from both a quantitative and a qualitative point of view. A long-standing area of interest in CALL, also relating to writing, has been the research and development in intelligent CALL (ICALL). One of the key goals in ICALL is to design computer algorithms that are capable of providing effective diagnostic feedback to language learners. In this regard, Sylvie Thouësny and Françoise Blin (Chapter 8) discuss language learner modeling and ways in which the computer may relate morpho-syntactic errors to the students' underlying knowledge of the grammatical system. In a somewhat similar vein, Karin Harbusch and Gerard Kempen (Chapter 9) consider the design of a natural-language paraphrase generator, and how and when this may be used for modeling and providing feedback on the grammatical structure of L2 sentences. The system is highly innovative in that it can provide feedback as the students actually construct a sentence. Concluding Part II, utilizing another well-established technology in CALL, Yuxia Wang and Suen Caesar Lun (Chapter 10) consider the application of corpus and concordancing techniques in language learning. In this chapter, the authors describe ways in which these technologies can provide learners with models that potentially can facilitate their acquisition of verb syntactic usage. These models are accompanied by pedagogical strategies associated with the learning task; implicit and explicit strategies, used in conjunction with the concordance program, are then compared and assessed.

The third part of this volume on materials design and development represents a well-established area of activity in CALL. As might be expected with contributions from different parts of the world, the scale, focus, goals, and technologies employed vary from project to project, although a focus on design and evaluation remains a constant throughout. In the first chapter of the part, Nathalie Ticheler and Itesh Sachdev (Chapter 11) describe the Flexi-Pack Project for languages of the wider world. This project aims to promote the learning of less frequently taught languages, such as Turkish, Bengali, and Nepali, using blended language learning that combines face-to-face learning and self-study with multimedia materials. The authors present the pedagogical rationale for the project and their findings from a preliminary evaluation covering staff and student responses to the materials and the learning experience. Chapter 12 by Ana Gimeno-Sanz also describes a course development project with its rationale, but in this instance with a particular focus on the design of authoring templates that facilitate the creation and integration of video, graphics, audio, and text into a web-enhanced language learning environment. This project also involves the design of an authoring shell or "content manager" which allows users to create a database of selected multimedia materials, including exercises and a wide range of resources. In the next chapter, Debbie Corder and Alice U-Mackey (Chapter 13) discuss social networking and such emerging technologies as wikis, blogs, and e-portfolios and the ways in which they may be effectively utilized in course design and development. A course in intercultural competence is described with its pedagogical rationale and assessment approaches and activities. A particular emphasis is given to the ways in which the various technological and pedagogical elements are combined to create a cohesive whole for students. In the final project of this part, Akiyoshi Suzuki and Teresa Kuwamura describe the E-Job 100 project, which involves the creation of a website that contains videos that show how people of various occupations read, write, listen to, and speak English at their workplaces. The design enables students to access language documents that are used in a real work environment and students are able to play different roles according to their chosen occupations. As with all projects described in this part, following implementation, the impact of the innovation is carefully evaluated.

The last two parts in this volume, on learner training and teacher education, in one important sense go hand in hand. Learner training in CALL, often undervalued or overlooked, helps ensure optimal value in any CALL activity, and therefore must form an important component in teacher preparation. Also, if introduced effectively, the teacher experience can be generative in that a thoughtful awareness of how the teacher is introduced and trained in a new application or technique can potentially be transferred when that same teacher is training students. For both teacher and student, knowing how to actively manage and control the learning environment is absolutely crucial to success. Part IV on learner training includes one chapter organized around a skill and another broader perspective structured around the design of a course. Kenneth Romeo and Philip Hubbard (Chapter 15) discuss the training required for students to use software and resources for listening effectively, although many of the ideas introduced here are readily transferable to other skills also. The chapter explains how to prepare students for the very considerable range of technology-mediated materials available, with guidelines covering technical, strategic, and pedagogical aspects. Then, in the next chapter, Maija Tammelin, Berit Peltonen, and Pasi Puranen (Chapter 16) present a rationale for learner guidance around four themes: orientation for e-learning; e-learning skills and the roles of an e-learner; the roles of an e-tutor; and interaction, peer reviewing, and feedback.

The final part of the book provides for perspectives on teacher education from different parts of the world, including South America, Europe, and Japan. Though the geographical regions are different, exerting different forces and influences that lead to varying priorities from region to region, there remain important commonalities across the contexts. Thus, in Chapter 17, Carla Barsotti and Claudia Martins provide a view from Brazil, where the majority of the population does not have access to ICTs. The chapter focuses on the design and evaluation of teacher education programs in this setting with a special emphasis on first understanding the diverse needs of language teachers in the region, and then using this information to provide practical ways to meet the requirements that are identified. Marie-Noëlle Lamy (Chapter 18) also takes a South American perspective, this time from Argentina. Again, great care is taken to research local needs and to establish the goals and priorities of the participant group as a basis for collaborative course development for in-service teacher education. An appreciation of the local context and setting along with cultural-historical factors is found to be crucial in the development of the course. This is followed in Chapter 19 by Salomi Papadima-Sophocleous, who reports on the design and evaluation of student e-portfolios used with a group of BA language and literature students studying CALL in Cyprus. The portfolios give students an opportunity to create digitized presentations of their work and stand as evidence of their current knowledge and abilities; they can also be used as a point of departure for further exploration and development. The final chapter of the book, from Japan, concludes the teacher education part. Here Seijiro Sumi argues for the importance of the teachers' voice in the context of "normalized" CALL activity, that is, where the technology has been integrated into the classroom to such a degree that its use is regarded as normal, everyday activity. In any teacher education exercise, listening to the teachers' voice is critical, and arguably this is the only way the course may be refined and improved to better meet the needs of its audience.

In considering this volume as a whole, and while it is recognized that the contexts may vary, an underlying theme through many of the chapters is the focus on design and evaluation. It is this recurring focus, widely evident in modern day CALL, that so often brings the local and the global together through a common interest. This focus upon design and evaluation reflects a commitment by individuals and groups globally to engage with new technology responsibly by creating robust pedagogical designs that are carefully and systematically evaluated. The latter two parts of the book on learner training and teacher education also show a commitment to communicate these ideas to others with the ultimate goal of making language learning with new technologies as effective as possible.

Mike Levy
Françoise Blin
Claire Bradin Siskin
Osamu Takeuchi

Part I
New Technologies, New Pedagogies

1 Blogging, Collaborative Writing, and Multimodal Literacy in an EFL Context

Hsien-Chin Liou

INTRODUCTION

Nowadays, the screen plays a more important role in modern society than ever before, although it may not immediately supplant paper. Scollon and Scollon (2004) make it clear that a dichotomized view of face-to-face and Internet-mediated life, and the difference between real and virtual, dissolves under examination of lived communicative practice (Thorne, 2005). Internet-mediated language education emphasizes participation in dialogue and development of the linguistic and meta-communicative resources necessary for carrying out such processes (Thorne, 2005). Tandem learning, reciprocity, and learner autonomy may evolve with Internet-mediated language education. Visual elements in the new medium, particularly with multimodal texts, have gained prominence. Multimodal texts integrate not only text-based writing, but also sound (music and speech) and images (still, animated, and video-based). The interest of readers dominates what brings sense of the (written) representation. Digital technologies offer new opportunities of literacy practice so that the reader can become author, perhaps even in the process of reading, in ways that were not possible with the book.

The advantages of setting up a blog-based language course lie in ease of use and collecting information, the communicative features, and enhancement of self-expression. We have commonly observed that young people are more fluent with multimedia than print, compared with those from older generations. As graphics, sound files, and video become common in online texts, multiple means of communication enable personal arguments (Nelson, 2006). How students make use of various modes of communication to make an argument and establish relationships with readers (Lin, 2008) is what researchers may want to know and what writing teachers may want to teach to their learners.

While collaborative learning has been advocated in the general education literature, the complexity and interactivity of online collaboration cannot be dismissed easily. In Hertz-Lazarowitz and Bar-Natan (2002), 599 children were surveyed on their perceptions of writing efficiency, self-regulation, and experiences of writing with computers. Computers and peers are the key element for students' writing development. Gollin (1999) studied a collaborative writing project at a private consultancy in Australia. Written and spoken products were documented to show the impact of their interactions with contributors and informants outside the team members. This study demonstrated the complexity and interactivity inherent in collaborative writing and the roles of personal and organizational power in the writing process. In a study on network-based collaborative projects among native and nonnative speakers of Spanish, Lee (2004) found that such online collaboration promoted scaffolding for composing meaning and form. Lee pointed out that learners' language proficiency, computer skills, and age differences were crucial factors that led to successful collaborative interaction.

In the project to be reported in this chapter, blogging is used as an instructional platform as it enables traditional writing pedagogy, online interaction, and multimodal expression. The target participants were 25 English-majoring undergraduate students who were taking a writing course in an English as a Foreign Language college context. Various blog assignments were designed that encouraged peer review, collaborative writing, and incorporation of multimedia. Specific cases of 8 participants' online works were examined in detail to investigate their use of multimodal texts on the blog with semiotic awareness through transduction and transformation (Kress, 2003). Before describing the details of the case study itself, a brief literature concerning online peer review and multimodal expressions will be discussed.

ONLINE PEER REVIEW

The advantages of online peer review and technology-enhanced assessment of writing have been thoroughly discussed in a volume by Breuch (2004) and supported by Anson (2003), Liou (2009), and Liou and Peng (2009), among others. Embedded commentary, online response after reading, conferencing, and streaming video are discussed in Anson. Liou (2009) examined the effects of using a web-based co-editing platform to help college EFL learners to write more accurate and better English essays. Based on a single group pre-test/post-test research design with three cycles of drafting, peer response, and revising in pair-work, a test on adverbial connectors and verb–noun collocation and a timed writing task were given before and after the three cycles, followed by an evaluation questionnaire. Additionally, students' learning processes were documented using their drafts and revised versions and the online discussion logs out of four representative peer dyads. Results showed that online peer response could foster learners' ability in both the use of collocations and connectors, and overall writing quality with students' satisfaction. Moreover, with explicit instruction and prior preparation for online peer collaboration, learners were found capable of using various language functions to scaffold their peers or to complement each other collaboratively during online peer response sessions. Liou and Peng (2009) supported the usefulness of teacher training for blog-enhanced peer reviews.

MULTIMODALITY, MULTIMEDIA, AND GENRE

We are in a multimedia age, and traditional means of reading and writing are enhanced or transformed dramatically. The soundtrack of a musical score, speech, and moving and still images of various kinds are prevalent when we surf online. In the past, we had the ability to deal with the stable social frames and resources for representation; now, we need the notion of design (Kress, 2003, 2005), which says:

> In this social and cultural environment, with these demands for communication of these materials, for that audience, with these resources, and given these interests of mine, what is the design that best meets these requirements? Design focuses forward; it assumes that resources are never entirely apt but will need to be transformed in relation to all the contingencies of this environment now and the demands made. (Kress, 2005, p. 20)

We should cultivate the type of EFL learners who are equipped with an agency: the agency of "the individual who has a social history, a present social location, an understanding of the potentials of the resources for communication, and who acts transformationally on the resources environment and, thereby, on self are requirements of communication" (Kress, 2005, p. 20). What Kress means by a process of learning involves "transformative engagement in the world, transformation constantly of the self in that engagement, transformation of the resources for representation outwardly and inwardly" (p. 21).

A theory of multimodal meaning-making must account for the complementary processes of *transformation* and *transduction*, which Kress (2003) explains as the purposive reshaping of semiotic resources *within* and *across* modes, respectively. They are the psychological machinery of synaesthesia. Kress (2005) argues that it is critical to explore the affordances of different modes and media at this point because we are in a period of rapid and radical social, economic, political, cultural, and technological change, change that is reorganizing and realigning the uses and effects of modes and media.

Synaesthesia is defined as the emergent creation of qualitatively new forms of meaning as a result of "shifting" ideas across semiotic modes (Kress, 2003, p. 36, cited in Nelson, 2006, p. 56). Nelson (2006) examined the process and product of five ESL freshman student writers taking a multimedia writing class. For course design, he used Adobe Photoshop for students to do digital storytelling by merging texts, sound (voice and music), and imagery (still and video). The process writing approach was adopted for the development of students' digital essays in the course with a theme on language, culture, and identity. Based on a tradition of design experiments, Nelson used empirical data drawn from interviews, student journals, and the digital story-related artifacts themselves, and demonstrated how synaesthetically derived meaning emerged in the process of creating multimodal texts. Through analyses, Nelson came up with categories of facilitators and hindrances to multimodal authorship (shown in the students' authorial voice): resemiotization through repetition, recognition of language topology, and amplification of authorship as facilitators. The analysis also acknowledged the influence of genre and over-accommodation of audience as hindrances.

It is argued that "synaesthesia can be the process and locus of 'much of what we regard as creativity' (Kress, 2003, p. 36) in multimodal communicative practice" (Nelson, 2006, p. 59). Particularly, this is true when one day in the future we all write with video, instead of texts. However, "synaesthesia may have both amplifying and limiting effects" (p. 56) on the projection of nonnative students' authorial intention and voice. Nelson reiterates the importance of semiotic awareness, which refers to an ability to look at and through media for decoding and designing multimodal meaning. For implications of L2 writing pedagogy, awareness of multimodal representation of meaning is important for learners, and so is an allowance of freedom of using multimodality for sense-making in writing instruction. In a Japanese EFL context, Nelson (2008) delivered a digital storytelling course and collected nine students' works for analysis of multimodal synthesis and the multimedia authors' voices. Controlling the polysemy of multimedia can let the students' voice be heard.

Exploring "how multilingual writers negotiate and express their identities visually in multimodal genres" (p. 319), Tardy (2005) examined how four graduate students used Microsoft PowerPoint presentation slides to project both disciplinarity and individuality. She found that their habitus was influenced by the discourse they met and their personal responses to those discourses. Along the line of inquiry on multimodal literacy, Wysocki (2004, p. 137) proposes an approach for analyzing the visual aspects of texts by asking us to (a) name the visual elements in a text, (b) name the designed relationships among those elements, and (c) consider how the elements and relations connect with different audiences, contexts, and arguments.

Addressing this trend of research on the use of computers and writing research, Lunsford (2006) expands the definition of writing to include epistemic, multivocal, multimodal, and multimediated practices in the computers and writing classroom. He further suggests that writing teachers should "create classroom experiences that allow students to compose in 'the most compelling discursive modalities of their generation'" (p. 169).

To sum up, a considerable amount of worldwide growth in weblogs in a variety of different contexts and languages has attracted second or foreign language teachers to explore their impact on various language skills. Using such features as archiving, hyperlinks, comments, and instant/self-publishing, several teaching projects or empirical studies have been conducted on the use of weblogs for language teaching. Among the research on second language writing, students' perceptions have been much examined concerning online participation or peer review; however, few studies have investigated both the students' perceptions and their writing products, or even the process. This chapter reports on a case study on blogging and writing instruction with contextual factors and student writing emphasized.

THE STUDY

A case study approach with mixed quantitative and qualitative methods was applied. The course context was a college third-year required "Reading & Writing II" class with 25 students who were mainly junior students with a smaller number of senior or older ones. The class met for two hours each week. A blog platform was set up to help the course delivery, while the students and the instructor met mostly in a traditional classroom with a PC and a projector to illustrate how the participants can do blogging, given their mature computer literacy. Periodical peer reviews were required as part of the course writing assignments, plus a pair essay, some take-home essays, a source-based paper, and some journal entries. Incorporation of multimedia was encouraged.

Design of Tasks

The syllabus was designed with individual and pair writing tasks. Two specific tasks were designed for pair writing. In the first round, one of the pair members served as the main author, while the other served as the contributor. They went through brainstorming, drafting, commenting, and revising. In the second round, the roles of the pair members were reversed. Blog entries were designed as individual journal writing. An individual source-based project was also included. Other assignment types included journal entries and individual essays. All students' writing was uploaded to the blog platform so that participants could view one another's essays. Peer comments were mandatory in some weeks to encourage online class interaction with reading and writing.

A 13-item evaluation questionnaire was designed to obtain the participants' perceptions on technology integration (such as privacy and blog writing, and comparison of writing on blogs and paper) and task design (see Appendix 1.1). Specific cases of 8 participants' online works were examined in detail to investigate their use of multimodal texts on the blog with semiotic awareness through transduction and transformation.

Questionnaire Data

It was found that over 90 percent of the students agreed that the peer review activity during the collaborative composing process was helpful, and 84 percent of them thought the collaborative essay was more effective than individual work. Among factors that may have an influence on the students' satisfaction, the collaborative process with their peers and the writing content were rated higher (4.54 out of 5.00) than other aspects of the essays. In the first pair writing task, online chat was implemented to assist discussion or interaction after class; however, it was not regarded as helpful and the students preferred face-to-face interaction. As for items related to blogging, 58.6 percent of them liked the experiences while the other half of them expressed unfamiliarity with the media or the need of adding media to their texts; 90 percent of them did not mind sharing blog entries with others; and over 70 percent of them indicated other benefits of keeping a blog entry regularly, such as going back to their blog entries to understand what they had learned in the semester, making a writing course more interesting, or viewing classmates' blog entries and giving comments.

In sum, the collaborative process was generally regarded as beneficial, although the collaborative essays were not necessarily better than individual works. Blogging was regarded as useful in terms of self-reflections on their writing performance over a semester and as motivating in a writing class, and it was also facilitative when combined with peer viewing and commenting.

Online Texts in 8 Cases

Randomly, 8 out of the 25 participants were chosen for examination of their online written works, due to the large volume of data involved. The summarized data of the 8 cases are shown in Table 1.1, which includes the participants' writing proficiency, sources they incorporated in their blog writing, and the types of media they had used for meaning representation. A wide range of multiple modes of online media was applied by most of the students, such as video, graphics, and mp3[1] files.

Some analytical categories following the approach by Nelson (2006) were developed to illustrate the writing and multimodal representations of the chosen cases through "iterative coding and analysis of the data" (p. 61). Collaboration was required when two students were involved in doing peer reviews: One served as the reader commenting on another's essay in order to enhance the textual quality. It was found that benefits from peer comments were recognized by most participants in blog writing, concerning both content and multimodal presentation styles of their online essays. Through reading peers' essays, gaining new knowledge (including cross-cultural understanding) and writing techniques were also pointed out. Constructive feedback on how multimedia could be incorporated appeared in some of the peer comments.

Table 1.1 A Summary of the 8 Cases

Participants	Sources used	Media use	English writing proficiency
1. Carol	Video clip with "Ars Electronica in Linz"	Limited with one video and one graphic	Good
2. Kelly	Coit Tower at San Francisco with a picture; a translation school at Paris with its URLs attached	Extensive use of graphics, one audio file	Good
3. Roberta	Songs, lyrics	Video, graphics, audio-mp3	Good
4. Kimberley	A Japanese film	Video, more graphics, audio-mp3 (style/color)	Intermediate
5. Gloria	US/Taiwan education	Extensive video clips (Madonna), graphics	Intermediate
6. Shirley	Video from friends (student club)	Video, extensive graphics	Intermediate to good
7. Lily	Writing to her mother in snail mail	Video, graphics, hyperlinks (*Life Is Beautiful*, *Schindler's List*)	Intermediate
8. Melissa	Graphics on bikes and food	Graphics	Intermediate to good

Note: All pseudonyms.

To illustrate, Kelly would relate her peer comments beyond the textual level and evaluate how a piece of writing on blogs demonstrates its organization and presentation style as in the following example:

> You have a clear format on her blog; she titles each blog by numbers and makes it very easy for professor, teaching assistant, and classmates to locate those blogs. And I think you write in a lucid way that viewers can learn your feelings towards various topics or events very easily. Pictures and video clips are interesting and well put.

Using sources in online writing with media was sometimes suggested in peer comments:

> I think it would be better to add some links or more images in your blog entries since you want to introduce some music or movies to us.

As a form of collaborative writing, peer response activities as implemented in such a blogging-assisted writing class encouraged more opportunities for interaction through reading and writing. Carol, in two blog posts, indicated:

> It is not only interesting but also inspiring to visit other classmates' blogs to know more about their opinions and ideas on certain subjects. For example, I find great pleasure in reading my classmates' future plans after graduating from Tsing Hua. I felt perplexed and uncertain about what to do in the future. However, after reading several classmates' blogs, I saw more possibilities of what I want and what I can do after graduation.

> [Another post] This post is informative and useful as a guideline for people who want to lose weight. I have to admit that I was strongly attracted by the title. After all, as female, who wouldn't want to be in a good shape? I am surprised to find that sleeping quality can affect the efficiency of losing weight. Before reading your article, I had no information about this. Besides, I cannot agree with you more that determination and perseverance are the most crucial elements that lead to the success of losing weight and staying in shape. I plan to try these tips you provide to make myself look fitter during the summer vacation. Wish me good luck!

In another case, Carol reflected how she had mastered the literacy of blog writing:

> Before entering collage, I had little knowledge about computer and the internet . . . While most of my friends and classmates made good use of the internet chatting and searching information, I remained a computer phobic. To me, writing blog is a new way of sharing life, opinions, and emotions with others. What distinguish blogging from other means of communication is that once you post an entry, you share it not only with your family and friends, but also the world since everyone online can easily get access to your blog by merely a simple click.

For Carol, the traditional private writing act was transformed through blogging into a public writing experience. Such new online writing experience enables new ways of self expression via new media:

> I used to consider that blogging is too much exposure of one's personal feelings. I guess I would have such idea because I read quite a lot blogs talking about the authors' most private feelings and lives. These experiences confused me and some entries were unbearable. Some wrote how they were angry with their friends. These bloggers' friends obviously

would know whom they were referring to, even the scolded targets could see the articles. Unbelievably, in real worlds they could pretend like nothing have ever happened. Isn't that wired? Isn't that deliberate? Moreover, some friends wrote about their feelings deep in the mind, which the readers could be sure that it is private and secret. As a friend, though having read those articles, it's offensive and embarrassed to ask more about the private incident in person. To me such situations are pretty strange. It seems like people doing so only want **to show off and attract others' attentions.**

However, recently an incident has provided me a new view on blogging. Several days after having the most important <u>volleyball competitions</u> among foreign languages and literature departments, my friend, Sharon, gave me some links to our teammates' blogs. At first I did not take it seriously. After reading, beyond my imagination, I was totally overwhelmed by these blogs. They were mostly written by our younger classmates. Though we did not get a prize, these new partners showed their determination of staying in our team and shared their love for playing volleyball in their blogs. As the leader of the team, I could not be happier knowing their true and positive feelings about the team and volleyball. Due to blogging, I had chance to know these precious emotions from my teammates, <u>which would be too embarrassing to tell when we were face to face.</u> **For the very first time I experienced the advantage and cleverness of blogging as a way of sharing emotions and of communication.** [Boldface and underlining effects made by participants on screen.]

As one case of cross-cultural understanding, Kimberley showed her liking for Japanese films, at great length explaining "Mushishi." For this group, some of them may take Japanese as their second foreign language. A full-time lecturer in this department also provided plenty of input into Japanese language and culture. Inherently, Taiwan is heavily influenced by and closely tied with Japanese due to its historical background and geographic affinity.

The first time I heard an anime "蟲師" [Chinese characters cited in student writing], I am not attracted to it name and even consider it a weird anime filled with grotesque and ridiculous scene. However, as an old proverb says: "never judge a book by it cover"; after watch one of parts of the anime, I found it is so creative, delicate, meaningful that I was totally fascinated.

"蟲師" is called "Mushishi" in Japanese. The anime "Mushishi" I watch on TV is adapted from its original comic books. "Mushi" is translated in Chinese as "蟲," it is a creature "often displaying supernatural powers. . . ." "Mushishi" means "mushi master"(蟲師), who travels from place to place to research Mushi (蟲) and assist people suffering from problems caused by them. . . .

Different from some of anime rough in production, the delicate style of sketch and mild color in "Mushishi" attract me much. Narrator in the stories always narrates some poetry-like sentences. . . .

Another student portrayed her experience of making an advertisement video for a student club:

Perhaps I had never thought that I can produce a video on my own before I did it for my dancing club . . . the annual Body Language Club (BLC) . . . there are four steps to create a short video if you want to have your own videos. First, before to search for the materials, I draw a sketch. Talking more specific, I had to think what kind of style I want to show. For example, the style should be funny, softly fragrant, or cold. As I decided what kind of style I want to show, I can think about the ways of beginning and ending. It was just like giving the sketch a skeleton and then I can give it blood and flesh.

Second, starting to seek for materials I needed in my video. For example, I need a short video for my introduction, so I cut a phrase from recorded video. And I wanted some pictures to show the performances in recent years so I picked several representative pictures as my materials.

Third, I started to connect the materials I had to a serial videos. Surely I had to add some special effects for every material to make coherence. Finally, the most importantly, I had to review the work once and once to ensure every detail were fine.

This is the video I did for advertising BLC club, and it really gave me a great sense of achievement.

In a journal entry, Melissa demonstrated creativity by merging online sources into her favorite hobby, biking, augmented with a picture in one of the journal entries (see Figure 1.1):

This activity is really interesting. It's not surprising to drive a car from Beijing to Paris, and someone already did that in 1907. Now it's really amazing to cycling from Beijing to Paris. Therefore, they plan to spend 4 months to accomplish this magnificent feat, and their goal. Everyone wants to save our world, but only a few people really set an example by personally taking part. Everyone including me all have to think about it.

Within the category of amplification of authorship in Nelson's study (2006), he describes instances in which participants' multimedia essays came to evidence a deeper, fuller quality of meaning through the synaesthetic process of shifting expression across modal boundaries, that is, transduction. Nelson showed how one female student wished to say what she wanted to express as a product of recreating an utterance in a different modal form.

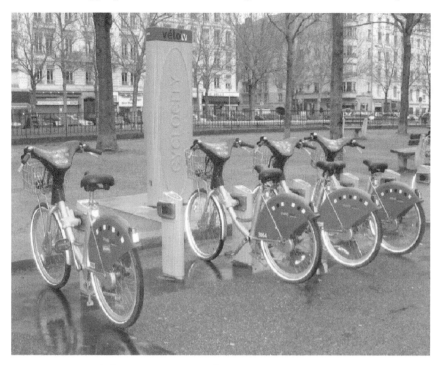

Figure 1.1   Bicycle hire station in Lyon.[2]

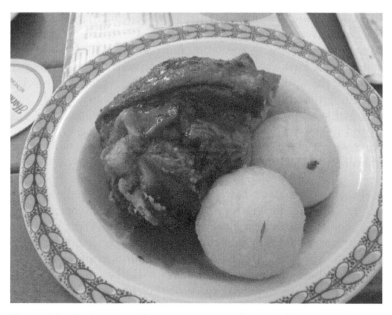

Figure 1.2   A picture can be more attractive than words.

The advantage of using YOUTUBE is that it's quick, easy and we don't have to upload video by ourselves and thus save space [commercial blog service providers usually have a limited space for users]. Also, I would use some pictures in my articles when I talk about food or beautiful scenery, and it will make people more into my writings. The following are examples which I mention above (see Figure 1.2).

This is a good example of a picture worth a thousand words.

Lily, another participant, attached new meaning to the traditional writing through letters. Is this transduction of media for writing from paper to screen, and screen to paper again? It is worth our reflections.

> Recently my mom and I started to write letters to each other. My mom said, "five dollars for delivery can not only reduce phone bills but also let the post officer have works."
>
> The beginning of our actions was impressive. I remembered it was Friday when I threw my letters written last night into the postbox. On Monday I received a letter from my mother, and the date of writing was on last Friday. That is, we did not tell each other before but we wrote letters almost the same time. How interesting it is! Perhaps that is why we are mother and daughter, who have connection in our sub-mind. I clearly remembered the first moment I read my mother's words, which from far away; I cannot help but crying. I felt upset toward my school work at that time, and the words from mother consulted my heart in time. I appreciated the letter's coming, which released me.
>
> Since the internet has been developing so fast, people use e-mail instead of hand-writing letters. There is no denying that sending e-mails is more convenient and cheaper for us; however, I think hand-writing letters sometimes bring special meaning for us indeed. There are several reasons. First, the hand-writing can represented a person's personality and the situation one's writing. Second, we can think much more in writing than typing words because it cost us much time in writing. Personal speaking, I reveal more emotion and become more sensitive when I am writing. Third, letters on paper can be easier to be stored. After we get older, these "writing documents" can be our memorable treasure.

As illustrated, various video clips were incorporated into student writing to enhance messages in their essays. For instance, video content included (a) the performance where a classmate went for a singing contest, (b) the performance of their favorite singers, (c) the video production a student joined through a student club organization, or (d) the cover of the album of a student's favorites with the mp3 sound files and lyrics included. With a journal entry of traveling from Peking to Paris with bikes, a student showed her creativity with English text and various modes of online media. It seems that some students in this generation have the awareness of living in a multimodal world and formed the habit of using multimedia for self-expressions. All these examples demonstrate the students' strong awareness of using various media for self-expression and their sense of synaesthesia.

DISCUSSION

For collaborative writing, blogging facilitates viewing of other students' writing and providing feedback. Students generally acknowledged the advantage of using weblogs as a collaborative writing platform.

Although some of the participants were unfamiliar with adding multimedia elements into their writing in the weblog platform, others demonstrated sophisticated use of various media for meaning representation with their writing assignments. They had incorporated video clips, audio files (in mp3 format), and various types of graphics for meaning representation. Unsurprisingly, with additional semiotic means such as graphics for the album cover of songs, bikes in Paris, or friends' contests on campus, students' self-expression was found to be greatly enhanced compared with traditional textual presentation on paper. Most of them demonstrated a certain degree of media literacy with selection and manipulation of various media. Transduction did happen in their blog writing. When multimodal texts were expressed and perceived through different modalities, for example, oral language and pictures, meaning in student writing was much more enhanced.

The experience of EFL multimodal authors was found to be closely accompanied by their semiotic awareness. Such awareness could have been inherently available before they took the current writing course or developed through experimenting with various blogging assignments. Synaesthesia, defined as the emergent creation of qualitatively new forms of meaning as a result of "shifting" ideas across semiotic modes (Kress, 2003, p. 36, cited in Nelson, 2006, p. 56), is evident in various cases in this study.

Mostly, the participants were satisfied with the integration of blogging into their writing class with the designed assignments. How about their English writing performance in terms of linguistic accuracy? In some cases, it could be weak enough to hinder the clarity of their expression. Perhaps, due to attentional resources being allocated to inclusion of different media with online searching and editing of the original sources, typographical mistakes were more often seen in blog writing and in-class writing on paper, compared with paper writing at home. If richness of self-expression is one key element for writing assessment, blog writing of this group was not inferior to their take-home writing on paper.

CONCLUSION

This chapter describes a case study with 25 third-year English-majoring college students who participated in a writing class enhanced by a blog environment. Their questionnaire responses on the overall course and two collaborative writing tasks were analyzed along with their online writing texts of multimodal representation from 8 cases. Blogging was useful in terms of enabling self-reflections on the students' writing performance and motivation in a writing class. It was also facilitative when combined with peer reviews and multimodal representation.

The use of weblogs can be helpful when designing collaborative activities such as peer review or co-writing with a likelihood of student satisfaction. In the future, writing teachers may explore specific features of weblogs in enhancing courses with their respective goals. With data on how the participants felt and what they did with their writing in a blog-enhanced course, the project can provide English teachers with pedagogical implications on writing instruction, and provide researchers with an understanding of how students construct multimodal representation and transfer traditional writing to multimedia representation with transduction and synaesthesia across several task designs. The findings in this study echo what Nelson (2006) maintains: "with respect to some contexts and curricular goals, keying up the *noticeability factor* through the practice of multimodal composition could represent a value-added direction in language and literacy education" (p. 71).

ACKNOWLEDGMENTS

The chapter is partially funded by the National Science Council under the project number NC96–2411–H007–033–MY3. Help from the participating students and the research assistant, Vivian Wu, is acknowledged.

NOTES

1. The mp3 is an audio-specific format that was designed by the Moving Picture Experts Group as part of its MPEG-1 standard (http://en.wikipedia.org/wiki/MP3).
2. The official website: http://www.beijingtoparis.com/ch-index.html. The participants' blog: http://www.deray.org/ (you really should see this one's blog, it's really interesting, and you may want to go cycling as well after reading his blog: http://www.crazyguyonabike.com/doc/HeatherB2P).

REFERENCES

Anson, C. M. (2003). Responding to and assessing student writing: The uses and limits of technology. In P. Takayoshi & B. Huot (Eds.), *Teaching writing with computers* (pp. 234–246). New York: Houghton Mifflin Co.

Breuch, L. K. (2004). *Virtual peer review: Teaching and learning about writing in online environments*. Albany: State University of New York Press.

Gollin, S. (1999). "Why? I thought we'd talked about it before": Collaborative writing in a professional workplace setting. In C. Candlin & K. Hyland (Eds.), *Writing: Texts, processes and practices* (pp. 267–290). Harlow: Longman.

Hertz-Lazarowitz, R., & Bar-Natan, I. (2002). Writing development of Arab and Jewish students using cooperative learning (CL) and computer-mediated communication (CMC). *Computers & Education, 39*, 19–36.

Kress, G. (2003). *Literacy in the new media age*. London: Routledge.

Kress, G. (2005). Gains and losses: New forms of texts, knowledge, and learning. *Computers and Composition, 22*, 5–22.

Lee, L. (2004). Learners' perspectives on networked collaborative interaction with native speakers of Spanish in the US. *Language Learning & Technology, 8*(1), 83–100.

Lin, Y. Y. (2008). *A preliminary study of English multimedia writing: Implementing weblog in a college composition class*. Unpublished master's thesis, Foreign Languages and Literature, National Tsing Hua University, Hsinchu.

Liou, H. C. (2009). A case study of web-based peer review for college English writing. *Curriculum and Instruction, 13*(1), 173–208.

Liou, H. C., & Peng, C. Y. (2009). Training effects on computer-mediated peer review. *System, 37*(3), 514–525.

Lunsford, A. A. (2006). Writing, technologies, and the fifth canon. *Computers and Composition, 23*, 169–177.

Nelson, M. E. (2006). Mode, meaning, and synaesthesia in multimedia L2 writing. *Language Learning & Technology, 10*(2), 56–76. Retrieved from http://llt.msu.edu/vol10num2/nelson/default.html

Nelson, M. E. (2008). Multimodal synthesis and the voice of the multimedia author in a Japanese EFL context. *Innovation in Language Learning and Teaching, 2*, 65–82.

Scollon, R., & Scollon, S. W. (2004). *Nexus analysis: Discourse and the emerging Internet*. New York: Routledge.

Tardy, C. M. (2005). Expressions of disciplinarity and individuality in a multimodal genre. *Computers and Composition, 22*, 319–336.

Thorne, S. L. (2005). Pedagogical and praxiological lessons from Internet-mediated intercultural foreign language education research. In J. A. Belz & S. L. Thorne (Eds.), *Internet-mediated intercultural foreign language education* (pp. 2–30). Boston: Thomson and Heinle.

Wysocki, A. F. (2004). The multiple media of texts: How onscreen and paper texts incorporate words, images, and other media. In C. Bazerman & P. Prior (Eds.), *What writing does and how it does it* (pp. 123–163). Mahwah, NJ: Lawrence Erlbaum Associates.

APPENDIX 1.1   THE EVALUATION QUESTIONNAIRE

Options: 5 strongly agree; 4 agree; 3 no opinion; 2 disagree; 1 strongly disagree

1. I don't mind sharing my blog entries with others.
       5   4   3   2   1

2. Uploading blog entries took me more time than writing using Microsoft *Word*.
       5   4   3   2   1

3. I like writing on blog than writing with Microsoft *Word* (submitting to the teacher).
       5   4   3   2   1

4. I like English writing on blog to record my reflection or as a personal diary for learning process.

      5   4   3   2   1

5. I can go back to my blog entries to understand what I learned this semester.

      5   4   3   2   1

6. I like to publish my English writing through blog entries.

      5   4   3   2   1

7. I will continue to write on blog for writing practice.

      5   4   3   2   1

8. To integrate a writing course with blogging makes such a course more interesting.

      5   4   3   2   1

9. I like to view classmates' blog entries and give comments.

      5   4   3   2   1

10. To integrate a writing course with blogging helps peer collaboration and peer interaction.

      5   4   3   2   1

11. Through blogging, I master more about Internet technology (if you were not good at blogging before).

      5   4   3   2   1

12. I don't like blog assignments this semester because _____.

    I don't like adding of multimedia into my writing (one example answer from participants).

13. I like blog assignments this semester, because _____ (if the above statements are not comprehensive for your reasons, state them here).

    I don't need to print the assignments on paper and remember to bring them for submission (one example answer from participants).

2 Podcasting in Foreign Language Learning

Insights for Podcast Design from a Developmental Research Project

Wai Meng Chan, Ing Ru Chen, and Martin G. Döpel

INTRODUCTION

Podcasting has seen phenomenal growth as a means of delivering content to listeners, be it for entertainment, commercial, or educational purposes. A recent marketing report (Lewin, 2009) put the size of the podcast audience worldwide in 2008 at 17.4 million (or 9 percent of all Internet users). This number is expected to reach 37.6 million (17 percent) by 2013.

A podcast is a media stream consisting of audio and/or video files, but it can also contain pdf files. The metadata of these files (URLs, titles, and descriptions) are stored in a file called an RSS feed, which is checked regularly by software called podcatchers and downloaded automatically. Thus, users do not have to visit a webpage to look for new content: Their computer does it all. By synchronizing their portable media players with their computers, the new content will be copied to these gadgets as well. A podcast can therefore be accessed either on the computer or on a portable media player, and listening can take place even on the move.

In view of this, it is not surprising that podcasting technology is now increasingly employed in higher education, especially in foreign language learning (see, e.g., Young, 2007), as ownership of portable media players among students increases by the day. Furthermore, podcasts are easy to produce, as there are convenient applications to record, edit, and publish podcasts (see, e.g., Döpel, 2007).

Findings from research into media-based learning would seem to support educational podcasting. Such research advocates the use of the auditory mode to complement the visual mode in the presentation of learning content (see Weidenmann, 2002). Much of today's learning materials are designed to be perceived through the visual mode (e.g., in the form of texts and pictures). In Weidenmann's view, the use of audio materials will aid the intake of information and learning, as the spoken language will (a) enhance retention in memory (Baddeley, 1986; Engelkamp, 1991), (b) arouse attention, and (c) come across as being more personal (because of the voice, intonation, and expression). The use of other sensory channels can prevent the overloading of the visual channel (Engelkamp & Zimmer, 1994) and help learners better comprehend complex content (Paechter, 1993). Research on learning styles–based instruction (see Dunn, 2000) has also long advocated the need for teachers to become more aware of learners' individual learning styles (Reid, 1987; Smith & Renzulli, 1984) and to promote the use of less developed sensory channels (Grinder, 1991). The use of podcasts thus appears beneficial in two ways: (a) It caters better to the needs of auditory learners, and (b) it exposes learners with other learning style preferences (visual, tactual, and/or kinesthetic; see Dunn & Dunn, 1999) to learning through the auditory mode.

Given the potential of educational podcasting, the authors initiated a project to design and produce a podcast to supplement the learning of German language beginners at a university in Singapore. In preparing the project, it became apparent that there have been few published studies on the design and use of podcasting in language learning (see also Young, 2007). Thus an accompanying research study was conducted to gather much needed data on how students access and use the German language podcast, as well as their perceptions about its design and usefulness. This chapter will report on both the development of the podcast—its design and contents—and the key findings from the accompanying study.

LITERATURE REVIEW

Podcasting in Foreign Language Teaching

Compared to the voluminous literature on CALL, academic publications on podcasting in language learning have thus far been relatively scarce. Much of the literature on podcasting has focused on technicalities such as podcast subscription and production (e.g., Stanley, 2006), emphasized the potential of podcasting for learning on the go (e.g., McCarty, 2005), or discussed its possible contribution to promoting meaningful and communicative use of the foreign language (e.g., Young, 2007). Monk, Ozawa, and Thomas (2006) described how English teachers at a Japanese university attempted to take advantage of the university's move to distribute iPods to all first-year students. They offered students a podcast with news from Voice of America and Breaking News English to facilitate the development of their listening comprehension. A survey conducted after the semester ascertained that students were apparently not aware of the podcast: 65.6 percent of them never or rarely downloaded the mp3 files, and only 4.2 percent did so very often. Furthermore, 45.3 percent of the students found them not at all useful or not useful, and only 15.2 percent believed the iPod was used effectively by the teachers.

Edirisingha, Rizzi, Nie, and Rothwell (2007) produced a podcast with six episodes for a module on intercultural communication. Each episode of approximately 10 minutes contained summaries of key concepts, interviews with students, discussions about assessment tasks, as well as tips on presentation and research skills. Fifty percent of the students did not make use of this additional offering, citing in most cases that they were too busy. However, Edirisingha et al. reported that, of the 35 respondents to their questionnaire, 53 percent found the podcast useful in providing more information about the course assessment and in preparing for their seminars and workshops. Forty percent stated that it stimulated their interest in the subject, while another 40 percent said it helped to motivate them.

In another study, Abdous, Camarena, and Facer (2009) described the use of podcasting in eight different courses for French, German, Japanese, Spanish Language and Literature, and World Literature with small enrollments of 8 to 34 at an American university. Students were classified in two groups, namely, those (80) enrolled in courses with podcasts that were integrated into the course curricula and were thus compulsory (PIC), and those (33) in courses with podcasts that were offered as noncompulsory, supplementary materials (PSM). While 72.5 percent of the PIC students listened to at least one unit, only 45.5 percent of the PSM students listened to at least one unit. However, the majority of the students apparently felt that podcasts were an attractive option, as 65 percent of the PIC and 54.5 percent of the PSM students said they were more likely to enroll in courses with a podcast. In general, students in both groups found the podcasts to be useful for developing listening, speaking, and vocabulary.

Podcast Design

Edirisingha et al. (2007) proposed a model with guidelines for the development of educational podcasts. In this model, they identified three key features that can facilitate students' learning: (a) learner choice and flexibility, (b) access to peers' tacit knowledge through discussions, and (c) informal learning.

With regard to the first feature, Edirisingha et al. (2007) advocated that podcasts should give learners sufficient choice and flexibility in approaching and organizing their learning. They listed four flexibility dimensions as planning guidelines:

1. Time: tempo or pace of studying
2. Content: learning material
3. Instructional approach and resources: learning resources, modality, and origin
4. Delivery and logistics: time, place, methods, technology, and delivery channel.

The second feature identified by Edirisingha et al. (2007) is based on their assumption that podcasts are well suited to capturing and conveying tacit knowledge of fellow students—both peers and senior students. They had included interviews and discussions in their podcast but did not discuss in detail how these can promote the acquisition of tacit knowledge or how explicit and tacit knowledge relate to each another. Lastly, based on the belief that informal learning can be more stimulating to students, they recommended using podcasts to provide opportunities for informal learning, which takes place outside of formal academic settings. However, while this model can provide a framework of reference for future theory-building, their model is based solely on data from their podcast projects and is strongly linked to the contexts of these projects, for example, the subjects that are taught through the podcasts.

In a separate paper, Edirisingha (2006) put forward the following design recommendations:

- Integrate podcasts into online courses with strong links to other activities and resources, especially if they encourage active and collaborative learning.
- Record them afresh each week and include up-to-date news and feedback.
- Make them partly reusable and recyclable with some sections that are independent of news or feedback from that week.
- Make sure the file size is small enough so that they are downloadable onto mobile devices.
- Follow a "radio magazine" style rather than a lecture.

The last guideline advocating an informal radio style was to find resonance among other scholars. Cebeci and Tekdal (2006) believed that podcasts should be designed as Wafer-Like Audio Learning Objects (WALOs), which they described as "an audio object that consists of any number of fragments of speech, music, and voice effects" (p. 50). They argued that WALOs will be more efficient in improving learning processes compared to ordinary audio objects or podcast files. Based on an unpublished survey of theirs, they further suggested that podcasts should be of a limited length and not longer than 15 minutes. A podcast should be mixed with music, which can increase its listenability and provide a logical marker between the podcast's different topics.

Rosell-Aguilar (2007, p. 489) reviewed a number of academic and commercial language learning podcasts and concluded that materials for podcasting should:

- provide exposure to the language and its characteristics;
- use a range of materials, including authentic materials;
- provide explicit learning outcomes with clear objectives within a defined syllabus;

- provide exposure to the culture of the areas where the target language is spoken;
- be engaging and of adequate length;
- have a clear consideration of the medium, including the portability and screen size.

He further suggested that podcasters should consider supporting learners by providing additional resources such as transcripts, grammar explanations, glossaries, online exercises, and forums.

PODCAST PROJECT

Project Background

Planning and preparations for the German 1 podcast project started in May 2007 and the podcast was broadcast between August and November 2007. The German 1 podcast was intended to:

- encourage students to learn outside the classroom and on the move;
- provide students with opportunities to review curriculum content;
- expose students to more listening texts in the target language;
- engage in further practice in other language skills/areas such as speaking, pronunciation, grammar, and vocabulary;
- provide learning strategy tips;
- provide students with information about the cultures of German-speaking countries to enhance their country knowledge and stimulate their interest in the target languages and societies.

A podcast homepage (http://courseware.nus.edu.sg/e-daf/podcast/) was created on the German language program's website to "house" the podcast lessons. The homepage provides the URL of the podcast's RSS feed and a link to an information flyer on hardware and software requirements. This flyer was also handed out to students in class and they were briefed about the necessary steps to subscribe to the podcast. Students were also informed about the alternative of downloading or playing the lessons from the podcast homepage where links had been created to access the mp3 files of all podcast lessons as well as the accompanying handouts and task solutions. Altogether 14 lessons were created for the semester. Some parts of the lessons were "blended" into the classroom instruction to boost students' interest and to enhance the integration between the podcast and the course curriculum.

German 1 is the first of two beginners' modules; 255 students from various faculties were enrolled in this elective module from August to November 2007. Among them, 173 (68 percent) were freshmen. Students enrolled in this module are typically motivated by a wide spectrum of reasons, for instance, an interest in the German language, culture, music, philosophy, and technology; the intention to travel in Germany; or the prospect of an exchange semester at universities in German-speaking countries.

Podcast Design and Production

Various aspects of the podcast's design—such as the number, length, and frequency of the lessons; the language and style of presentation; the contents and types of exercises/tasks—were carefully considered, taking into consideration the authors' expectations of students' needs and interests, proficiency level, general workload at the university, and concentration span. It was decided to script and record weekly bilingual lessons of 10 to 15 minutes, with English as the main presentation language, especially in the initial lessons. More texts in German were added incrementally during the course of the semester. A radio magazine style was adopted as the style of presentation and musical elements were added at the beginning and the end of each lesson ("intro" and "extro") to provide a framework. Brief musical interludes were also inserted to mark the transition between individual lesson segments. The decision to adopt a radio magazine style was consistent with Cebeci and Tekdal's (2006) and Edirisingha's (2006) recommendations.

The contents of each lesson were designed in line with the objectives mentioned earlier. An accompanying handout was created in pdf format for each lesson to incorporate task types that are not easily reproducible in a spoken form, links to other relevant resources on the German program's website, as well as learning support such as glossaries, transcripts, and illustrations. The handout was also intended to provide some form of scaffolding for learners with other dominant perceptual styles, especially those with a preference for visual learning.

Recording took place in a recording studio on campus with technical assistance. The lessons were then created from the audio recordings using Audacity, and uploaded to the university's courseware server. The RSS feed was updated regularly as each lesson was published.

Structure and Contents of the Podcast Lessons

The podcast lessons had an average length of 13 minutes. The pie charts in Figure 2.1 provide a breakdown of lessons 3 and 13, and the proportion of time allotted to the individual components of each lesson. The term "meta" refers to meta-information such as greetings and the content overview at the beginning of each lesson as well as transitional texts and summaries between individual segments and at the end of the lesson.

The weighting of the components varied from lesson to lesson, depending on the topics and focus of each lesson. Nevertheless, in general, in line with

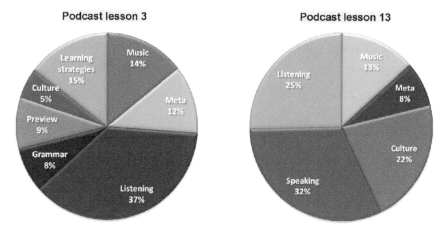

Figure 2.1 Weighting of individual components in podcast lessons 3 and 13.

the objective of providing students with more listening practice, listening tasks constituted a major component of most lessons. In the first half of the semester (e.g., in lesson 3), more emphasis was given to grammar review and practice as well as to instruction in useful learning strategies, which were vital at this initial stage. In the latter half (e.g., in lesson 13), the emphasis shifted towards providing more listening and speaking exercises as well as culture and country information relevant to the weekly course topics.

Figure 2.2 shows the structure of lesson 13. As with all lessons, it is framed by an introduction and an overview at the beginning as well as a concluding section ("signing off") and an extro at the end of the lesson.

Complementing the textbook topic of that week, the culture segment talked about environmental consciousness in Germany. It explained how a deposit is charged for recyclable and disposable packaging, and how consumers can have these refunded at shops and supermarkets. The handout contained a collage of photographs showing typical forms of recyclable and disposable packaging in Germany, and a glossary of relevant new vocabulary. Following the culture segment were two listening tasks, on conversations at the marketplace and in a restaurant. The gapfill and multiple-choice exercises to test comprehension of these conversations were

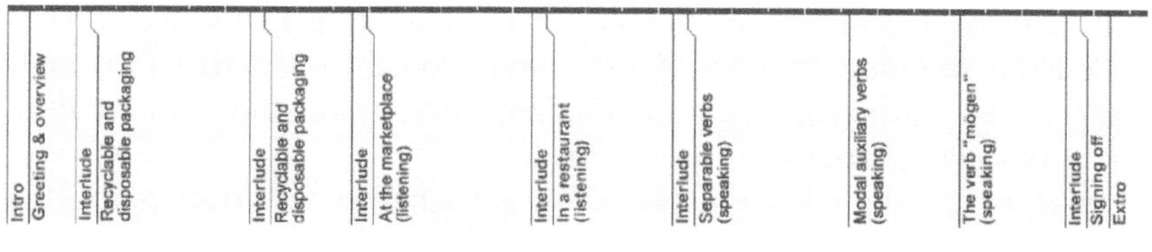

Figure 2.2 Structure of podcast lesson 13.

printed in the handout. In addition, there were three speaking exercises that were designed for students to apply newly introduced grammar structures (separable verbs and modal auxiliary verbs) in speaking. These exercise tasks were also included in the handout.

THE STUDY

As mentioned earlier, an accompanying study was conducted to address the lack of empirical data on the use of podcasting in foreign language learning. Specifically, the study was intended to achieve the following objectives:

- To gather data on the Internet, hardware, and software resources available to students for podcast access as well as their previous experience with podcasts.
- To investigate students' use of the German 1 podcast and their patterns of use.
- To ascertain students' perceptions of the usefulness and quality of the German 1 podcast.

Procedure

Qualitative and quantitative data were collected through three anonymous questionnaires administered in weeks 2, 8, and 13 of the 13-week semester, respectively, to 225 German 1 students who consented to participating in the study. Questionnaire 1 was designed to elicit data on the respondents' demographic background. It also sought to collect data on Internet, hardware, and software resources available to students for podcast access. All 225 copies of Questionnaire 1 were returned to the researchers. Questionnaires 2 and 3 were almost identical and each consisted of three parts. Multiple-choice and multiple-response items were used in Part 1 to elicit data on the respondents' podcast access and use (including the hardware and software used), and their patterns of use. Part 2 comprised 5-point Likert-scale items designed to gauge students' perceptions of the usefulness and quality of the podcast, including its contents and technical quality. Open-ended questions were included in Part 3 to elicit qualitative evaluations of the podcast as well as suggestions for future additions and improvements. For Questionnaire 2, 182 copies were returned, and for Questionnaire 3, 203 copies.

The data were analyzed using SPSS Version 16. For the multiple-choice and multiple-response items, frequency analyses were performed. Likert-scale items in Questionnaires 2 and 3 were coded from 1 to 5 ("strongly disagree" to "strongly agree") and the frequency, mean, and standard deviations of the responses were ascertained.

In reporting the results of the study, this chapter will restrict itself to the most salient results from the analysis of the data from Questionnaires

1 and 3. The results of Questionnaire 2 were near identical to those of Questionnaire 3 and did not show any significant differences. Furthermore, as Questionnaire 3 was administered in the last week of the semester and covered 13 of the 14 podcast lessons, it provided a more complete picture of students' podcast use and perceptions.

Questionnaire 1 Results

The average age of the 225 respondents was 20 and 68.6 percent were female. About 68 percent of them were freshmen in that semester. The respondents were from various faculties at the university, with the largest groups being from Arts (43.1 percent), Engineering (20.9 percent), and Science (18.2 percent).

All respondents owned a laptop and/or a desktop computer. In addition, all respondents had broadband Internet access at home and/or on campus; 91.4 percent had broadband access at home, while 71.4 percent reported using the campus network. The respondents were apparently vastly exposed to the Internet, with 89.2 percent using the Internet daily. More than three-quarters (77 percent) owned an mp3 player. It would thus appear that students had the necessary hardware and Internet resources necessary for podcast access.

However, only slightly more than a quarter (27 percent) subscribed to podcasts, with only 10.3 percent subscribing to educational podcasts. Hence, the statistics seem to suggest that the majority of the students had little or no previous experience with podcasts, especially with educational podcasts. Most of the students (67.7 percent) reported usually listening to podcasts at home and only 11.3 percent said they did so on the go. Ninety-three percent were reportedly prepared to spend 10 minutes or more listening to a German-language learning podcast. Of these, the largest group of 43.3 percent indicated their willingness to spend 15 to 30 minutes doing so.

Questionnaire 3 Results

Podcast Access

Figure 2.3 shows the number of podcast lessons students accessed, according to Questionnaire 3 data. The majority of the students, 40.4 percent, listened to at least 11 to 13 lessons. A further 15.3 percent reported accessing 8 to 10 lessons. This means that over half of the students surveyed listened to eight or more lessons in the course of the semester. Only 6 students (3 percent) did not listen to any podcast lesson at all. Five of these 6 students volunteered a reason for not listening: While one said he/she could not be bothered, the others stated technology-related reasons, such as the following:

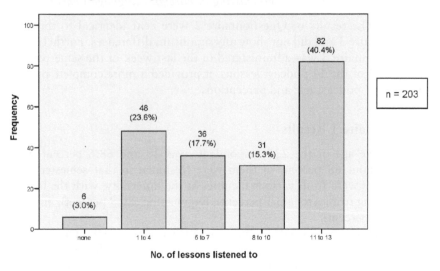

Figure 2.3   Number of podcast lessons listened to by students.

I had problems with downloading them.

My laptop could not open the podcasts even after I downloaded the software required.

Patterns of Podcast Use

Only 9.1 percent of the 197 respondents who accessed the podcast listened to the lessons as they were published, that is, on a weekly basis. The majority listened to the lessons only occasionally, that is, less than once every fortnight (35 percent) or only before the semester tests (45.7 percent).

Most students (80.7 percent) reported listening to the podcast at home. However, a considerable number also reported listening at locations outside their homes (36 percent on campus and 12.2 percent on the move). In addition, a handful (2.5 percent) listened at other locations (e.g., in cafés). Not surprisingly, as most respondents reported listening at home, the majority (70.1 percent) used only their computers to listen to the lessons. Nevertheless, nearly 30 percent indicated using an mp3 player to access the podcast, with 5.6 percent using it solely, while 24.3 percent used it in addition to a computer.

The most frequently used software was iTunes, reported by 42.6 percent of the students. This may perhaps be attributed to the fact that it was one of the podcatchers recommended by the course instructors. In addition, iPod users would have to use iTunes to synchronize their iPods. Of the non-podcatcher software used by 55 percent of the respondents, Windows

Media Player was the most frequently used, apparently by those who listened using their computers.

Students' Perceptions of the Quality and Usefulness of the Podcast

The data presented in the following stemmed from 197 students, as 6 of the 203 respondents to Questionnaire 3 did not listen to the podcast. Table 2.1 shows the frequency distribution and mean scores for items pertaining to students' overall assessment of the podcast, including its frequency, length, learning content, and technical quality, as well as the degree of their enjoyment.

The students' overall assessment was generally positive, as the frequency distribution and mean scores indicate. The majority of respondents agreed or strongly agreed with the statements given in Table 2.1. The positive quantitative scores are corroborated by the respondents' qualitative comments, numbering over 50, about the podcast's contents and quality. The following are a few representative examples:

The podcasts are very interesting and helpful.

I really appreciate the effort put into creating such wonderful podcasts to aid us in learning German, especially at LAG1201. The contents and quality had been very satisfactory.

Table 2.1　Students' Overall Assessment of the Podcast (in Descending Order by Mean Score)

Item	Statement	Frequency (Percentages)					Mean	StD
		D	N	SD	SA	A		
12	I find the podcast to be useful.	0.5	0.0	5.1	62.9	31.5	4.25	.593
27	I find the overall technical quality to be good.	1.5	0.5	6.6	66.5	24.9	4.13	.677
21	I find the topics to be relevant to the course.	0.5	1.0	7.1	70.6	20.8	4.10	.597
10	I find the frequency of the podcast lessons to be appropriate.	1.0	2.0	9.6	68.0	19.3	4.03	.681
11	I enjoy listening to the podcast.	0.5	4.1	12.2	64.5	17.8	3.96	.717
25	I find the length of the podcast lessons to be appropriate.	1.0	3.6	11.2	71.6	12.7	3.91	.683

N.B. n = 197; SD—strongly disagree, D—disagree, N—neither agree nor disagree, A—agree, SA–strongly agree; StD—standard deviation.

It's a great effort, and a very up-to-date and fun way to help students learn more about the German language and culture. Thank you!

The quality is good as the content is useful and the sound quality is good as well.

The highest mean score was registered for Item 12 pertaining to the podcast's usefulness. This is consistent with the students' perceptions of the podcasts' individual components, as the statistics in Table 2.2 indicate.

The frequency distribution and mean scores for the items in Table 2.2 suggest that, with the exception of the sneak previews, the students perceived the various kinds of information and practice included in the podcast to be useful. They appeared to be most satisfied with the listening exercises, the grammar information and exercises, and also the country and culture information. The students' appreciation of the country and cultural information was confirmed by comments such as the following:

Table 2.2   Students' Assessment of Individual Aspects of the Podcast's Learning Contents (in Descending Order by Mean Score)

Item	Statement	Frequency (Percentages)					Mean	StD
		D	N	SD	SA	A		
14	I find the listening exercises to be useful.	0.5	0.5	8.1	58.4	32.5	4.22	.653
17	I find the grammar information and exercises to be useful.	0.5	1.0	9.6	66.0	22.8	4.10	.636
13	I find the information about German-speaking countries and their cultures to be useful.	1.5	0.5	17.8	53.8	26.4	4.03	.775
18	I find the vocabulary information and exercises to be useful.	0.5	1.5	15.7	65.0	17.3	3.97	.662
16	I find the pronunciation tips and exercises to be useful.	0.5	3.6	15.2	64.5	16.2	3.92	.707
15	I find the speaking exercises to be useful.	1.0	5.6	19.3	59.5	14.2	3.81	.785
19	I find the strategy tips to be useful.	1.0	1.5	25.9	60.4	11.2	3.79	.694
20	I find the sneak previews to be useful.	2.5	8.6	42.1	39.1	7.6	3.41	.850

N.B. n = 197; SD—strongly disagree, D—disagree, N—neither agree nor disagree, A—agree, SA–strongly agree; StD—standard deviation

Information about German culture is interesting.

More interesting and lighthearted + cultural specific stuff, e.g.: the day-light saving topics.

More about the different places in Germany and to introduce the culture in Germany. I find it very interesting to know more about the country of Germany, including its food, people, etc.

The students found the handout to be helpful (mean = 4.09, 90.3 percent agreeing or strongly agreeing) and well designed (mean = 3.97, 84.2 percent agreeing or strongly agreeing); 26.9 percent reported reading it most of the time, and 42.1 percent said they always read it (mean = 3.95). Yet, interestingly, many students did not print the handout (mean = 3.10), with 34.2 percent stating that they never or rarely printed it. This implies that a large number of students read the handout only on-screen on their computers.

Open-ended questions regarding improvements to the podcast yielded a multitude of different suggestions, with most calling for more practice in various language areas/skills (including listening, speaking, phonetics and pronunciation, vocabulary, and strategy tips). Though it was difficult to see a general trend, it should be noted there were a considerable number of suggestions for the inclusion of more grammar topics. For some of the students, this interest in grammar was apparently linked to a strong achievement motivation and was a reflection of their concern with test performances and grades, as the following statements seem to indicate:

Well-organized and nicely planned. Very useful for semester test.

The vocab/grammar revision and listening parts are useful, especially before the semester tests.

Maybe a pre-semester test podcast to help us revise.

This explanation would be consistent with the fact that a large number of students (45.7 percent) reported listening to the lessons only before the semester tests.

DISCUSSION

The results from Questionnaire 1 reveal that the respondents had the necessary hardware and Internet access to receive and listen to the German 1 podcast, as the overwhelming majority had a broadband connection at home and also used the campus network to access the Internet. In addition, more than three-quarters owned an mp3 player. The availability of such hardware and Internet resources gave students a potentially high degree of flexibility and mobility in accessing the podcast.

Considering that only relatively few respondents were subscribed to educational podcasts (10.3 percent) at the beginning of the semester, the access rate was remarkably high. By the end of the semester, 97 percent had listened to at least one lesson, and 55 percent had accessed at least 8 out of 13 lessons. The access rate was thus considerably higher than that reported by Edirisingha et al. (2007) and Abdous et al. (2009). In the former study, 50 percent of the respondents did not access any podcast unit at all, while only 45.5 percent of the students offered supplementary podcasts in the latter study listened to one unit or more. Edirisingha's students cited their busy schedule and a lack of time as reasons for not accessing their course podcast. In the present study, 4 of the 6 students who reported not listening to any lesson at all complained about technical difficulties or said they were unfamiliar with technology. Judging from their responses, it would appear that they had developed negative attitudes towards technology-based learning because of a lack of technological knowledge. Perhaps, conversely, their negative attitudes had created an aversion towards technology-assisted materials. While the number of such learners was extremely low, one should nevertheless contemplate means to provide learners with the necessary training and motivation for technology-based learning. Such efforts will have to go beyond merely informing students about hardware and software requirements or the URLs of the podcast homepage and RSS feed. Nevertheless, the high access rate provides a clear indication that preparedness levels for learning through podcasts were generally high among the German 1 students.

An interesting but not unexpected finding is that most students accessed the podcast using their computers at home. One reason for this may be that many students were not accustomed to learning through using their mp3 players or on the move. This would be consistent with the fact that only 10.3 percent had previous podcast learning experience. Edirisingha et al. (2007) also reported that 31 percent of their subjects preferred to use mp3 players only to listen to music and speculated that these students might have considered listening to academic materials on their mp3 players to be an intrusion in their personal lives. In the present study, another reason may have been the inclusion of a handout, which necessitated the use of a computer with a pdf reader. In another podcast project at the same university, many students, in explaining their preference for specific locations, indicated that they preferred listening at home because of the comfort, the quieter environment, and the desire to take notes while listening (Chan, in press).

Nevertheless, the fact that almost 30 percent of the students used their mp3 players to listen to at least part of the podcast provides an indication for the potential that podcasting holds for more mobile learning. In fact, nearly 15 percent accessed the podcast on the move as well as in places like fast-food restaurants and cafés. The German 1 podcast had thus encouraged some to make informal "classrooms" out of buses, trains, and cafés, and to maximize learning time while on the move.

The podcast lessons and their contents were well received by the students, who apparently found them to be both useful and enjoyable. There is, however, some evidence to suggest that their perceptions of the podcast's usefulness may be linked to a strong achievement motivation. For instance, many students reported listening to the lessons only before the semester tests and were apparently seeking to use them for test preparation. A further indication can be found in the suggestions of students to link the podcast more closely to the course assessment and to provide explicit test practice. Such suggestions should, however, be treated carefully and critically, lest students' podcast use becomes even more extrinsically motivated.

Podcasts were designed originally to deliver audio content and are thus commonly associated in language learning with the development of listening. The medium's natural advantage in delivering listening materials may account for the fact that respondents gave the listening exercises in the German 1 podcast the highest rating of all.

One vital finding lies in the recognition that students had a strong interest in the culture of German-speaking countries. This is evidenced by (a) the high quantitative rating given by students for the country and culture information, and (b) the many positive qualitative comments highlighting the culture segments and suggesting a wider coverage of culture topics in future podcasts. The data collected thus support Rosell-Aguilar's (2007) call to provide cultural exposure.

With regard to the handout, it was found that a third or 34.6 percent of the students apparently never or rarely printed the handout. However, interestingly, 88 percent read the handouts at least some of the time, with 42.1 percent reporting always reading it. The handout served as a form of scaffolding for those who were more accustomed to visual and text-based learning materials such as textbooks and worksheets. In addition, the handout allowed the authors to design and include exercise types not suitable for oral presentation or an exclusively audio delivery. It also made possible the inclusion of glossaries and transcripts as learning support. As many students apparently read the handout on-screen and did not print it, one could consider using advanced pdf features to create interactive worksheets (e.g., with input fields, checkboxes, and hyperlinks), or to use enhanced podcasting technologies to deliver the handout information to students' mobile devices (e.g., by including notes as mp3 file tags that can be accessed on-screen on an iPod or iPhone).

IMPLICATIONS

Implications for Practice

The study reported earlier has produced some insights for educational podcast design. In the following are considerations arising from these insights.

Content

Listening Tasks and Exercises

The subjects of the study seemed to perceive that podcasting is most suited for the development of their listening. This is most likely attributable to the auditory nature of this medium. Listening tasks and exercises should thus constitute a core feature of a language learning podcast.

Country and Culture Information

The inclusion of information on culture, society, and lifestyle in German-speaking countries was apparently well received by the students. The many positive qualitative statements indicate that there was considerable interest among students in these aspects. We argue that this is more likely to apply to languages other than English, because these are usually closely associated with or viewed as integral elements of specific cultures. With regard to English, there are many who dispute its ownership and claim that it does not belong to any one country or culture. Furthermore, because of its status as lingua franca of the business and technological sectors, many learn it essentially for its utilitarian value. In contrast, for most other languages, many learners are motivated by a distinct interest in the cultures behind them.

Providing Variety in Content and Developing Other Language Skills

The results of this study suggest that a podcast can also support students' learning not just in listening but in other language skills and areas as well. The respondents apparently also perceived the podcast's other components on grammar, pronunciation, vocabulary, speaking, and learning strategies to be useful. In fact, providing a variety of content would enhance a podcast's appeal for a wider audience with varying needs, interests, and preferences. The inclusion of materials such as a handout, on-screen notes, illustrations, and transcripts can extend learners' learning experience and provide some form of differentiation for learners of different abilities.

Design

Mode of Presentation

The German 1 podcast was presented in the informal, conversational style of a radio magazine, as advocated in other studies (e.g., Cebeci & Tekdal, 2006; Edirisingha, 2006). This was well received by the majority of the German 1 audience, who reported enjoying the podcast. Greeting the audience and addressing them directly in providing task instructions or grammar explanations constitute useful means of personalizing the podcast, enthusing learners, and conveying to them the instructors' commitment to the podcast.

Language of Presentation and Instructions

Listening to a podcast is an individual activity that typically takes place without the support of the teacher. Furthermore, if learners are on the move, they are unlikely to have access to a dictionary or other aids. Thus, especially for beginning learners, the podcast may have to be scripted to some extent in their first language or in a mixture of the first and target languages. Care should be taken to ensure that instructions are comprehensible. Nothing can be more frustrating and discouraging to learners than a podcast that is largely incomprehensible, especially when they cannot call upon a teacher for guidance and support. As learners gain greater proficiency and familiarity with the podcast and its task instructions, the target language can successively replace the first language as the language of presentation.

Task Design

Podcast tasks should generally be designed for two-way use, that is, for use with a computer as well as a mobile device. This implies, for instance, that instructions and perhaps even task solutions should be included not just in a handout but also in the audio recording itself. The tasks will have to be of limited complexity and length if learners are to be able to accomplish them even without the support of visual materials. For speaking tasks, sufficient response time should be given to learners.

Integration with Classroom Instruction

Blending Podcast and Classroom Instruction

Blending the podcast or individual podcast lessons with classroom instruction in a meaningful manner will motivate learners to listen. Such exposure may help them to see the relevance of the podcast for the course curriculum. For instance, students may be asked to listen to a podcast's culture segment in preparation for a subsequent discussion in class.

Preparation of Learners

Particularly for learners with little podcast learning experience, a demonstration of the podcast and its features in class is recommended. Instructors could take learners through the technical steps necessary to subscribe to the podcast. This appears vital in view of the finding that technical problems and an aversion to technology-based learning prevented some from accessing the German 1 podcast. If a computer classroom is available, students may be given actual hands-on experience in subscribing to the podcast.

Implications for Research

As mentioned earlier in this chapter, there is little published empirical research on podcasting in foreign language learning. While the data and insights from the present study may advance our understanding of podcast design and learners' podcast use, we are still far from being able to present a complete picture of how podcasts can contribute to meaningful and effective language learning. Further research is necessary to develop a comprehensive model of podcast-based language learning, and such research should survey learners of different proficiency levels and contexts as well as examine podcast projects of varying designs.

Furthermore, currently published research has tended to assess the effectiveness and usefulness of podcasts based on learners' perceptions. Such research will have to be complemented by experimental studies involving more objective measures of a podcast's effectiveness and students' proficiency gains.

Future research could also focus on how learners process tasks in a podcast lesson. Which strategies do they use or which are required for effective processing of podcast tasks? If indeed effective podcast learning strategies can be identified, how can a program be devised to instruct learners in the use of these strategies? A qualitative research design, involving instruments such as stimulated recall, interviews, and learner journals, will most likely afford a more complete and differentiated understanding of these processes.

CONCLUSION

This chapter reported on a project to produce a weekly podcast for German language beginners. It also presented findings from an accompanying study that investigated how students used the podcast as well as their perceptions of its usefulness and quality. The results indicate that students evaluated the podcast's design and technical quality positively. They rated it as especially useful in exposing them to authentic listening materials, helping them review and practice grammar, and providing country and culture information. While many did not embrace the possibility of listening to the podcast on the move, there were nevertheless signs that the podcast encouraged and enabled some to extend their learning beyond the confines of their classrooms and homes to public places such as buses, subway trains, or fast-food restaurants.

REFERENCES

Abdous, M., Camarena, M. M., & Facer, B. R. (2009). MALL technology: Use of academic podcasting in the foreign language classroom. *ReCALL, 21*(1), 76–95.

Baddeley, A. D. (1986). *Working memory.* Oxford: Oxford University Press.

Cebeci, Z., & Tekdal, M. (2006). Using podcasts as audio learning objects. *Interdisciplinary Journal of Knowledge and Learning Objects, 2,* 47–57.

Chan, W. M. (in press). Der Einsatz vom Podcast im DaF-Unterricht: Ein Vehikel zur Landeskundevermittlung [Podcasting in German as a foreign language: A vehicle for the transmission of country and culture information]. In R. Maeda (Ed.), *Transkulturalität: Identitäten in neuem Licht.* Munich: Iudicium.

Döpel, M. G. (2007). Review of "Audacity" and "Propaganda": Two applications for podcasting. *Electronic Journal of Foreign Language Teaching, 4*(1), 159–164.

Dunn, R. (2000). Capitalizing on college students' learning styles: Theory, practice, and research. In R. Dunn & S. A. Griggs (Eds.), *Practical approaches to using learning styles in higher education* (pp. 3–18). Westport, CT: Bergin and Garvey.

Dunn, R., & Dunn, K. (1999). *The complete guide to the learning-style inservice system.* Needham Heights, MA: Allyn and Bacon.

Edirisingha, P. (2006). *The "double life" of an i-Pod: A case study of the educational potential of new technologies.* Paper presented at Online Educa 2006, Berlin, Germany. Retrieved from http://hdl.handle.net/2381/406

Edirisingha, P., Rizzi, C., Nie, M., & Rothwell, L. (2007). Podcasting to provide teaching and learning support for an undergraduate module on English language and communication, *Turkish Online Journal of Distance Education, 8*(3), 87–107.

Engelkamp, J. (1991). Bild und Ton aus der Sicht der kognitiven Psychologie [Picture and sound from the perspective of cognitive psychology]. *Medienpsychologie, 3,* 278–299.

Engelkamp, J., & Zimmer, H. (1994). *The human memory—A multi-modal approach.* Göttingen/Bern: Hofgrefe and Huber.

Grinder, M. (1991). *The educational conveyor belt.* Portland, OR: Metamorphous.

Lewin, J. (2009, March 4). Podcasting goes mainstream. *Podcasting News: New Media Update.* Retrieved from http://www.podcastingnews.com/2009/03/04/podcasting-goes-mainstream/

McCarty, S. (2005). Spoken Internet to go: Popularization through podcasting. *The JALT CALL Journal, 1*(2), 67–74.

Monk, B., Ozawa, K., & Thomas, M. (2006). iPods in English language Education: A case study of English listening and reading students. *NUCB Journal of Language Culture and Communication, 8*(3), 85–102.

Paechter, M. (1993). *Sprechende Computer in CBT: Eine didaktische Konzeption* [Speaking computers in CBT: A pedagogical conceptual plan] (Arbeiten aus dem Seminar für Pädagogik. Bericht 1/93). Braunschweig: Technische Universität Braunschweig.

Reid, J. M. (1987). The learning style preferences of ESL students. *TESOL Quarterly, 21*(1), 87–111.

Rosell-Aguilar, F. (2007). Top of the pods—In search of a podcasting "podagogy" for language learning. *Computer Assisted Language Learning, 20*(5), 471–492.

Smith, L. H., & Renzulli, J. S. (1984). Learning style preferences: A practical approach for teachers. *Theory into Practice, 23,* 44–50.

Stanley, G. (2006). Podcasting: Audio on the internet comes of age. *TESL-EJ, 9*(4), 1–7.

Weidenmann, B. (2002). Multicodierung und Multimodalität im Lernprozess [Multicoding and multimodality in the learning process]. In L.J. Issing & P. Klimsa (Eds.), *Information und Lernen mit Multimedia und Internet* (pp. 45–62). Weinheim: Beltz.

Young, D. J. (2007). iPods, MP3 players and podcasts for FL learning: Current practices and future considerations. *The NECTFL Review, 60,* 39–49.

3 Mobile Technologies and Language Learning in Japan
Learn Anywhere, Anytime

Midori Kimura, Hiroyuki Obari, and Yoshiko Goda

INTRODUCTION

Over the past decade, mobile technologies and communication devices have become essential tools in higher education, and mobile learning (m-learning) has been acknowledged as a successful means of raising awareness of the importance of "anywhere, anytime" learning in an increasingly connected world (Metcalf II, 2006). M-learning encourages "self-access," and emphasizes the importance of learner independence and learner development. Learning is more effective when learners are active in the learning process, assuming responsibility for their learning and participating in the decisions that affect it. Therefore, "self-access language learning" is now often used as a synonym for "autonomous language learning" (Benson & Voller, 1997, p. 54). Holec (1981, p. 3) describes autonomy as "the ability to take charge of one's learning," and contemporary language-teaching methodologies make the assumption that taking an active, independent attitude to learning—that is, becoming an autonomous learner—is beneficial to learning (Benson, 2001; Little, 1991; Wenden, 1991). However, the presence of self-access facilities does not necessarily ensure that independent learning is taking place (Sheerin, 1997). Simply having students use technology does not raise achievement. The impact depends on the ways the technology is used and the conditions under which applications are implemented (Roblyer & Doering, 2007). Sturtridge (1997), based on her experience as a consultant to self-access projects in various parts of the world, has identified a number of factors contributing to the success or failure of self-access centers: management, facilities, staff training and development, learner training and development, learner culture, and materials. To appreciate the full potential of mobile technologies, educators must look beyond the use of individual devices, embedding them in the classroom or as a part of an outside-of-classroom learning experience (Wilen-Daugenti, 2007).

LEARNING BY MOBILE PHONE (M-LEARNING)

A review of m-learning projects funded by the European Union since 2001 (Pęcherzewska & Knot, 2007) confirms that mobile phones are the most frequently used device in m-learning projects. Research focused on language learning using mobile phones has become varied with a range of tools, activities, and language learning objectives, including e-mail (Kiernan & Aizawa, 2004), reading (Cavanaugh, 2007), Internet browsers (Taylor & Gitsaki, 2003), listening practice using the wireless application protocol (WAP) (Nah, White, & Sussex, 2008), quizzes and surveys (Levy & Kennedy, 2005; McNicol, 2005; Norbrook & Scott, 2003; Stockwell, 2008), and text messaging for vocabulary learning (Andrews, 2003; Levy & Kennedy, 2005; McNicol, 2005; Norbrook & Scott, 2003; Pincas, 2004; Stockwell, 2007, 2008; Thorton & Houser, 2005). All of the preceding involved one-way teacher-to-learner communication, although Nah et al. tried a student-centered collaborative learning approach using a WAP site to provide a mobile discussion board for listening.

Further specialized research projects include coaching for improving oral communication competence using mobile phones (Cooney & Keogh, 2007), and gathering oral or visual information using mobile phones with inbuilt cameras and voice recording facilities, a project conducted by City College, Southampton (see JISC, 2005).

STRENGTHS AND LIMITATIONS OF LEARNING BY MOBILE PHONES

Strengths and limitations appear repeatedly when reflecting upon the diverse range of research studies involving mobile phones covered in the previous section. Prevailing strengths are associated with qualities inherent in the device itself, that is, compactness, fast connection, individuality, and easy usage. Mobile phones provide high-speed Internet access, a rich mix of data, CD-quality music, and high-quality still and motion pictures. They can transmit video suitable for m-learning as well. These data can be saved in the device or in a memory stick (SD card), or micro SD card, which holds up to 32GB.

Limitations concern the small, non-user-friendly keypad, small display screen (resulting in constant scrolling), low screen resolution, slow processing, limited storage capacities, high costs, and risks (theft, breakages). Stockwell (2008) confessed that 60 percent of his students did not use the mobile phone at all and only 13.9 percent used it for more than half of the activities, adding that some felt unsure how to do the activities on the mobile phone, besides the aforementioned shortcomings. Nah et al. (2008) support his findings in that some assignments clearly were not suited to students' study habits; for example, they might prefer studying in a quiet place, or they did not like studying on short time-slices in public places, and other students did not take the assignment seriously due to the reason that each mark was not crucial to their overall course mark.

As a result of these technological limitations and differences in learning styles, the authors believe greater attention should be paid to m-learning program design, and students' individual differences (IDs).

LEARNING ENVIRONMENTS AND MOBILE PHONES IN JAPAN

In Japan, where people own more mobile phones than PCs, the mobile phone often functions as the most widely used mobile device. According to data collected by our m-learning research group, Task Force 26 (TF26), from 685 students from various universities in Tokyo, 90 percent of university students use the mobile phone far more often than they use computers (Kogure, Shimoyama, & Obari, 2009). In Japan, the context of use is also very important. For example, the cost structure is an issue, and telephone companies are trying to solve it by offering attractive discount services; students' responses also revealed that 95 percent of them were using the services. This implies that the infrastructure for m-learning environments has been established and we could develop the contents without being concerned about the financial burden on the students. Positive feedback from students indicated that mobile phones were more efficient than computers for sending text messages, and 63.1 percent were interested in such short-term training programs as studying English vocabulary by mobile phone.

The biggest challenge that course material designers confront in Japan is not so much the cost, but the variety of operating systems. Different carrier systems (Docomo, Softbank, and AU) require different formatting of course materials. Content needs to be specifically formatted for particular models of mobile phones to accommodate their restricted screen size and memory. Also, particular carriers have a lack of network connectivity standards and in addition there can be geographical limitations.

M-LEARNING AND LEARNING THEORY

Learners differ in their learning styles and preferences in terms of types of activity, and they may have particular language requirements arising from their studies. Research on IDs is significant, because the outcome of learning efforts is influenced by a variety of individual psychological variables (Benson, 2002; Ellis, 1994). Ellis emphasizes that IDs have been considered among the most important elements for L2 acquisition, and beliefs, affective states, and general factors (age, sex, aptitude, learning style, motivation, and personality) are interrelated (Thomas & Harri-Augstein, 1995).

Two factors that have traditionally been treated as key IDs are learning styles and language learning strategies (Dörnyei, 2005), and these are interrelated. Learning styles are internally based characteristics, often not perceived or used consciously, that are the basis for the intake and understanding of new information; students can identify their preferred learning styles and stretch those styles by examining and practicing various learning strategies. There are numerous studies on IDs in strategy use, especially on working memory (Bray, Saarnio, & Hawk, 1994; Fletcher & Bray, 1995; Mackey, Philp, Ego, Fujii, & Tatsumi, 2002; Osaka & Osaka, 2002). A mnemonic strategy is defined as "a set of behaviors specifically initiated to cope with the problem of remembering," and their research investigated an important way of overcoming memory limitations, which is essential to help learners acquire languages, especially vocabulary learning.

OVERARCHING RESEARCH QUESTIONS

The aim of the studies reported here was to investigate the effectiveness of learning by mobile phones with integration of e-learning and m-learning and to address the following research questions:

1. How can learning by mobile phones enhance English language learning?
   a. How effectively can a mobile group learn compared with a PC group?
   b. How do IDs contribute to improving English proficiency?
2. How can mobile technology support learners and foster autonomous learning in the English language classroom?
3. How can integration of e-learning and m-learning help EFL learners to improve their overall English proficiency?

THE THREE STUDIES: THE PROMISE OF
ENGLISH STUDY BY MOBILE PHONES

This chapter describes three projects that involved English study via mobile phone. The first project was TOEIC (Test of English for International Communication) test preparation by mobile phone; experiments for this project were conducted over a five-month period in 2003. The second and most recent project focused upon vocabulary learning using flashcards via mobile phone. The third study focused upon the integration of e-learning and m-learning. Each project will now be described in turn.

Study 1: The TOEIC Preparation Study

In Japan, TOEIC is very popular because the test score is used by a wide range of companies as well as government agencies to make significant personnel decisions. The preparation program mainly consisted of drill-and-practice programs for vocabulary study and grammar practice, and the learning management system provided immediate feedback to the learners.

Method

Participants

The subjects in the first project consisted of 98 business majors at university who were divided into two groups according to their own learning preferences: The m-learning group was made up of 41 students (mobile group; $n = 41$), and the computer-network learning group was made up of 57 students (PC group; $n = 57$).

Procedure

We uploaded 1,183 TOEIC questions (Part V and VI vocabulary and grammar) on a website that contained an online English-language study program service consisting of multiple-choice questions with answers and answer keys. Both groups could download and solve as many questions as they wished. For the mobile group, a set of three questions was sent each time the service was accessed, and when a student solved the questions, their answers were sent through the Internet, scored, and the results returned immediately.

Both groups of learners were asked to take a test before the project (pre-test). The pre-test consisted of 50 questions. The same test was given as a post-test at the end of the project. The study lasted five months. We compared the pre- and post-test scores and conducted a survey at the end of the project. The survey questionnaire consisted of 14 questions that had "yes," "no," and "neither" answers. These questions were aimed at providing information on aptitude, gender, personality, learning style preferences, and motivation. The responses from the questionnaire on IDs and test results were compiled and compared statistically to analyze the differences between the two groups.

Technologies

The mobile Internet included the Learning Management System (LMS), which monitored the students' learning progress and listed the incorrect answers. In this study, we wanted to see statistically if learners would really study English with a mobile phone in their spare time, and to ascertain the effectiveness of mobile technologies in language learning. The students were informed by e-mail of the results of their performance as well as the assignments on the website that were to be practiced every day.

Results

To the question of when and where the learners used their mobile phones to study TOEIC questions, more than 50 percent of the students responded, "While waiting for a friend" and "During my commute." They made good use of the short time available to study by mobile phone. The students became more proactive concerning the conduct and conditions of the project, requesting that they be allowed to choose the delivery time, frequency, and quantity of practice materials. As to the question of how they like using IT devices, more than 60 percent of both the PC and the mobile group answered that they used computers often, they favored learning with IT devices, and were interested in e-learning and m-learning. Of particular interest is the figure (80.5 percent) of the mobile group, who responded "Use mobile phone often," indicating very clearly that the groups were formed along the lines of their preferences.

Survey results also found that the mobile group preferred a "multiple-choice test style" and a "study little by little every day" learning strategy, and students in the mobile group seemed more planned in their study. Test results were compared between the two groups. Test scores (full mark = 50) of the PC group was 30.2 (pre-test) and 32.9 (post-test), and for the mobile group, 29.4 (pre-test) and 32.6 (post-test) respectively. We statistically confirmed that both groups improved in their scores and there was a significant difference between pre-test scores and post-test scores in both groups ($p < 0.0001$); however, there was not a significant difference ($p = 0.8$) in the test score improvement between the two groups, although the mean score of the mobile phone group (*Mean* = 3.17) is higher than the PC's (*Mean* = 2.86). This means that students learn well either by PC or by mobile phone.

Study 2: Vocabulary Learning by Mobile Phones

The second and most recent project focused upon vocabulary learning using flashcards via the mobile phone. We found in the survey (Kogure et al., 2009) that many students were interested in learning vocabulary by mobile phones, and that as far as the students were concerned, vocabulary was the most important level of L2 knowledge for all learners (Harp & Mayer, 1998); therefore, the authors advise that this should be one of the compulsory items to choose for an m-learning project. It was conducted for six weeks in October and November 2007.

Method

Procedure and Participants

The vocabulary items were chosen according to what were considered to be useful words for daily life, and 150 words were selected from two vocabulary lists (JACET 8,000 word list, and ALC 12,000 word list). Those were divided into three groups considering the part of speech and the meaning, and each group of words was used for three types of the contents respectively. According to Kadota and Ikemura (2006), it is possible to activate vocabulary learning by showing words in different forms. They refer to five forms: translation, illustration, example sentences, oral introduction with sound, and appropriate amount of words. To identify the effectiveness of vocabulary learning with mobile phones, the first were selected for learning by mobile phones. These were (a) an English word with Japanese translation, which is the traditional Japanese way of learning vocabulary; (b) an English word with a picture clue, which combines a word with images; and (c) an English word to memorize highlighted in red in a sentence and the Japanese translation (see Figure 3.1). We compared the test scores between the pre-test and post-test.

The participants were undergraduate students living in/around Tokyo in Japan. In total, 137 students majoring in seven different fields joined the experiment. The experiment extended across six weeks in autumn in 2007. In the first week, a pre-test and a pre-questionnaire were conducted. The pre-test consisted of 30 words out of 150 words. The pre-questionnaire was organized to describe the vocabulary learning styles and strategies of the participants. Students' feedback was used from the viewpoint of three strategies (O'Malley & Chamot, 1990; Oxford, 1990): (a) meta-cognitive (planning, monitoring); (b) cognitive (memorization, practice); and (c) affective (communication with others).

The post-test was composed of the same words as the pre-test to measure the effect of mobile vocabulary learning. The questionnaire was organized to investigate the preference for the type of content and the strategies the students used.

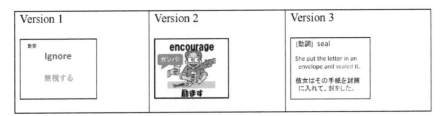

Figure 3.1 Three kinds of vocabulary.

Technologies

We created an application called "Flashcard activity"—the most basic drill-and-practice functions, arising from the popularity of real-world flashcards. Digital flashcards were uploaded on the Internet and students downloaded them into the memory card (SD card) in their mobile phone, so that they did not have to access the Internet every time they studied. Students could make a list of difficult words with sound in their card, which encouraged efficient study and economical battery use.

Results

The best test score was achieved in version 1 (an English word with Japanese translation), 21.4 (full mark = 30); followed by version 3 (an English word in example sentences with the Japanese translation), 20.3; and version 2 (an English word with a picture clue), 17.3. However, most students preferred version 3 (68 percent) to the other two (version 1, 51 percent; version 2, 41 percent). They commented that studying words in sentences helped them understand how to use words in real communication. Many students appeciated "anytime, anywhere learning" style (72.5 percent), and wanted to study vocabulary periodically using example sentences to review class lessons (65.2 percent). Actually, students' time spent studying while commuting increased dramatically among the following majors, due to the introduction of vocabulary learning by mobile phones: English (from 65 percent to 82 percent), Business (from 71 percent to 92 percent), and Pharmacology (from 73 percent to 100 percent), and this is valuable evidence that learning by mobile phone fits their study habits and lifestyles. There was a big change in strategy use during the project: The popular memory strategies, "making a word list" decreased from 83.2 percent to 50 percent, "writing words many times" decreased from 80.6 percent to 27 percent, and "reading words aloud" decreased from 76.2 percent to 30.2 percent. Those were their favorite memory strategies, but the study tool changed their learning strategy usage, and many high-achieving students commented that they preferred to have writing exercises to memorize vocabulary spelling.

Study 3: Integration of E-Learning and M-Learning

Background and Context

Blended Learning

The successful integration of e-learning and m-learning is a further example of blended learning, which usually simply refers to face-to-face learning combined with some form of e-learning. Some benefits of blended learning are as follows:

- Blended learning prevents learner isolation and saves cases of dropouts.
- Stanford University reported that they succeeded in raising students' self-pace course completion rate from a little over 50 percent to 94 percent by incorporating elements of BL (Singh & Reed, 2005).
- In a blended learning best practice survey, 73.6 percent of respondents reported blended learning to be more effective than non-blended approaches (Wilson & Smilanich, 2005).

Simply sitting in front of the computer or using the mobile technologies all the time is not likely to greatly motivate students learning English. If students feel isolated, many of them will give up the course early. However, in blending face-to-face learning in a classroom setting with e-learning, it is expected that we can complement some, if not all, of these setbacks (Macdonald, 2008). On the other hand, face-to-face learning has its advantages too, such as sustaining motivation, morale, and good study habits through regular meetings at the same time and place; socializing with other classmates; and receiving inspiration/advice from a knowledgeable teacher.

The Integrated Language Learning System

For Study 3, an integrated university system was used. This comprised the Aoyama Gakuin University Cyber Campus System (AGU-CCS) combined with the CaLabo EX CALL system, thereby creating an integrated learning environment that was launched in April 2003 specifically to teach English as a foreign language. The AGU-CCS, which is an e-learning system in our campus, supports various kinds of study forms, such as self-learning, live learning for large numbers of students, and collaborative learning. Once the student's computer is connected to the Internet, it is possible to access CCS from anywhere, whether at home or studying at the university or working at the office, and at any time of the day or night, by logging on with user ID and a password. It is easy to access AGU-CCS with smart phones. It is also capable of providing podcasting, and enables m-learning using an iPod or other mp3 device, including the mobile phone (see Figure 3.2). Online Computerized Assessment System for English Communication (CASEC, see http://casec.evidus.com/english/) has been implemented since April 2004 to check the progress that the students made, with the comparison of pre-tests and post-tests.

In 2008 a survey was conducted involving about 150 students who were asked their views on using the AGU-CCS. Of these participants, about 77 percent found that using CCS integrated with CaLabo EX CALL system and m-learning was very useful for studying English. If students used the AGU-CCS systems integrated with CaLabo EX CALL, they could take full advantages of learning EFL that had been combined with ICTs.

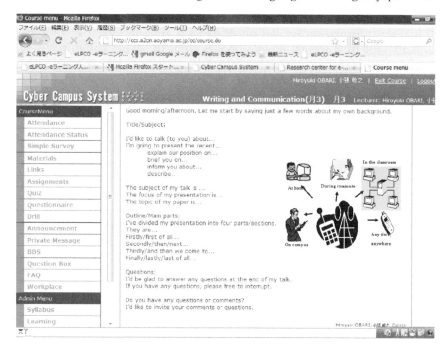

Figure 3.2   An integration of e-learning and m-learning.

Method

Participants and Procedure

Sixty-three students enrolled as Economics majors participated in this learning activity using mobile phones for class. There were three learning activities, divided broadly into pre-activities, main-activities, and post-activities. Students used the mobile phone as pre-learning activities and post-learning activities to learn English words and phrases related to the textbook, world heritage sites, and English presentation expressions during their commuting hours or during their free time. Important English key words and phrases were prepared in advance for mobile use, and sometimes these words and phrases were directly sent to students' mobile phones from the cyber campus system.

To check the students' progress in English proficiency, the following factors were considered: (a) improvements of CASEC scores, and (b) analyses of speech prosody in comparison with the prosody of native speakers. The CASEC computer test was administered in order to assess English proficiency as a pre-test in April 2008 and as a post-test in January 2009. Pre- and post-recorded data of participants were collected and analyzed in terms of fundamental frequency (F0), speech duration, and speech power.

Technologies

Whatever information we put on AGU-CCS announcement section was directly sent to students' mobile phones from the cyber campus system. Multimedia learning materials with many formats such as mp3, mp4, wmv (Windows Media Video), avi, and mpeg4 were uploaded on CCS so that students could download multimedia learning materials into their mobile phones for viewing or listening purposes; these materials were then used in the classroom as pre-activities and post-activities. Online English speech training software was also available to learn English pronunciation.

Results

As a result of the integration of e-learning and m-learning, students made steady progress in the English proficiency test, which significantly improved the average score of 63 students from 539 ($SD = 93$) in the pre-test in April of 2008, to 586 ($SD = 76$) in the post-test in January of 2009 after 24 weeks of lessons.

Several parameters—fundamental frequency (F0), speech duration, and speech power—were used to analyze prosody of Japanese English speakers before and after 24 weeks of lessons with integration of e-learning and m-learning. The speech duration was shortened between pre- and post-reading as it was indicated from 5,383 ms to 4,872 ms ($p < 0.01$). The students could speak English a little faster than they could before and their speech rate became faster and better. Vowel duration/sentence duration, ratio of vowel duration over sentence duration, decreased from 0.51 to 0.49 ($p < 0.01$). Japanese speakers tend to be influenced by five main Japanese vowels when speaking English. However, due to the effect of the integrated lesson, vowel ratio over sentence duration became shorter to get closer to the English prosody.

Ratio of consonant power over vowel power increased from 0.32 to 0.39 ($p < 0.01$). When Japanese English speakers speak English, they tend to pronounce consonants with less stressed accent. However, these Japanese English speakers produced consonants better than they did previously after 24 weeks of lessons. In the ratio of maximum F0 over minimum F0, there is no significant difference between before and after lessons. However, only 46 percent of participants improved the ratio of F0. This is because this English pronunciation software put more emphasis upon training segmental features, rather than on prosody.

The differences of scores between pre- and post-recorded readings indicated that integration of e-learning and m-learning encouraged self-learning and autonomous learning, and it led to the improvement of overall English proficiency (Obari, 2009).

DISCUSSION

In the first project, the survey on IDs in the TOEIC preparation study disclosed several interesting factors regarding effective m-learning. Students who prefer m-learning were already exercising the meta-cognitive learning strategy of planning, and they were studying little by little every day to achieve their goal; the PC group students did not practice to the same extent. Although there was not a significant difference in the test scores between the two groups, the mobile group students seemed to become more proactive than the PC group, by often requesting more questions. Therefore, for the TOEIC study, we are able to confirm that learning by mobile phones is effective for a kind of multiple-choice drill activity.

In the second project on vocabulary learning via mobile phones, and where they were obliged to study using their phones, students' study time increased, at least during the experiment when they were learning with mobile phones. Study times in three areas increased as follows: English majors (from 65 percent to 82 percent), Business majors (from 71 percent to 92 percent), and Pharmacology majors (from 73 percent to 100 percent). This provides valuable evidence to support the idea that learning by mobile phone fits students' study habits and lifestyles. Lehner, Nosekabel, and Lehmann (2002) also reported that mobile devices gave commuter students the ability to use their spare time wisely to finish homework and prepare for lessons. However, there is an issue that needs to be addressed for the next project concerning memory strategy use. The students decreased their usage frequencies of some of their favorite memory strategies, including "writing words many times" and "underlining or highlighting the important parts." Students reported they have been using these strategies for more than 10 years and they are essential memory strategies for Japanese students; therefore, we believe we need to develop a program to include some writing-in-vocabulary exercises for the future.

In the third project of the integration of e-learning and m-learning, this research indicated, from the results of improvements of CASEC score and prosody analyses, that the integration of AGUCCS, CaLabo EX, English pronunciation software, and mobile technologies is useful in learning EFL. The CASEC test has been helpful to check the progress of each student from pre-test and post-test. Students seemed to be more motivated to target the certain score of CASEC while they tried to make effective English presentations with PowerPoint using various ICT tools, including mobile devices. In the very near future, many more mobile devices such as iPad and smart phones will be available for these learning devices.

Broadening out the discussion now beyond the three studies, we would like to discuss how mobile technology can support learners and foster autonomous learning in English language classrooms. Benson and Voller (1997) emphasized that learning is more effective when learners are active in the learning process, assuming responsibility for their learning. Therefore, learner development is not something that teachers "do" to learners, but that learners develop themselves. However, some students might not be able to find the way to be an independent learner unless teachers give them a chance of being trained, and we believe that the results from these projects can contribute to that purpose. By actually using mobile phones for pre-activities and post-activities in class, the participating students came to realize the effectiveness of m-learning through the experience and the outcome—good test scores—and this experience provides a practical introduction and guide to self-learning and autonomous learning.

Summarizing our projects, we consider that they were successful overall in facilitating English learning, and there were some common factors among them:

- Information on the screen was very simple and short.
- Each task could be learned in a few minutes.
- They matched students' study habits and lifestyles.
- Study contents met students' needs.
- They were successfully integrated in the curriculum.

Factors that differed among them were caused by the technology and the system. The TOEIC program with LMS was a "ready-made" lesson, programmed by a professional engineer, and it therefore provided immediate feedback by LMS; however, learning contents were not customized for learners, and telephone bills were expensive at the time of the project in 2002 (although this would not be such a big issue today because of a special discount telephone bill service). On the other hand, vocabulary learning was prepared by the teachers. It was a custom-made project in the sense that students' English proficiency and IDs were also taken into consideration; however, it placed a heavy burden on teachers in preparing learning contents.

We have seen the success in self-learning with mobile phones so far; however, we should emphasize that our project could not have been so successful without the existence of the Research Center for e-Learning Professional Competency (eLPCO). They collaboratively worked with e-learning professionals and offered us educational support and system implementation so that teachers could develop a flexible learning environment. They shared Sturtridge's (1997) idea and contributed to developing independent learning environments for teachers and students.

Improvement in English education was accomplished as a result of the development of ICTs, which established a cyber community for learning in Japan. Now learners can study anywhere, anytime, and any topic according to their interests, time allowance, or their abilities using mobile technologies. This has opened up new opportunities for communication between both learners and teachers, and among English-language users themselves. Many English teachers see a great potential in learning in a cyber community, because it encourages self-learning and a learner-oriented approach to English education, and fosters autonomous learners.

RESEARCH CENTER TO SUPPORT MOBILE LEARNING

In order to create a flexible learning environment and encourage anywhere, anytime learning, an organizational support system comprised of e-learning professionals is essential for both faculties and students. We further believe such an environment will foster autonomous learners.

The eLPCO in Aoyama Gakuin University (AGU) has been researching around the theme of e-learning professionals for both Japanese higher education and corporate needs for about 10 years. eLPCO is a part of the Research Institute, AGU, and has four main research domains: General Affairs, Research Dissemination and Educational Support, Research Development, and System Implementation Domains. Our m-learning research group TF26 belongs to the Educational Contents field in the research and development domain. eLPCO is researching the potential use not only of computers but also of other mobile devices for educational applications. Combinations of existing and emerging technology are also studied to integrate the technology into learning environments.

Major duties of the ICT specialist of eLPCO are managing and implementing the CCS, LMS, as well as other ICT systems. They monitor the CCS and if any problem occurs, they have to handle it and to minimize its negative effects on students' learning. They are providing not only the necessary system support directly related to the CCS, but also useful information and tips on how to integrate the latest technologies into teachers' classes. They also offer some free seminars regularly through the school year to teachers who do not have basic IT skills or literacy. If a teacher has some inquiry about the system or technology, one of the specialists will helpfully consult with him or her. This kind of help or support gives teachers confidence and creative ideas on how to use technology effectively in language learning.

If new technology is available, then the ICT specialists are able to collect information and test features and capabilities in cooperation with other faculties and researchers. When the ICT specialists consider improvements of the system, TF26 gives some advice and opinions based on their research results and experiences. This collaboration among researchers, teachers, and eLPCO's ICT specialists enables the development of a flexible learning environment for users, including teachers, students, and administrators.

CONCLUSION

Our research results have shown that mobile technologies introduced in our projects were effectively integrated into the language learning class to meet the needs of students. Learners could access the learning materials whenever they wanted to learn, and study them at their own pace, thereby encouraging learner autonomy. We should also emphasize that m-learning became effective with the support of eLPCO, which provided an organizational support system to encourage anywhere, anytime learning. We believe such an environment will foster autonomous learners.

We found many advantages in m-learning; however, we must also pay attention to some disadvantages. As we could see in the case of Stockwell (2008), although using mobile phones is generally easy, when complicated programs are introduced, students show negative attitudes. The most important factor in learning with technologies is that projects should be learner-friendly. "Technically possible" does not equal "desirable, feasible, or inevitable." Our projects did not require a heavy burden on learners, either in terms of technology demands or content. Besides, bite-size study seemed to have attracted students who otherwise would not have been so interested in learning itself. Effective learning should take IDs into consideration, and learning materials should be carefully designed considering the students' learning strategies. Although we often hear complaints from nonmobile learners about the mobile phone's limited screen size, it is the combination of miniaturization, mobility, and power that grabs today's mobile phone users. We have been working to ensure that our students extracted maximum understanding and benefit when learning via mobile phones.

At the time this research was conducted the mobile technology infrastructure was limited. It has since improved greatly with high-speed Internet access, a rich mix of data, expansion of memory storage capacity, CD-quality music, and high-quality still and motion pictures. We can expect changes and improvements to continue; however, what is important is that the research on the application of mobile technologies to learning and teaching continues also. Further studies with a wider range of participants and more variety in content would be advantageous and potentially the results would lead to better curriculum design and programs that are more learner-oriented in the future.

With the help of eLPCO, it has become possible to fully utilize the potential of mobile technology and integrate e-learning and m-learning in the classroom as well as outside-of-classroom learning, and achieve a proficiency improvement.

ACKNOWLEDGMENTS

This research project was supported by the Good Practice Project of Ministry of Education, Culture, Sports and Science in Japan. We wish to thank all the members of TF26 at eLPCO at Aoyama Gakuin University.

REFERENCES

Andrews, R. (2003). Lrn Welsh by txt msg. *BBC News World Edition*. Retrieved from http://news.bbc.co.uk/2/hi/uk_news/wales/2798701.stm
Benson, P. (2001). *Teaching and researching autonomy in language learning*. London: Longman.

Benson, P. (2002). Autonomy as a learner's and teacher's right. In B. Sinclair., G. Ellis, D. Little, I. McGrath, & R. Ravindran (Eds.), *Learner autonomy, teacher autonomy: Future directions* (pp. 111–117). London: Longman.

Benson, H., & Voller, P. (Eds.). (1997). *Autonomy & independence in language learning.* New York: Longman.

Bray, N. W., Saarnio, D. A., & Hawk, L. W. (1994). A context for understanding intellectual and developmental differences in strategy competencies. *American Journal of Mental Retardation, 99,* 44–49.

Cavanaugh, T. (2007). Using the cell phone for class content: An exploration. In R. Carlsen, K. McFerrin, J. Price, R. Weber & D. A. Willis. (Eds.), *Proceedings of Society for Information Technology & Teacher Education International Conference 2007* (pp. 1931–1936). Chesapeake, VA: AACE.

Cooney, G., & Keogh, H. (2007). *Use of mobile phones for language learning and assessment for learning.* Paper presented at MLearn 2007. Retrieved from http://www.learnosity,com/files/learnosity-use-of-mobile-hones-for-language-learning-and-assessment-for-learning.pdf

Dörnyei, Z. (2005). *The psychology of the language learner. Individual differences in second language acquisition.* Mahwah, New Jersey: Laurence Erlbaum Associates.

Ellis, R. (1994). *The study of second language acquisition.* Oxford: Oxford University Press.

Fletcher, K. L., & Bray, N. W. (1995). External and verbal strategies in children with and without mental retardation. *American Journal of Mental Retardation, 99,* 363–375.

Harp, S. F., & Mayer, R. E. (1998). How seductive details do their damage: A theory of cognitive interest in science learning. *Journal of Educational Psychology, 90,* 414–434.

Holec, H. (1981). *Autonomy in foreign language learning.* Oxford: Pergamon.

JISC. (2005). Multimedia learning with mobile phones. Innovative practices with e-learning. Case Studies: Anytime, any place learning. Retrieved from http://www.jisc.ac.uk/uploaded_documents/southampton.pdf

Kadota, S., & Ikemura, T. (2006). *Eigo goi shido handbook.* Tokyo: Taishukan Shoten.

Kiernan, P., & Aizawa, K. (2004). Cell phones in task based learning. Are cell phones useful language learning tools? *ReCALL, 16*(1), 71–84.

Kogure, Y., Shimoyama, Y., & Obari, H. (2009). *Mobile literacy of university students.* Paper presented at Japan Engineering Education Association, Tokyo University.

Lehner, F., Nosekabel, F., & Lehmann, L. (2002). Wireless e-learning and communication environment: WELCOME at the University of Regensburg. *e-Service Journal, 2*(3), 23–41.

Levy, M., & Kennedy, C. (2005). Learning Italian via mobile SMS. In A. Kukulska-Hulme & J. Traxler (Eds.), *Mobile learning: A handbook for educators and trainers* (pp. 76–83). London: Taylor and Francis.

Little, D. (1991). *Learner autonomy. 1: Definitions, issues and problems.* Dublin: Authentik.

Macdonald, J. (2008). *Blended learning and online tutoring.* Burlington, VT: Gower Publishing.

Mackey, A., Philp, J., Ego, T., Fujii, A., & Tatsumi, T. (2002). Individual differences in working memory, noticing of interactional feedback and L2 development. In P. Robinson (Ed.), *Individual differences and instructed language learning* (pp. 181–209). Amsterdam: John Benjamins Publishing Co.

McNicol, T. (2005). Language e-learning on the move. *Japan media review.* Retrieved January 22, 2010, from http://ojr.org/japan/wireless/1080854640.php

Metcalf II, D. (2006). *mLearning. Mobile learning and performance in the palm of your hand.* Amherst, MA: HRD Press.

Nah, K., White, P., & Sussex, R. (2008). The potential of using a mobile phone to access the Internet for learning EFL listening skills within a Korean context. *ReCALL, 20*(3), 331–347.

Norbrook, H., & Scott, P. (2003). Motivation in mobile modern foreign language learning. In J. Attewell, G. Da Bormida, M. Sharples, & C. Savill-Smith (Eds.), *MLEARN 2003: Learning with mobile devices* (pp. 50–51). London: Learning and Skills Development Agency.

Obari, H. (2009). Integration of e-learning and m-learning in teaching EFL in Japan. In T. Bastiaens, J. Dron, & C. Xin (Eds.), *Proceedings of World Conference on E-Learning in Corporate, Government, Healthcare, and Higher Education 2009* (pp. 1009–1015). Chesapeake, VA: AACE.

O'Malley, M. J., & Chamot, A. U. (1990). *Learning strategies in second language acquisition.* Cambridge: Cambridge University Press.

Osaka, M., & Osaka, N. (2002). The effect of focusing on a sentence in Japanese reading span test. In E. Witruk, A. D. Friederici, & T. Lachmann (Eds.), *Basic functions of language, reading and reading disability (Neuropsychology and cognition)* (pp. 155–162). Boston: Kluwer Academic Publishing.

Oxford, R. (1990). *Language learning strategies: What every teacher should know.* Boston: Heinle and Heinle Publisher.

Pęcherzewska, A., & Knot, S. (2007). *Review of existing EU projects dedicated to dyslexia, gaming in education and m-learning* (WR08 Report to CallDysMProject. June 2007).

Pincas, A. (2004). *Using mobile support for use of Greek during the Olympic Games 2004.* Paper presented at M-Learn Conference 2004, Rome, Italy.

Roblyer, M. D., & Doering, A. H. (2007). *Integrating educational technology into teaching.* Upper Saddle River, N.J.: Pearson/Merrill Prentice Hall.

Sheerin, S. (1997). An exploration of the relationship between self-access and independent learning. In P. Benson & P. Voller (Eds.), *Autonomy and independence in language learning* (pp. 54–65). London: Longman.

Singh, H., & Reed, C. (2005). Achieving success with synchronous blended learning solutions, In L. Bielawski & D. Metcalf (Eds.), *Blended eLearning* (pp. x–x). Amherst: HRD Press.

Stockwell, G. (2007). Vocabulary on the move: Investigating an intelligent mobile phone-based vocabulary tutor. *Computer Assisted Language Learning, 20*(4), 365–383.

Stockwell, G. (2008). Investigating learner preparedness for and usage patterns of mobile learning. *ReCALL, 20*(3), 253–270.

Sturtridge, G. (1997). Teaching and language learning in self-access centres: Changing roles? In P. Benson & P. Voller (Eds), *Autonomy and independence in language learning* (pp. 66–78). London: Longman.

Taylor, R. P., & Gitsaki, C. (2003). Teaching WEKK in a computerless classroom. *Computer Assisted Language Learning, 16*(4), 275–294.

Thomas, L., & Harri-Augstein, S. (1995). *Self-organized learning: Foundations of a conversational science for psychology.* London: Routledge and Kegan Paul.

Thorton, P., & Houser, C. (2005). Using mobile phones in English education in Japan. *Journal of Computer Assisted Learning, 21*(3), 217–228.

Wenden, A. (1991). *Learner strategies for learner autonomy.* London: Prentice Hall International.

Wilen-Daugenti, T. (2007).*Technology and learning environments in higher education.* New York: Peter Lang Publishing Inc.

Wilson, D., & Smilanich, E. (2005). *The other blended learning.* San Francisco: Pfeiffer.

4 EFL Students' Metalinguistic Awareness in E-Mail Tandem

Akihiko Sasaki and Osamu Takeuchi

INTRODUCTION

Due to the rapid development of telecommunication technology, the use of computer-mediated communication (CMC) in language education has become widespread. Different types of CMC activities, including both synchronous (i.e., real time) and asynchronous (i.e., time delayed) modes of communication, have been increasingly introduced in language classrooms in an attempt to facilitate learners' authentic communication with the native speakers of the target language (L2) (Levy & Stockwell, 2006; Warschauer & Kern, 2000). This study focuses on e-mail tandem language learning, which is one type of asynchronous activity among various types of CMC activities.

E-MAIL TANDEM LANGUAGE LEARNING

When applied in the field of language education, the term *tandem* is "used to refer to organized language exchanges between two language learners, each of whom wishes to improve his or her proficiency in the other's native language (L1)" (Appel & Mullen, 2000, p. 291). Students on both sides use their L2 (i.e., the partner's L1) to talk about topics that focus on their needs and interests, and offer occasional assistance to the partner's L2 use by correcting linguistic mistakes, suggesting alternative expressions, assisting comprehension of the text, and so forth. Occasionally, students use their L1 (i.e., the partner's L2) in some parts of the communication so that learners have opportunities to practice not only producing L2 but also receiving its models provided by their native-speaking partner (Brammerts, 2003).

The original form of tandem language learning was conducted in face-to-face interaction, with the main channel of communication being oral (Appel & Mullen, 2000). This is, however, difficult to implement in foreign language (FL) learning settings, where the access to native L2 speakers is inevitably limited. E-mail tandem has an advantage over the original face-to-face format in this regard since the telecommunication technology allows FL students to remotely communicate with native L2 speakers living in other countries across different time zones (Appel & Mullen, 2000). Moreover, its asynchronous mode of communication provides students with more time to attend to and reflect on the form and content of the message, compared to dynamic and fast-paced face-to-face interaction (Arnold & Ducate, 2006). E-mail tandem, therefore, is thought to be a practical and suitable alternative approach for FL learners, even for beginners, who need sufficient time to read, comprehend, and produce their L2.

According to Brammerts (2003), the goals of tandem exchange include improving the learners' L2 communicative and linguistic abilities, as well as learning from each other's cultural background, knowledge, and experiences. The pedagogical benefits of e-mail tandem activity highlighted in previous studies vary, but they have included raising students' cultural awareness (Dodd, 2001; Woodin, 2001), increasing motivation (Appel & Gilabert, 2002; Ushioda, 2000), developing language learning skills (Braga, 2007), enhancing learner autonomy (Little, 2003; Ushioda, 2000), and providing opportunities for repeated attempts at producing comprehensible output and noticing the gap (McPartland, 2003). Edasawa and Kabata (2007) and Kabata and Edasawa (2008, August) also found that, in their e-mail tandem projects between Japanese and Canadian universities, students extended vocabulary, grammar, and phrase/sentence expressions through collaborative communication.

Important among these earlier investigations on e-mail tandem is Appel's (1999) study that addressed the question of raising learners' metalinguistic awareness (MA). She reported that her e-mail tandem students had developed their MA by correcting their partners' language. Raising students' MA is one of the major themes of this chapter, and in the next section, the significance of MA in language learning will be discussed in terms of its theoretical basis.

METALINGUISTIC AWARENESS

According to van Lier (1996), MA is a person's ability to objectify language. More specifically, it is one's capacity to shift his/her attention from the meaning conveyed in the language to the properties of the language, together with an ability to analyze the structural and functional aspects of language (Kuo & Anderson, 2008). It thus includes a person's sensitivity to certain linguistic patterns, such as parts of speech, word order, inflection, agreement, number, and so on. Similarly, MA may include translating one language into another, judging whether a given sentence is grammatical, or making explicit an intuitive knowledge of L1. Appel's (1999) students mentioned that they were more and more aware of the grammar rules of their L1 when they corrected their partners' L2 use.

This cognitive process is regarded as development of their MA (Bialystok, 2001; Kuo & Anderson, 2008).

In empirical SLA studies, MA has been traditionally operationalized as a learner's ability to identify and correct an error, and to provide the rule governing the correction (Renou, 2000), and many researchers now agree that MA plays a facilitative role in additional language learning (e.g., Bialystok, 2001; Cenoz & Jessner, 2000). Van Lier (1996) explained that, while young L1 learners naturally attend to language features in the input necessary for their linguistic development, L2 learners do not have such innate devices available and need other kinds of support. He suggested that it is MA that may help guide L2 learners to focus attention on linguistic input effectively.

Among the previous studies that investigated the relationship between MA and L2 proficiency, some studies measured learners' MA in L2 (Elder & Manwaring, 2004; Roehr, 2007), while others focused on MA in L1 and suggested its positive correlation with L2 proficiency (Cummins, 2000; Lasagabaster, 2001; Otsu, 2008, May). Considering that MA in itself is regarded as part of neither L1 nor L2, but as one integrated source of linguistic ability that a person can have access to in using and learning languages (Jessner, 1999; Yamada, 2006), it is assumed that MA can be measured in any language in which the person is functioning. In this chapter, therefore, students' MA is assessed by their abilities in identifying and correcting errors that their e-mail tandem partners have made, and providing L1 linguistic rules for them.

In Appel's (1999) paper, she presented excerpts from some of her students' comments, which illustrated that the analysis of their partners' language in the feedback phase made them aware of their L1 linguistic features and affected their L2 knowledge and use. Her paper, however, did not refer to specific linguistic features of L1 that her students analyzed, and did not show in detail how such explicit L1 knowledge was subsequently utilized for their further L2 learning.

Admitting the theoretical benefit of MA in L2 learning, the authors of this study believe that detailed examination of the development of tandem learners' MA and its relationship with their L2 proficiency would be beneficial for illustrating a practical advantage of e-mail tandem learning. The present study therefore attempts to investigate the following research questions:

1. In the feedback phase, what L1 features do Japanese tandem learners notice in their partner's language use and analyze to explain linguistic rules to their partner?
2. How does their heightened MA affect L2 knowledge?
3. Do EFL learners with a higher degree of MA possess higher L2 proficiency?

METHOD

The E-Mail Tandem Project

The authors of this study have conducted a series of e-mail tandem projects between Japanese and American secondary school students commencing each fall since 2003. The Japanese students belong to a junior high school affiliated to a private university located near the Osaka metropolitan area. The partner school in America is a public high school located in San Jose, California. Both schools have a considerable reputation for academic excellence, and are well known for their families' high educational and socioeconomic status. In order to carry out the project, students of both sides have access to computers in their schools' PC labs, as well as home PCs. The data for this chapter were collected from the 2006 and 2007 projects.

Participants

The 2006 and 2007 projects included 10 and 7 Japanese students respectively. They were members of an English elective course taught by the first author of this chapter. The students were all boys, aged 14 to 15 (ninth grade), learning English as a foreign language. Their English proficiency level was from high beginner to low intermediate. The average score of GTEC for Students, an English proficiency test,[1] was 537.5 in 2006 and 485.3 in 2007. According to the summary of the 2006–2008 test administration, the national average score was 408 for 10th grade, 445 for 11th, and 463 for 12th. Given these figures, the English ability of the students of this study was considerably higher when compared with that of other Japanese students of the same age.

On the American side, a total of 35 and 27 students joined the 2006 and 2007 projects respectively. Since the American students outnumbered Japanese students, the authors formed small groups of 3 to 4 American students and required one Japanese student to exchange e-mails with each American student of the assigned group. Although Japanese students carried the burden of reading and writing more e-mail messages than American students, they were convinced by the authors that it would provide them with more language learning opportunities.

American students included both male and female, aged 15 to 17. Their L1 was English, and all of them learned Japanese as a foreign language in an elective course. According to their Japanese teacher, their Japanese proficiency level was from high beginner to low intermediate.

Procedure

In both the 2006 and 2007 projects, each Japanese student used a webmail account that the authors had created in advance, while American students used their private e-mail accounts. For Japanese students, a 90-minute workshop was held at the outset of the course to ensure their technical and typing skills were up to the level necessary to carry out the project. In the remaining course period, most of the class time was used for the project, but the students were also encouraged to work out of class, such as in the school's PC lab and on home PCs.

Both Japanese and American students were notified in advance that the goals of the project were to deepen their understanding of a different culture and to assist the partner's L2 learning. They were told to investigate different aspects of each other's culture, such as school life, holidays, and family events, by asking and answering questions. Students were also instructed that, in providing feedback on their partner's L2 language use, they should pick up and address serious errors that hindered their comprehension, while omitting comment on minor and infrequent errors. This more selected approach was generated from the authors' experiences in past projects, where students were constantly faced with various types of errors made by their partners and they could not deal with all of them within the allotted project period. Also, it was expected that students, being allowed to handle the limited number of L1 errors, would have more time to attend to and analyze L1 features, and thereby make their implicit L1 knowledge explicit, which is thought to facilitate their MA development.

Every e-mail exchanged between Japanese and American students consisted of four parts: (a) small talk, (b) feedback on their partner's language use, (c) answers to their partner's questions, and (d) questions to their partner. Students of both countries were instructed to use their L1 in Parts B and C, and L2 in Parts A and D. It was considered that the feedback and answer provision phases (i.e., Parts B and C) should be cognitively and linguistically demanding because these activities would require students to construct and express their complicated thoughts. In contrast, in the small talk and question-posing phases (i.e., Parts A and D), they could resort to formulaic expressions (e.g., "How are you?") and basic structures (e.g., "What kinds of music do you . . . ?") that they regularly learn in L2 classes. Therefore, it was thought to be appropriate for students to use their L1, where their language was stronger and they had more confidence, in such challenging phases as Parts B and C.

The project lasted eight weeks in both 2006 and 2007, and students were told to create and send at least four e-mail messages to each partner during the period. Each dyad in the 2006 and 2007 projects had 4.6 and 4.4 e-mail exchanges on average respectively. The length of the e-mail messages students wrote varied, but they wrote at least one letter-sized page each time.

Data Collection and Analysis

Since this study attempted to investigate Japanese tandem learners' MA development and its influence on their English knowledge, the authors focused on the data only from the Japanese side. Three kinds of data were collected from Japanese students and analyzed in this study: post-project questionnaire, oral interview,[2] and e-mail logs. The post-project questionnaire required them to write (a) any linguistic features of their partners' Japanese use that they had noticed and analyzed in the feedback phase, and (b) any thoughts they had obtained from their L1 analysis that they could apply to their English learning. Students answered these questions while reading the whole e-mail logs to recall their past thoughts. After this session, the first author of this study had oral interviews with each student to collect more detailed information about their responses on the questionnaire. All of these comments were backed up by the analysis of their e-mail logs.

RESULTS AND DISCUSSION

Research Question 1

The results of the questionnaire and interview sessions showed that not every student provided comments on MA. Each of them described strong and weak points of their partners' language use, but, in most cases, they did not go into further L1 linguistic analysis. Compared to Appel's (1999) subjects, the junior high school students of this study might have been insufficiently cognitively or linguistically mature to analyze their L1 in an explicit manner. Kabata and Edasawa (2008, August) reported that even university students tended to avoid such linguistic considerations. It might be that it is highly demanding for ordinary learners (as opposed to linguists) to make L1 explicit, infer grammatical rules, or make linguistic generalizations or extrapolations.

There were, however, comments collected from 7 students that illustrated their MA development (i.e., identifying and correcting L1 errors, and explaining L1 rules), and their attempts to apply these rules to their own L2 knowledge. In the following section, these students' MA comments are presented. Students A–E were the participants of the 2006 projects, and Students F and G were from 2007.

Student A

Student A noticed that his female partner always placed causal adverbial clauses after the main clause, as in Example 1. He said that it was grammatical but, as she repeatedly used causal clauses in the sentence-final position, it sounded a little strange to him because in Japanese, people usually put them before the main clause (Example 2).

Ex. 1   Watashi-wa nihongo-no kouza-wo torimashita. <u>Nazenara nihon-no bunka-ni kyoumi-ga aru-kara desu.</u> [I took the Japanese course <u>because I am interested in Japanese culture.</u>]

Ex. 2 <u>Nihon-no bunka-ni kyoumi-ga aru-node</u> watashi-wa nihongo-no kouza-wo torimashita. [<u>Because I am interested in Japanese culture</u>, I took the Japanese course.]

(English translations and underlines used in this and subsequent quotations are the authors'.)

English adverbial clauses occur sentence-finally more often than sentence-initially, and causal adverbials especially tend to occur finally (Celce-Murcia & Larsen-Freeman, 1999). Student A remembered this English norm he had learned in his regular English class and hypothesized that his partner's Japanese was affected by her L1 custom. He then introspectively contrasted positional differences of causal clauses between English and Japanese, reflected on his own English writing, and realized that he himself had placed causal clauses sentence-initially because of his L1 transfer. He concluded that he would be careful when he expressed causal clauses in English.

Student B

Student B reported that his female partner repeatedly made errors in using two of the Japanese postpositional particles, "*-wa*" and "*-ga.*" In Example 3, it is appropriate to use "*kafeteria-<u>ga</u>*" instead of "*kafeteria-<u>wa</u>,*" and "*Watashi-<u>ga</u>*" in Example 4 should be "*Watashi-<u>wa</u>.*"

Ex. 3 Watashi-no gakkou-niwa, kafeteria-<u>wa</u> arimasu. [There is a cafeteria in our school.]

Ex. 4 Watashi-<u>ga</u> futsuu 6ji-ni okimasu. [I usually get up at six.]

The Japanese language has a rich system of postpositional particles that immediately follow a noun phrase and indicate its grammatical and/or semantic roles within a sentence. Both "*-wa*" and "*-ga*" mark a subject of a sentence, and learners of L2 Japanese frequently have trouble distinguishing these particles (Ichikawa, 1997). The dominant view to grammatically account for their difference is that "WA has thematic and contrastive functions providing old information, while GA has neutral descriptive and exhaustive listing functions providing new information" (Nariyama, 2002, p. 370).[3] Native Japanese speakers, although they use these particles properly to the context, are seldom aware of such rules.

Student B corrected all the "*-wa*" and "*-ga*" errors his partner had made, but did not provide grammatical accounts explicitly. In the interview, he recalled her tough question and said:

In her response, my partner asked me, "How can I distinguish '-wa' and '-ga'? They both mark the subject of the sentence!" I felt she was irritated, and I understood her feeling. But I couldn't answer right away. I noticed it was very difficult to teach the language even though we can intuitively use it.

He said that he felt obliged to generate good linguistic explanations for her. One day in his regular English class, when students were working on Japanese–English translation activity, the teacher instructed that the firstly introduced common noun needs the indefinite article (i.e., *a*), and the identical noun subsequently used needs the definite article (i.e., *the*). Student B then associated English indefinite and definite articles with Japanese "-*ga*" and "-*wa*," and inferred that "-*ga*" might mark first mention and "-*wa*" might be used for subsequent mention, which corresponds to the general Japanese grammatical accounts mentioned earlier.

Student B, by his long and undaunted analysis, realized that both English and Japanese have the same function using different linguistic systems. This is regarded as a significant finding made through contrasting the linguistic systems of two languages, which is a distinct advantage of the feedback phase in e-mail tandem activity.

Student C

As was the case with Student B, Student C also pointed out his male partner's misuse of postpositional particles. In Example 5, "-*ga*" (subject marker) should be "-*wo*" (direct object marker), and "-*no*" (possessive marker) and "-*wo*" in Example 6 should be "-*wo*" and "-*e*" (directional marker). Student C stated in the questionnaire that he was "annoyed" by these errors his partner frequently made.

Ex. 5 Watashi-no nihongo-ga naoshite arigatou gozaimashita. [Thank you for correcting my Japanese.]

Ex. 6 Otousan-wa watashi-to otouto-no gakkou-wo kuruma-de okurimasu. [My father drives me and my brother to school.]

Other than the subject marking particles (i.e., "-*wa*" and "-*ga*"), Japanese postpositional particles include ones that assign other cases (e.g., direct/indirect object, possessive, directional, locative, etc.). One of the prominent linguistic features of the Japanese language is that, due to the rich inflectional system utilizing the full range of particles, word order within a sentence is more flexible than in English (Nagata, 1997). For instance, Example 7 represents the basic word order both in Japanese and English.

Ex. 7 John-wa [John] Kathi-ni [Kathi] uma-wo [horse] katta [bought]. [John bought Kathy a horse.]

Although Japanese has a subject-object-verb (SOV) order, the word order before a verb is relatively flexible because the grammatical function of each noun phrase is indicated by case marking particles (Ex. 7a–7e). In other words, postpositional particles free Japanese sentences from canonical word order.

Ex. 7a   John-wa [John] uma-wo [horse] Kathi-ni [Kathi] katta [bought].
    7b   Kathi-ni [Kathi] John-wa [John] uma-wo [horse] katta [bought].
    7c   Kathi-ni [Kathi] uma-wo [horse] John-wa [John] katta [bought].
    7d   uma-wo [horse] John-wa [John] Kathi-ni [Kathi] katta [bought].
    7e   uma-wo [horse] Kathi-ni [Kathi] John-wa [John] katta [bought].

In the interview, Student C said that he had advised his partner to select particles correctly when writing Japanese because the Japanese language relies on the particles to distinguish cases in a sentence. Student C then referred to his English teacher's continuous emphasis on the significance of word order in English, and said:

> In analyzing my partner's particle errors, I came to realize that English has no particle system, and, therefore, English relies on word order to make the sentence understandable. I finally recognized the reason my regular English class teacher always says to us, "Word order is very important in English."

As Student B had demonstrated, Student C also discovered that English and Japanese employ quite different linguistic systems (i.e., word order in English and postpositional particles in Japanese), but both fulfill the same language function (i.e., marking grammatical and/or semantic roles of each noun phrase). It is thus also reasonable to say that this remarkable finding was made possible through contrastive analysis of the linguistic systems between L1 and L2, which could be an outcome of e-mail tandem activity.

Students D and E

Both Students D and E gave similar comments in the questionnaires. They wrote that their partners' Japanese was fairly understandable, but some expressions sounded unnatural because of the wrong word choice.

Ex. 8   Okaasan-ga bento-wo <u>ryouri shimasu</u>. [Mom <u>cooks</u> lunch.]
Ex. 9   Sensei-wa tanoshii hanashi-wo <u>iimasu</u>. [Our teacher <u>tells</u> funny stories.]

In Example 8, the literal translation of *ryouri shimasu* is *cook*, and *iimasu* in Example 9 is *say* or *tell*, so their partners' Japanese word choice is semantically reasonable. However, native Japanese speakers use *tsukuri-masu* when *bento-wo* precedes the verb as a direct object, and *shimasu* is used for *hanashi-wo*.

In the interview, Students D and E were asked if they had had similar experiences in their English learning. Student D said that he was a little confused when he learned English phrases such as *take a bath* and *make a mistake* because the literal Japanese translations of these expressions go *furo-ni hairu* [enter a bath] and *machigai-wo suru* [do a mistake]. Student E mentioned that he once wrote *I did an effort* in a writing assignment in his English class, and it was corrected by the teacher saying that he should have used *made* instead of *did*. He remembered that he then did not understand why it was so because in Japanese, *doryoku-wo* [effort] is followed by *suru* [do] as a verb, but not by *tsukuru* [make].

Following these retrospective comments, Students D and E recognized that both languages have conventional patterns of object–verb combination, that is, what linguists call collocation.

Student F

Student F noticed that his female partner had overused "*-no*" to every pre-noun adjective. Since "*-no*," one of the Japanese postpositional particles, can be used as a modifier particle, it is often the case that adult learners of L2 Japanese put "*-no*" to every word that modifies or shows the attributes of the following noun (Ichikawa, 1997). Japanese adjectives, however, are not always inflected in this way. For example, "*-no*"s in Examples 10 and 11 are not required because *yasui* [inexpensive] and *oishii* [fine] are both independent adjectives (i.e., adjectives that directly modify nouns without any particle).

Ex. 10   yasui-no fuku [inexpensive clothes]
Ex. 11   oishii-no restaurant [fine restaurant]

In the interview, the author encouraged Student F to recall the similar type of L2 error he had made. Then he recollected that he once wrote "longly" in his writing test and was corrected by the grader. He said that he had consulted a dictionary since then to avoid such overuse of a basic morphological rule (i.e., overgeneralization).

Student G

Student G noticed that his female partner spelled "*mu*" in place of "*n*." He explained to her that, in Japanese, all the nasal sounds are spelled with "*n*," not "*mu*." Thus, "*mu*"s in Examples 12 and 13 should be replaced with "*n*."

Ex. 12   kyamupu [camp]
Ex. 13   shimuboru [symbol]

In the interview, the first author asked Student G in which context his partner made such misspellings. He reexamined his e-mail log collaboratively with the interviewer and found that she used "mu" where it is spelled "m" in English. He then learned that "m" represents the nasal sound produced with two lips closed before "p" and "b," and recognized that there are two types of nasal sounds, [n] and [m], and English distinguishes them in writing, while there is no distinction in Japanese.

Table 4.1 Linguistic Features Analyzed by Students A–G

Student	L1 linguistic features	Category
A	Position of causal adverbial clause	Syntax
B	Function of subject marking particles	Morphology
C	Function of postpositional particles	Morphology
D and E	Combination of words (Collocation)	Vocabulary
F	Inflectional rule (Overgeneralization)	Morphology
G	Phonics	Phonology/Graphology

In the cases of Students D–G, their contrastive analyses between L1 and L2 were facilitated by the interviewer's prompts. In conducting e-mail tandem activity, therefore, teacher intervention of this sort may be necessary, especially for adolescent EFL students, to provoke their metalinguistic thought.

The L1 linguistic features that Students A–G analyzed are presented in Table 4.1. The categories that each linguistic feature falls into are syntax, morphology, vocabulary, phonology, and graphology. These are the knowledge of Grammatical Competence, which is one of the components of Bachman's (1990) Language Competence. According to these results, tandem learners participating in this study focused on linguistic aspects of language, rather than on pragmatic ones such as register, honorifics, and genre.

Research Question 2

An intriguing cognitive process was observed in analyzing the second research question. Students A–G attended to their partner's ungrammatical use of Japanese, analyzed the linguistic features to generate explicit L1 explanations, and eventually developed MA, which otherwise might not have been obtained. Then, either spontaneously or encouraged by the interviewer's prompts, they contrasted L1 and L2, looking for commonalities or differences of the linguistic systems they had analyzed. Student A, for example, contrasted the positional differences of causal adverbial clauses between English and Japanese, and learned that English causal clauses take sentence-final position, while those in Japanese come sentence-initially. Student B found that both English and Japanese have the same function to denote first and subsequent mention, but use different linguistic systems (i.e., "*a*" and "*the*" in English, and "*-ga*" and "*-wa*" in Japanese). Student C discovered that, in order for the language to signal grammatical cases within a sentence, Japanese utilizes postpositional particles while English relies on word order. Some researchers have insisted that this cognitive effort, that is, linguistic contrasts between L1 and L2, can be seen as an activity driven by learner's MA, and eventually helps facilitate the development of L2 proficiency. For example, Yamada (2006) suggested that MA entails ability to compare and contrast two languages to discover commonalities as well as differences, which would bring success in L2 learning. Jessner (1999) stated that MA assists learners to perceive similarities or differences between L1 and L2, which can activate their prior linguistic knowledge and guide them in the development of the L2 system.

In sum, the results of this study illustrated the process of MA development and its role in L2 learning: Students developed their MA by making implicit L1 knowledge explicit through linguistically thought-provoking experiences (e.g., the feedback phase in e-mail tandem), and subsequently compared and contrasted the systems and functions between the two languages to discover commonalities and differences, which would eventually reduce the difficulties involved in their L2 learning. According to these arguments, learners' metalinguistic analysis of L1 and contrasts between the two languages might be one key factor in making e-mail tandem successful in terms of their L2 development.

Research Question 3

In order to answer the third research question, the authors plotted all the students' scores on the English proficiency test, and identified the scores of Students A–G, who successfully reported their MA comments (see Figure 4.1). The figure shows an overall tendency between students' MA and

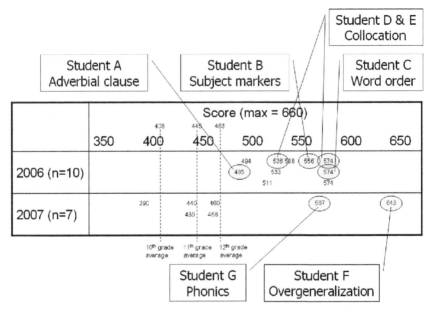

Figure 4.1 Plotted scores of the GTEC English proficiency test.

English proficiency: Students who could induce L1 explicit knowledge and identify similarities and differences between L1 and L2 tended to perform better in the test than those who did not. Put differently, Japanese learners with a higher level of MA are likely to be more successful in English learning.

CONCLUSION

The current study showed that not every participant reported MA comments in e-mail tandem activities. This result seems to suggest that it was very demanding for junior high school students to make such a linguistic analysis by themselves. Interestingly, students who successfully demonstrated metalinguistic analysis said that they had been guided to develop their MA by several aspects of the e-mail tandem project. Students B and C said that they were obliged to find good linguistic explanations of the L1 features with which their partners had trouble, and worked hard throughout the project. Students D–G stated that their MA comments and L1 and L2 contrast would not have occurred without the post-project questionnaire and interview sessions. From these comments, the feedback phase and the post-project session of e-mail tandem seem to play a vital role in developing learners' MA: The former generates a feeling of obligation in tandem learners to support their partner's language learning, and the latter provides them with opportunities to make retrospective metalinguistic analysis. It should be noted that, in both cases, tandem administrator's intervention to assist learners' metalinguistic consideration is needed to facilitate their MA development.

Another finding of the study was that those who reported MA comments were successful English learners. This result supports past studies: MA and L2 proficiency positively correlate with each other (Bialystok, 2001; Cenoz & Jessner, 2000; Cummins, 2000; Lasagabaster, 2001; Otsu, 2008, May). It is not certain, however, whether high L2 proficiency enhances MA or high MA promotes L2 (Otsu, 2008, May).

If MA is proved to precede L2, then MA-raising activities should be employed in language education, and e-mail tandem could be utilized for this purpose because it has a feedback phase that triggers or obliges students to notice and analyze L1 features appearing in their partner's e-mail. Also, we should be aware that their noticing is promoted by the written nature of the e-mail discourse. Furthermore, it is the asynchronous mode of communication that allows them more time to analyze the language. These advantages of e-mail tandem are expected to lead students to develop their MA and contrast linguistic systems and functions between L1 and L2, examining similarities and differences between the two languages. This contrast will eventually contribute to the development of their L2 proficiency.

NOTES

1. "GTEC (Global Test of English Communication) for Students" was developed by Benesse Corporation, with the main focus on assessing the English communication skills of secondary school students, and is widely administered in Japan. Japanese students of this study took the BASIC level of the test (score range: 0–660, test reliability: $\alpha = 0.752$–0.791).
2. Both the questionnaire and interview were conducted in the students' L1 (Japanese), their stronger language.
3. Nariyama (2002) stated, "However, these functions by no means constitute an exhaustive and satisfactory description" (p. 370).

REFERENCES

Appel, C. (1999). *Tandem language learning by e-mail: Some basic principles and a case study (CLCS Occasional Paper No. 54)*. Dublin: Trinity College, Centre for Language and Communication Studies.

Appel, C., & Gilabert, R. (2002). Motivation and task performance in a task-based web-based tandem project. *ReCALL, 14*, 16–31.

Appel, C., & Mullen, T. (2000). Pedagogical considerations for a web-based tandem language learning environment. *Computers & Education, 34*, 291–308.

Arnold, N., & Ducate, L. (2006). Future foreign language teachers' social and cognitive collaboration in an online environment. *Language Learning & Technology, 10*, 42–66.

Bachman, L. (1990). *Fundamental considerations in language testing*. Oxford: Oxford University Press.

Bialystok, E. (2001). *Bilingualism in development: Language, literacy and cognition*. Cambridge: Cambridge University Press.

Braga, J. (2007). E-tandem learning for language and culture. *Essential Teacher, 4*, 33–35.

Brammerts, H. (2003). Autonomous language learning in tandem: The development of a concept. In T. Lewis & L. Walker (Eds.), *Autonomous language learning in tandem* (pp. 27–36). Sheffield, UK: Academy Electronic Publications.

Celce-Murcia, M., & Larsen-Freeman, D. (1999). *The grammar book: An ESL/EFL teacher's course* (2nd ed.). Boston: Heinle and Heinle.

Cenoz, J., & Jessner, U. (Eds.). (2000). *English in Europe: The acquisition of a third language*. Clevedon: Multilingual Matters.

Cummins, J. (2000). *Language, power and pedagogy: Bilingual children in the crossfire*. Clevedon: Multilingual Matters.

Dodd, C. (2001). Working in tandem: An Anglo-French project. In M. Byram, A. Nichols, & D. Stevens (Eds.), *Developing intercultural competence in practice* (pp. 162–175). Clevedon: Multilingual Matters.

Edasawa, Y., & Kabata, K. (2007). An ethnographic study of a key-pal project: Learning a foreign language through bilingual communication. *Computer Assisted Language Learning, 20*, 189–207.

Elder, C., & Manwaring, D. (2004). The relationship between metalinguistic knowledge and learning outcomes among undergraduate students of Chinese. *Language Awareness, 13*, 145–162.

Ichikawa, Y. (1997). *Nihongo Goyo Reibun Sho-jiten* [A dictionary of Japanese language learners' errors]. Tokyo: Bonjinsha.

Jessner, U. (1999). Metalinguistic awareness in multilinguals: Cognitive aspects of third language learning. *Language Awareness, 8*, 201–209.

Kabata, K., & Edasawa, Y. (2008, August). *Patterns of language learning in a cross-cultural bilingual keypal project.* Paper presented at the World CALL 2008 international conference, Fukuoka, Japan.

Kuo, L., & Anderson, C. (2008). Conceptual and methodological issues in comparing metalinguistic awareness across languages. In K. Koda & A. M. Zehler (Eds.), *Learning to read across languages: Cross-linguistic relationships in first- and second-language literacy development* (pp. 39–67). New York: Routledge.

Lasagabaster, D. (2001). The effect of knowledge about the L1 on foreign language skills and grammar. *International Journal of Bilingual Education and Bilingualism, 4,* 310–331.

Levy, M., & Stockwell, G. (2006). *CALL dimensions: Options and issues in computer-assisted language learning.* Mahwah, NJ: Lawrence Erlbaum.

Little, D. (2003). Tandem language learning and learner autonomy. In L. Walker & T. Lewis (Eds.), *Autonomous language learning in tandem* (pp. 37–44). Sheffield: Academy Electronic Publications.

McPartland, J. (2003). Language learning in tandem via email. In L. Walker & T. Lewis (Eds.), *Autonomous language learning in tandem* (pp. 195–202). Sheffield: Academy Electronic Publications.

Nagata, N. (1997). The effectiveness of computer-assisted metalinguistic instruction: A case study in Japanese. *Foreign Language Annals, 30,* 187–200.

Nariyama, S. (2002). The WA/GA distinction and switch-reference for ellipted subject identification in Japanese complex sentences. *Studies in Language, 26,* 369–431.

Otsu, Y. (2008, May). *Gaikokugo gakushu: Futatsu no nazo* [Foreign language learning: Two mysterious issues]. Plenary Address at the 2008 Conference of the Kansai Chapter, the Association of Language Education & Technology, Kobe, Japan.

Renou, M. (2000). Learner accuracy and learner performance: The quest for a link. *Foreign Language Annals, 33,* 168–177.

Roehr, K. (2007). Metalinguistic knowledge and language ability in university-level L2 learners. *Applied Linguistics, 29,* 173–199.

Ushioda, E. (2000). Tandem language learning via e-mail: From motivation to autonomy. *ReCALL, 12,* 121–128.

van Lier, L. (1996). *Interaction in the language curriculum: Awareness, autonomy & authenticity.* New York: Longman.

Warschauer, M., & Kern, R. (Eds.). (2000). *Network-based language teaching: Concepts and practice.* Cambridge: Cambridge University Press.

Woodin, J. (2001). Tandem learning as an intercultural activity. In M. Byram, A. Nichols, & D. Stevens (Eds.), *Developing intercultural competence in practice* (pp. 189–202). Clevedon: Multilingual Matters.

Yamada, Y. (2006). *Eigo ryoku towa nani ka* [What is the English ability?]. Tokyo: Taishukan.

5 Facilitating Collaborative Language Learning in a Multicultural Distance Class over Broadband Networks

Learner Awareness to Cross-Cultural Understanding

Yuri Nishihori

INTRODUCTION

Network technology has enabled us to realize multipoint connections on the Internet using video-conferencing systems that are blended with classroom activities. Assessing the use of this kind of integrative technology, however, has not been surveyed sufficiently to inform and facilitate language learning in a multicultural distance class over broadband networks. This chapter discusses different pedagogical effects concerning learners' awareness of cross-cultural understanding by comparing a two-point connection environment and a three-point connection environment. The analysis, based on questionnaires put to the participants, indicates that when placed in a three-point connection environment as opposed to a two-point connection environment, students with certain characteristics tend to participate more positively and with more awareness of cross-cultural understanding.

LITERATURE REVIEW

The role of networking technologies has become increasingly important with the employment of IP networks or the Internet, which can facilitate cross-cultural communication and, potentially at least, understanding, anywhere around the globe. In the 1980s, the major means for distance learning of this type was ISDN, which did not offer distance language learners sufficient technological devices for interactional skills, especially speaking skills. In the 1990s, video-conferencing began to become more sophisticated by utilizing early broadband networks. Experimental projects were carried out as a studio-based type of interaction with high costs and sophisticated technological solutions. Huge projects were undertaken to accumulate understanding and experience in this field (Buckett & Stringer,

1997, September; Buckett, Stringer, & Datta, 1999; McAndrew, Foubister, & Mayes, 1996; Wang, 2004a; Wong & Fauverge, 1999).

As a matter of course, costly video-conferencing was limited to lecture-type activities in educational settings. It was natural that interaction tended to be limited between a lecturer and distance learners. In essence, it was similar to a teacher-centered situation, which does not encourage peer interaction. This led to severe criticism regarding learners' poor achievement of communication skills (Goodfellow, Manning, & Lamy, 1999; Hampel & Hauck, 2004; Kötter, 2001; Wang & Sun, 2000; Wong & Fauverge, 1999).

Around the turn of the century, a radical breakthrough was made through the rapid development of technologies that made it possible for us to send voice, images, and text data simultaneously. Language learners became able to interact with teachers and peers both visually and orally through Internet devices in an authentic situation. A variety of video-conferencing tools were used in education such as NetMeeting, Yahoo! Messenger, and MSN Messenger. Since their introduction, research using these new tools has been conducted extensively because it was straightforward to introduce into language learning. This desktop style of conferencing system could be readily introduced to educational institutions without prohibitive cost (Wang, 2004b). It was even possible to connect individual peer students who use this type of desktop video-conferencing, although it was limited to a small window on a PC.

To facilitate learning, however, we still need to create a class online that is able to accommodate students and a teacher in one "visual" class, with other classes viewed on the screen in life size. The rapid development of technology has enabled us to connect classes inexpensively by constructing high-quality video-conferencing over an IP transmission system using consumer camcorders, PCs, and software, together with a high-definition (HD) camera.

To date there have been a number of studies conducted in this area, with a focus on the data accumulated between educational institutions in two countries (Fernandez et al., 2001; Kishida, Maeda, & Kohno, 2003; Simonson, Smaldino, Albright, & Zvacek, 2005; Yamada & Akahori, 2006). These developments are of great importance for language teaching, since they can be effectively utilized in the field of Teaching English as a Foreign Language (TEFL). It enables us to realize multipoint connections on the Internet using video-conferencing systems that are blended with classroom activities in multicultural language learning (Nishinaga et al., 2008). Computer Support for Collaborative Learning (CSCL) also plays a meaningful role in this authentic global class setting, because we need a rationale for online activities.

There is, however, still some way to go for individuals using desktop video-conferencing, as discussed by Wang (2004b). For authentic multicultural classes on the screen, it is still a challenge to develop educational software on the Internet. Our project promoted synchronous and symmetric communication using high-quality video-conferencing in multicultural language classrooms where nonverbal communication plays an important role for mutual understanding (Nishihori et al., 2004). It is important to accumulate data in order to evaluate what benefits this network enlargement can give to students (Nishihori et al., 2006) and how we can integrate technologies and learning flow into classroom activities (Barr, 2004). This chapter compares the data of Japanese students experiencing a change of setting from a two-point connection to a three-point or even a four-point connection. The results of our project, which relied on the cooperation of two to four countries, led us to the conclusion that interactive collaborative activities can be successful, especially in terms of how they have impacted on students' awareness of cross-cultural understanding. This success will advance current knowledge and elicit protocols required to support effective multicultural language learning in the future.

Our project involved investigating how a multicultural distance class could be facilitated between two to four countries through the use of interactive communication tools, including a high-quality video-conferencing system, a text-based discussion system, and a network-based display sharing system. The main objectives of our project were to implement high-quality, high-fidelity environments over long-distance broadband networks, and to provide students with better opportunities for cross-cultural understanding.

DISTANCE CLASS AND NETWORK CONFIGURATIONS

Distance Class Overview

This project was implemented in an English writing class at Hokkaido University, Japan, from 2000 to 2007 with an emphasis on computer-mediated communication. Interactive communication was achieved by means of a text-based chat application called Chat'n'Debate and a web-based voting system called Culture Box, along with a full-specification HD digital video-conferencing system called Ruff-HDV. Classes were initially conducted with students in Seoul, Korea, and Shanghai, China. In 2006, this was expanded to include Thailand as well.

In each year, about 25 participants, mainly freshmen at the Faculty of Engineering, took part in an afternoon class. As an experimental class, the two-point connection class was linked to some afternoon or evening classes from the previous day due to the respective time difference either at Stanford University or the University of Alaska, Fairbanks (UAF). To overcome time differences, and to give more opportunities for students to speak up, the main focus was placed on classes in East Asia. In the case of the three-point connection class, Shanghai Jiao Tong University (12:30 to 13:30) and Ewha Women's University (13:30 to 14:30) joined the experiment. With regard to the four-point connection carried out in 2006, the class was conducted with students from Thammasat University in Thailand, in addition to the students from Shanghai Jiao Tong University and Ewha Women's University.

Two-Country Project: The US (Alaska) and Japan

This project was organized in an English writing class at Hokkaido University, Japan, during the second semester of 2004, with an emphasis on computer-mediated communication after some initial preparation with Stanford University. Twenty-four freshmen took part in the experimental class on site from 13:00 to 14:00 on January 18, 2005. Eleven participants and six visitors took part at the UAF site in the US from 19:00 to 20:00 on January 17, 2005. They were students who were studying Japanese as part of a course, JPN 293 Virtual Study Abroad: Language, Culture and Geography of Japan. Although there was an 18-hour time difference, the experiment was able to be organized during regular classroom hours on both sides (Nishihori et al., 2005).

In the actual classroom, students faced the other group as life-size figures projected onto a large screen. Three activities were organized for this class: chat, an on-the-spot questionnaire with voting and comments, and an object lesson for students to ask other students unexpectedly to show an object they were carrying. This became an object lesson to show cultural difference in its true colors. These activities were conducted in English, since the UAF students were beginners in Japanese.

As it is impossible to hear all the students in a face-to-face situation, a collaborative space such as Culture Box (see Figure 5.1) or Chat'n'Debate, which were devised to foster collaborative interaction between both sets of students, played an important role. Culture Box simultaneously played

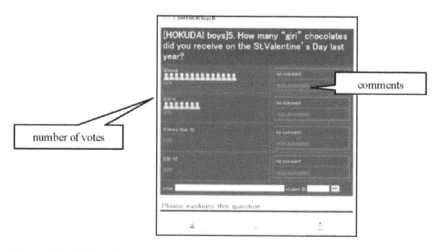

Figure 5.1   Culture Box.

the roles of both a questionnaire to students and an opinion poll. Students wrote comments in the Culture Box space to each of the answers provided by the other group. Changes in the number of votes were instantaneously displayed in graph form after every vote.

It is thrilling to see these changes being made on the screen. Students enjoy both voting to form a class opinion and contributing by commenting on answers. Topics of this particular experiment included names used to address parents, and the Japanese custom such as chocolates on St. Valentine's Day, both requested by UAF students who study Japanese culture. This gave a good exercise for Japanese students to offer some authentic information about their own culture to those in the same age group.

Topics in the object lesson also covered one's personal space while talking to someone else and personal effects carried by students on campus. Participants observed how close a pair of students would stand while talking, both in Japan and the US. They also observed the kinesics of both cultures: fingertip distance for the Japanese and wrist distance for the Americans. Students were asked to take out what they had from their pocket or bag on the spot. They all enjoyed the visible cultural differences shown on the screen.

Three-Country Project: China, Korea, and Japan

This project was planned to solve two problems: time difference and unbalanced language ability. Foreign language learners find it difficult to speak up with their native-speaker peers. It was felt that they would feel freer to communicate with peers who are in the same situation using their common language, English. Inviting two other countries in the same region, this project was implemented in an English writing class at Hokkaido University during the second semester of 2005. Twenty-four participants who were freshmen at the Faculty of Engineering took part in the experimental class at Hokkaido University from 13:30 to 14:30 on October 25, 2005. Eleven participants took part at Jiao Tong University from 12:30 to 13:30, and 11 participants at Ewha Women's University from 12:30 to 13:30.

Multi-Culture Box, which was developed from Culture Box, played a very important role in fostering collaborative interaction among the three sets of students. It also played the roles of both questionnaire and opinion poll. Compared to the single column in Culture Box, Multi-Culture Box had three columns to indicate each country. It was very exciting indeed to be able to see these changes being made in real time by the students in each country. Students enjoyed both voting to form a "cross-border class opinion" as well as commenting on answers from other countries. What made reading these answers particularly interesting was the fact that students were able to compare three countries at a glance to find similarities and differences.

The topic in the object lesson was mobile phones and their straps. The participants all enjoyed these object lessons by showing what they actually had on the spot. Similarities and differences in Asia were observed effectively through the variety of straps people were able to show through the medium of a broadband network.

Network Configuration and Software

An HD video-conferencing system, whose images were projected onto large screens rendering them life-size, was introduced to establish high-fidelity communication for this project. The HDV standard was designed to focus on recording HDTV (HD television) formatted signals on digital video (DV) tape. Having developed a new 1080/60i HDV conferencing system, this was subsequently implemented as software running on the Microsoft Windows XP operating system.

There is a great difference in the angular view distance between HDTV and SDTV. Since HDTV has three or six times more pixels than SDTV, the HDTV system can cover more students than SDTV by fixing the number of pixels per subject. Only one student and the immediate surrounding space can be captured by using the SDTV system. By using HDTV, however, five or eight students can be shown with the same precision. On top of this, there is also a wide field angle shooting camera without the need for panning. One of the most important features of a video-conferencing system like this for distance learning is the fidelity of its reproduced life-size image and sound which is instrumental in creating a high-fidelity environment (Nishinaga et al., 2008).

The network can be divided into two areas, Japanese domestic, and the Internet. The Japan Gigabit Network (JGN) 2, operated by National Institute of Information and Communications Technology (NICT), was used for the domestic network. JGN 2 is one of the open network test beds founded by the Japanese government, and its layer-two protocol is the Ethernet. Its maximum bandwidth reaches 10 Gbps, and the network itself provides a best-effort service to users.

DATA COLLECTION AND ANALYSIS

This chapter discusses different pedagogical effects concerning learners' awareness as to the usefulness of this type of distance class, as well as to cross-cultural understanding. The results of our projects were obtained through questionnaires to students. Students perceived the usefulness of this type of multilateral distance class from five different perspectives: whether this class was (a) enjoyable, (b) informative, (c) better than ordinary language classes, (d) preferable in terms of its activities, and (e) successful in meeting students' expectations.

After this experimental class, an anonymous questionnaire in English was distributed to students who awarded a numerical score from 5 (strongly agree) to 1 (strongly disagree) on the 5-point Likert scale to the following four statements and a question, each of which represented the aforementioned five perspectives respectively:

1. The class was fun!
2. The class was informative.
3. I learned something that I would not have in a regular classroom.
4. A language class should include this kind of activity more often.
5. Overall, did the class meet your expectations?

The data analysis based on this questionnaire provided us with a variety of information with regard to students' reaction to video-conferencing with collaborative interactions.

Data Analysis of the Two-Country Project: The US (Alaska) and Japan

Questionnaires were distributed to participants at both universities for them to evaluate the effects. The surveys indicated that there was a high degree of agreement among participants that this type of activity was meaningful and valuable. We found a high correlation between Hokkaido University students' and UAF students' opinions. It should be noted that the average evaluation exceeded 4 points in all the questions.

Data Analysis of the Three-Country Project: China, Korea, and Japan

Again, these results indicated that there was a high degree of agreement among participants in three countries. They were very positive in actively involving themselves in the real-time exchange of opinions. Also, it should be noted that the average evaluation exceeded 4 points in all the questions except Item 5. In particular, Item 3 showed the highest agreement among three countries about this new type of learning (see Figure 5.2).

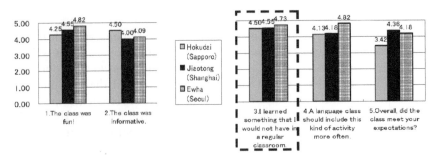

Figure 5.2 Questionnaire results (three-country project).

Data Analysis of the Three-Country Project:
Multicultural Reactions at a Glance

It is essential to capture and compare the exact nature of the students' reactions, which were simultaneously coming in from three separate countries, although we did in fact notice a high degree of agreement among them. In order to obtain this multidimensional data, principal component analysis (PCA) was employed in our study. PCA involves a mathematical procedure that transforms a number of possibly correlated variables into a smaller number of uncorrelated variables. In order to promote multicultural connections for educational purposes such as ours, we needed to develop a method to analyze data and capture a clear image of multicultural reactions at a glance. Principal components obtained by this method can project the multivariate data vectors in a graph in order to visualize three-way reactions.

In order to grasp the correlations within a multilateral context, a number of correlated variables are transformed into a small number of uncorrelated variables, called principal components, by utilizing the PCA (Jolliffe, 2002). With regard to PC1, questions 1, 3, 4 and 5 indicate that the loading is large, but for question 2, it is small. We can conclude that PC1 shows the perspective (1) "enjoyable." With regard to PC2, the loading of questions 2, 3, and 4 is relatively large, but for questions 1 and 5, it is small. We can further assume that PC2 concerns itself with the perspective (2) "informative." The cumulative proportion is a combination of PC1 and PC2. According to this analysis, the obtained principal components can project the multivariate data vectors onto a graph using PC1 and PC2.

By using a plot of the new data points, we are now able to grasp the relative reaction of students in each country at a glance (see Figure 5.3).

According to the preceding plot and labels of each PC, we can conclude that Japanese students found the multicultural class informative, but not

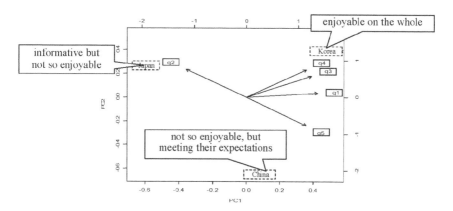

Figure 5.3 PCA analysis.

so enjoyable; Chinese students found it not so enjoyable, but meeting their expectations; Korean students found it enjoyable on the whole. In this way, we can grasp an overall picture of the reactions in each country, even though they occur simultaneously within our multicultural class. This is rather significant, as it is quite essential to capture the transient differences in the attitude of students in multicultural classes.

Data Analysis of Students' Reactions from Two to Three Connections

In order to compare the effects between two-point and three-point connections, a questionnaire was distributed only to Japanese students who participated in both a two-country connection and a three-country connection. Students awarded a numerical score from 5 (very much) to 1 (not at all) on the 5-point Likert scale to the five questions concerning awareness of being watched (or listened to), learning anything, efforts to watch the other classes, efforts to listen to the class, and efforts to participate actively (see Appendix 5.1).

Figure 5.4 shows the comparison of average scores of these five questions for both types of connections. The results of Question 5 show that there is a significant difference in efforts to participate actively in the case of the three-country connection compared to those for the two-country connection ($t = 2.453$; df = 43; $p < 0.05$; Nishihori et al., 2007).

These data indicate that the three-country connection has a more positive impact in the following areas, compared to those of the two-country connection: (a) awareness of being watched (or listened to) by other class(es), (b) efforts to watch other class(es), and (c) efforts to participate actively. There is no significant difference between the two types of connections. However, we can see a difference between the two groups of students in the three-point connection. This will be explained by comparing the class attitude of the two groups of students: those who answered that

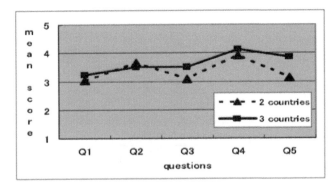

Figure 5.4   Comparison of the mean score from Q1 to Q5.

they learned much, that is, the positive evaluation (PE) group; and those who answered that they learned less, that is, the negative evaluation (NE) group in response to Question 2. The PE group participated in the class more actively than the NE group. In particular, there is a valid significance concerning Question 1 (t = 2.441; df = 18; p < 0.05).

The students were asked about their preference with regard to the number of participating countries. The PE group chose three countries more than did the NE group (which did not choose four countries at all). With regard to Question 8 concerning preferred modes, in the NE group there were many students who chose the answer "chat" only, whereas in the PE group, many students chose both chat and visual images. Most of them backed this up with the reason, "It gives us information." It is interesting to see that students included cultural factors in their reasons for choosing the three countries for Question 7. Students chose (d) and (f) from the six multiple choice answers (see Appendix 5.1), which shows a strong tendency to include various participants in order to appreciate various viewpoints.

CONCLUSIONS AND FUTURE CONSIDERATIONS

We have described the global classes in the two-country and three-country projects with a focus on TEFL. The aim of our project has been to investigate the pros and cons of this type of collaborative environment envisioned to strengthen cross-cultural communication. We have discussed how the use of a high-quality video-conferencing system and a web-based voting system promoted the establishment of effective multicultural environments for interaction on the Internet.

According to our survey, the classroom setting in the multipoint connection will have a positive impact in cross-cultural communication on those who are highly aware of learning. Our study has also shown that the development from two-country to three-country connections will be an educational development of great promise since it was successful in motivating students to participate in cross-cultural communication. There is no doubt that the utilization of video-conferencing with multipoint connections is of great importance in creating a life-size classroom for authentic interaction on the Internet.

It is our ultimate goal to create learning communities that closely resemble the real world through the utilization of Internet communication tools, including a high-quality video-conferencing system, a text-based discussion system, and a network-based display sharing system. We believe that this is most successfully achieved in second language learning by giving the language learner the role of the cross-cultural informant. We plan to further develop a system that supports multicultural language learning in a global network environment, adding a new dimension to collaborative language learning.

ACKNOWLEDGMENTS

This study was supported by Grant-in-Aid for Scientific Research (B) No. 17300275 and No. 20300274 from the Japan Society for the Promotion of Science. I am extremely grateful to the chief of this research group, Dr. Keizo Nagaoka, Waseda University, who kindly permitted me to compile our work over these years and to publish this chapter on behalf of all the members of this team: Dr. Nozomu Nishinaga, Dr. Yuichi Yamamoto, Dr. Takako Akakura, Dr. Maomi Ueno, Dr. Haruhiko Sato, and overseas researchers who helped us realize this global class.

REFERENCES

Barr, D. (2004). *ICT-integrating computers in teaching: Creating a computer-based language learning environment.* Bern: Peter Lang Publications.

Buckett, J., & Stringer, G. (1997, September). *ReLaTe (Remote Language Teaching): Progress, problems and potential.* Paper presented at CALL'97, London.

Buckett, J., Stringer, G., & Datta, J. (1999). Life after ReLaTe: Internet videoconferencing's growing pains. In K. Cameron (Ed.), *CALL and the learning community* (pp. 31–38). Exeter: Elm Bank Publications.

Fernandez, D., Garcia, A. B., Larrabeiti, D., Azcorra, A., Pacyna, P., & Papir, Z. (2001). Multimedia services for distant work and education in an IP/ATM environment. *IEEE Multimedia, 8*(3), 68–77.

Goodfellow, R., Manning, P., & Lamy, M. (1999). Building an online open and distance language learning environment. In R. Debski & M. Levy (Eds.), *WORDCALL: Global perspective on computer-assisted language learning* (pp. 267–286). Lisse, the Netherlands: Swets and Zeitlinger.

Hampel, R., & Hauck, M. (2004). Towards an effective use of audio conferencing in distance language courses. *Language Learning & Technology, 8*(1), 66–82.

Jolliffe, I. T. (2002). *Principal component analysis.* New York: Springer-Verlag.

Kishida, T., Maeda, K., & Kohno, E. (2003). Realization of active collaboration in distance-learning on the internet. *Information and Systems in Education, 2*, 77–84.

Kötter, M. (2001). Developing distance language learners' interactive competence—Can synchronous audio do the trick? *International Journal of Educational Telecommunications, 7*(4), 327–353.

McAndrew, P., Foubister, S. P., & Mayes, T. (1996). Videoconferencing in a language learning application. *Interacting with Computers, 8*(2), 207–217.

Nishihori, Y., Akakura, T., Nagaoka, K., Nishinaga, N., Tanaka, K., Yamamoto, Y., et al. (2007). A comparative analysis of learner awareness between multipoint connections in a videoconferencing class. *The Supplementary Proceedings of ICCE2007 Poster Papers,* 45–46.

Nishihori, Y., Nagaoka, K., Nishinaga, N., Tanaka, K., Yamamoto, Y., Sato, H., et al. (2006). Enabling a multilateral distance class between China, Korea and Japan. In R. Mizuguchi, P. Dillenbourg, & Z. Zhu (Eds.), *Effective utilization of technologies: Facilitating intercultural understanding* (pp. 383–386). Amsterdam: IOS Press.

Nishihori, Y., Nishinaga, N., Nagaoka, K., Collier-Sanuki, Y., Tanaka, K., Yamamoto, Y., et al. (2005). Effectiveness of collaborative learning in the network-based language communities. In C. Looi, D. Jonassen, & M. Ikeda (Eds.),

Towards sustainable and scalable educational innovations informed by the learning societies (pp. 836–839). Amsterdam: IOS Press.

Nishihori, Y., Nishinaga, N., Nagaoka, K., Tanaka, K., Okabe, S., & Yamamoto, Y. (2004). Enabling cross-cultural learning communities—Collaborative networking technologies and their pedagogical implications. *Information and Systems in Education, 3*(1), 57–66.

Nishinaga, N., Nishihori, Y., Nagaoka, K., Tanaka, K., Yamamoto, Y., Ueno, M., et al. (2008). Developments in networking technologies to create a multilateral class in the internet. *International Journal of Internet Education, 3*, 78–85.

Simonson, M., Smaldino, S. E., Albright, M. J., & Zvacek, S. (2005). *Teaching and learning at a distance: Foundations of distance education.* Upper Saddle River, NJ: Prentice Hall.

Wang, Y. (2004a). Distance language learning: Interactivity and fourth generation Internet-based videoconferencing. *CALICO Journal, 21*(2), 373–395.

Wang, Y. (2004b). Supporting synchronous distance language learning with desktop videoconferencing. *Language Learning & Technology, 8*(3), 90–121. Retrieved February 3, 2010, from http://llt.msu.edu/vol8num3/wang/

Wang, Y., & Sun, C. (2000). Synchronous distance education: Enhancing speaking skills via Internet based real time technology. In X. Zhou, J. Fong, X. Jia, Y. Kambayashi, & Y. Zhang (Eds.), *Proceedings of the first international conference on Web information systems engineering* (pp. 168–172). Los Alamitos, CA: IEE Computer Society.

Wong, J., & Fauverge, A. (1999). LEVERAGE—Reciprocal peer tutoring over broadband networks. *ReCALL, 11*(1), 133–142.

Yamada, M., & Akahori, K. (2006). Presenting information to assist learners in learner-centered communicative language learning using videoconferencing. *Information and Systems in Education, 5*(1), 5–16.

APPENDIX 5.1 QUESTIONNAIRE TO THE JAPANESE STUDENTS

Japanese students who participated in both classes awarded a numerical score from 5 (very much) to 1 (not at all) on the 5-point Likert scale to Q1 to Q6, except Q2-sub question.

Q1   Were you aware of being watched (or, listened to) by other class(es)?
Q2   Did you learn anything?
Q2-sub Give as many reasons as you like from the list below.
        a. the importance of a positive attitude for participating in the class
        b. the importance of a positive attitude for communicating with students of other countries
        c. specific matters such as the way to greet
        d. the cultural background of students from other countries
        e. other
Q3   Did you make efforts to watch other class(es)?
Q4   Did you make efforts to listen to others?
Q5   Did you make efforts to participate actively?
Q6*   Did you make equal efforts to watch the other classes?
Q7   How many countries do you think should participate?
        1. two 2. three 3. four 4. more than five
Q7-sub Give as many reasons as you like from the list below.

a. too many participants for us to take time to think about

b. too many participants for us to take time physically to read the results of voting, read chat conversations, and to watch others

c. too many participants who turn us into onlookers instead of participants

d. a variety of participants will make it possible for us to understand various cultures and ways of thinking

e. a variety of participants will make it possible for us to adopt various viewpoints

f. a variety of participants will make the class lively and fun

Q8   Which do you prefer?

1. only chat; 2. only screen images; 3. both of them; 4. neither of them

Q8-sub   Give as many reasons as you like from the list below.

a. It gives us information.

b. It takes up a lot of time.

c. It cannot give us enough information.

d. Screen images can give us information.

e. Screen images are information in the second dimension, not a direct experience like meeting someone.

f. Screen images are not so easy to see.

g. Other.

Part II

Developing Language Skills through Technology

6 Improving Pronunciation via Accent Reduction and Text-to-Speech Software

Ferit Kılıçkaya

INTRODUCTION

There is a common belief that proper pronunciation is an indispensable part of successful communication, which reflects an important current direction of teaching foreign languages in schools. The ultimate goal of language learning in most cases is communication, both written and oral; however, many language teachers often neglect or are forced to neglect pronunciation throughout the entire teaching process. One of the reasons for this is certainly lack of time, resulting from a focus on grammar and lexical aspects of teaching English more than on its pronunciation. It may also be the case that less experienced teachers, who show a great interest in this subject, prioritize their aims in such a way that grammar and vocabulary remain at the top of their agenda. As a result, although pronunciation receives interest both on the part of the teacher and the learner, it is often neglected due to the stated reasons. Furthermore, there is no denying that teachers often lack proper preparation for teaching pronunciation and do not take any measures to receive extra training in this field.

Pronunciation is important not only to communicate ideas easily but also to understand other speakers, given that listening comprehension and pronunciation are interdependent, as contended by Gilbert (1995): Learners of a language can be "cut off" from language if they cannot understand what is being said and cannot be understood by others speaking or learning that language. It is particularly important to integrate pronunciation into beginner classes as it will, from the very beginning, help avoid the risks of fossilization and stabilization of pronunciation habits (Ritchie & Bhatia, 2008). This integration can be achieved through various activities such as drills, listen and imitate, and computer-assisted pronunciation teaching (Kılıçkaya, 2006; Levis, 2007; Seferoğlu, 2005).

The goal of teaching pronunciation is not to make learners sound like native speakers of English, as only few highly gifted and motivated individuals can achieve this (Jenkins, 2005). A more realistic approach is to enable the learners to pronounce the language so that s/he can be understood (Celce-Murcia, Brinton, & Goodwin, 1996). In order to increase this ability, exposure to the target language is vital as learners acquire language mainly from the input they receive. A significant amount of exposure to the target language might help learners to practice the pronunciation and increase their ability to comprehend and express ideas (Tench, 1981). Consequently, the significance of the teacher's role is commonly acknowledged in maximizing their students' exposure to the target language as much as possible. In order to achieve this aim, most language teachers try to use mainly L2 during their lessons to promote the development of the communicative abilities needed to deal with real-life contexts requiring the target language or L2. Moreover, most try to take advantage of technology and provide their students with listening texts in the classroom via CD player, radio, TV, computer, and the Internet, as well as trying to encourage them to listen to English outside the classroom. They recommend English films to watch or even provide students with the DVDs, encourage them to visit particular EFL/ESL websites, or podcast the materials from the websites on their own and deliver them to students.

A BRIEF REVIEW OF TECHNOLOGICAL DEVICES USED IN PRONUNCIATION ACTIVITIES

Looking back to the past, the tape recorder (latterly the audiocassette player) was the first foreign language classroom device through which a classroom might be called technology assisted. As claimed by Kiely (2005), it "brought sound to the classroom for nearly half a century" and was particularly favored during the era when the audio-lingual method was popular around the world. Audiocassettes were mainly used to repeat words or sentences provided in coursebook materials and the main aim was to imitate the way these words or sentences were spoken. Today, audiocassette players have been increasingly replaced by CD/DVD/mp3 players due to their sound quality and their having the functions that traditional audiocassette players lack, such as easily finding the recording or going backward to locate previous tracks.

Another very popular and useful device that provides students not only with the audio input but also with the visual support is a videocassette player. In pronunciation classes, teachers used or still use videocassette players to present movement of articulatory organs while pronouncing particular sounds. In such presentations, using the materials available on the videocassettes, students can be "guided to relax their vocal apparatus, practicing the tensing and flexing of various speech organs" (Celce-Murcia et al., 1996, p. 314). Unfortunately, few such programs are available and video is used mostly as a feedback tool, focusing either only on sounds, or on speech organs' movement. Additionally, the teacher may slow down the pace of speech delivery or freeze the picture to make students focus on the speech organs when pronouncing a particular sound or word.

Following the advances in the technology, videocassettes have been replaced by CD/DVD videos, due to the high picture quality and the functions enabling finding and/or viewing part of the video easily. In addition to this, accent reduction software such as Pronunciation Power has come into the market with full functions and features that videocassettes do not have. Although each piece of software has different features and functions, most provide the presentation of each sound through auditory and visual activities. They aim to identify the deviations of a learner's current speech, such as pronunciation, and to change the way s/he uses her/his mouth to produce the sounds together with intonation and stress. Pronunciation Power I, marketed by the Canadian company English Computerized Learning Inc. (ECL) and developed by Blackstone Multimedia Corporation, focuses on the practice of the 52 English sounds and contains S.T.A.I.R. (Stress, Timing, Articulation, Intonation, and Rhythm). Moreover, it provides real-time visual illustrations of articulatory movements (both a side and a front view) for the production of each sound to accompany the recordings of these sounds' pronunciation. The front view is presented by a video clip of a jaw, lip, and tongue movement of a real person. The side view uses animated drawings providing an X-rayed image of the complete articulatory mechanics (including manner and location of airflow, placement and movement of lips and tongue, velum movement, etc.). A graphic representation of the sound utterance as a waveform is also available. Furthermore, a phonetic transcription of the sounds that were either read on one's own or listened to is included. The types of activities include identifying the target sound in minimal pairs with text and audio files, listening and recording the difficult word, and identifying a word through audio and spelling as well as in sentences with examples of the target sound. Considering these features and the types of activities provided in Pronunciation Power and similar products, language learners have been provided with activities, which especially empower them with both audio and video representations.

However, the main problem with these tools is that they only deal with some fixed sounds or words in isolation and do not provide opportunities for practicing the words in sample sentences or context. In order to overcome the problem of pronunciation of a limited number of words, CD/DVD dictionaries, such as the *Longman Dictionary of Contemporary English* (LDOCE5—http://www.longman.com/ldoce) have come into use, providing fast access to words in hyperlinked word entries with advanced searching capabilities and a wide coverage of words together with their pronunciations. Moreover, Internet-based dictionaries come into the picture also to provide definitions and example sentences with sound files for pronunciation, such as *Cambridge Dictionaries Online* (http://dictionary.cambridge.org/) and other meta-dictionaries giving access to multiple dictionaries and thesauri. In spite of these resources, the problem of using the words in sentences still prevails and teachers have referred to computers with Internet access to provide their students with real uses. The Internet is a great source of materials for meeting the challenge of leading pronunciation classes, presenting language, and benefiting from a source of teaching, listening, and pronunciation materials. The freely available websites such as Voice of America (http://wwww.voanews.com), Randall's ESL Cyber Listening Lab (http://www.esl-lab.com), English Listening Online (http://www.elllo.org), and Breaking News English (http://www. breakingnewsenglish.com) have been invaluable websites from which language teachers can download many audio files created for the purpose of teaching EFL. The huge amount of streaming audio and video materials on the Internet, CD/DVD/online dictionaries, and software for pronunciation has promoted pronunciation. However, as most EFL listening materials cover a limited range of topics and the level of materials is generally targeted towards learners with higher levels of English, selecting materials for the learners' level and interest has become another issue for teachers. Recently, text-to-speech technology, or speech synthesis, has drawn attention from some researchers such as Azuma (2008), Kataoka, Funakoshi, and Kitamura (2007) and Kılıçkaya (2006), as it can read and convert any document provided whether it comes from a website, a newspaper article, or a book.

Text-to-Speech Technology

Text-to-speech technology or speech synthesis is the conversion of text to speech through special computer applications called Text To Speech software (TTS). This technology works with voices, digitally created and trained to read any text. Each sentence is individually generated instead of being played from a previously recorded sentence, text, or document. TTS systems are primarily developed to address the needs of companies and organizations and appear to be invaluable tools for the visually impaired, enabling them to read anything on the computer, such as newspapers. However, in recent years, TTS has been widely used in audiobooks, dictionaries, and computer voice interfaces and it has been given much attention from researchers (see, for example, Azuma, 2008; Kataoka et al., 2007; and Kılıçkaya, 2006). Studies of TTS as a tool for foreign language education have generally focused on the suitability of this technology in language classrooms (Azuma, 2008), and whether students noticed that the voices produced are artificial (Kataoka et al., 2007). According to Azuma (2008), TTS speech has enough quality to be used as audio materials especially for listening for Japanese EFL learners. Kataoka et al. (2007) stressed that the students in their studies did not notice that the dialogues or the sentences were produced by TTS speech. Furthermore, in a study conducted by Kataoka (2007, December), high school students in Japan better memorized the words and phrases with the voices produced by text-to-speech technology, and learned and memorized more English words, than without using this technology. Although there is little research on TTS technology, preliminary results show that it has an important role, especially in listening and pronunciation in language classrooms.

This role has been put forward by Kılıçkaya (2006), who lists the advantages of text to-speech technology as follows:

- You can listen to any text and any topic (most EFL listening materials cover a limited range of topics and some of them are rather expensive).
- You can adjust the speed of reading according to your own needs.
- You can create audio versions from any text (wav or mp3 files).
- You can create pronunciation exercises for yourself (a single word can also be read).
- You can create mini-dialogues (changing speakers at run times is possible).

However, as nothing is without pitfalls, Sha (2009), regarding the disadvantage of TTS, argues that "[a] vital disadvantage of TTS is its limitations in naturalness, pleasantness and expressiveness (TTS voices can never be used in automated dialogue replacement in film making, at least up to now) though intelligibility seems a lesser problem" (p. 640).

In summary, the pronunciation skill in any target language is a crucial part of communication and language learners should be provided with pronunciation practice that is well incorporated in the classroom materials or activities. To help learners achieve intelligible pronunciation for better understanding and for being understood by native speakers, learners, or speakers of the target language, tools provided by accent reduction software and TTS in addition to CD/DVD materials can be of significant help by allowing learners to study at their own pace and exploit visual elements. The purpose of this study is to find out whether integrating accent reduction and text-to-speech software in elementary language classes would result in improvements in learners' pronunciation and to explore their opinions on accent reduction and TTS technology. Hence, this study tries to answer the following research questions:

1. Do accent reduction and text-to-speech technology result in better improvements in learners' pronunciation considering the scores on the tests given?
2. What are the learners' opinions regarding the use of accent reduction and text-to-speech technology?

METHOD

The Turkish Context for English as a Foreign Language (EFL)

Turkish students, though there might be some exceptions in some schools or institutions, mostly follow an English curriculum, in which pronunciation is not regarded as an integral part of language teaching and learning.

Language exams conducted in Turkey lack the assessment of oral skills and focus mainly on grammar, vocabulary, and reading. In other words, the receptive skills are preferred over the productive skills. Therefore, teachers do not regard pronunciation as an integral part of language teaching. The result is that Turkish students have problems with pronunciation, especially with plural and past tense ending, and differentiating between final /ʃ/ and /tʃ/ both in perception and production. However, language acquisition does not depend on the teacher and the teaching process only. Kenworthy (1990) argues that there are also other factors that affect pronunciation acquisition such as the native language—the problem of L1 interference and divergence of L1 and L2, and the amount of exposure—how much the learner is "surrounded" by English, and motivation and concern for good pronunciation. In Turkish, the relationship between the phonemes and the letters are one-to-one and each phoneme consists of just one letter, whereas each English phoneme can be represented in many different ways. Therefore, it can be said that the difficulties of Turkish speakers, resulting from L1 interference, can also be attributed to the irregular spelling in English. When we add the lack of practice in pronunciation in the curriculum, pronunciation becomes a real problem.

Participants

The participants of this study were 35 Turkish EFL students enrolled in a General English course. Students from three elementary classes at a private language institution in Turkey, aged between 22 and 28 with an average age of 23.5, participated in the study. Of the 35 participants, 25 were female and 10 were male. All were freshman students at various universities in Ankara, the capital of Turkey. They were graduates of high schools where English is a compulsory subject. Age and gender were not taken into consideration. The participants were chosen using purposive sampling; it did not include random assignment as the availability of participants was limited. However, before the course began, the participants took a placement test to specify their level of English and participants having similar scores were assigned to three groups. They were also given a pre-test to ensure that there were no statistically significant differences between the groups. The sample consisted of 10 students in the control group, 13 students in experimental group one, and 12 students in experimental group two.

Research Design and Instruments

During the course, the Total English Elementary Student's Book and DVD Pack was used as the main coursebook, which is based on the objectives of the Common European Framework of Reference (CEFR) and includes teacher support material, DVD with authentic clips from film and TV, and a "catch up" CD-ROM with practice for students who miss lessons. DVD and

CD-ROM materials were used in class after classroom lectures and activities, using a laptop, data projector, and speakers. The pre/post-test method was used for the study. Pronunciation questions were developed from the book *Tree or Three?* by Baker (2006), a pronunciation course for beginner and elementary students of English that provides practice in the pronunciation of English sounds, word stress, and intonation through a variety of interesting exercises and activities. Pre- and post-tests consisted of three sections: The first section consisted of 20 most frequently mispronounced words, the second consisted of 10 affirmative and declarative sentences including these words, and the last section presented a picture that portrayed a picnic where some children are busy with activities such as playing with a football and eating. Answers for both the pre- and post-tests were rated according to a 5-point Likert scale for responses. Before administering the pre- and post-tests, three instructors in the ELT department were asked to comment on the items presented in the test in terms of clarity and content. These tests were later given to 30 randomly selected students who were in the preparatory school of Middle East Technical University. The questions were then analyzed taking the Kuder-Richardson scale into consideration. According to the results, *the reliability level* was .89 on the Kuder-Richardson scale, showing that these tests could be used as standardized tests. In addition to the quantitative analysis, semi-structured interviews were conducted with the participants in experimental group two, who were asked to provide feedback on their use of text-to-speech technology in pronunciation activities. The participants were interviewed one by one. The interviews were recorded, with the learners' consent, and the researcher took notes. The participants were interviewed in their mother tongue, Turkish. The main questions were related to whether the students enjoyed the activities undertaken during their class hours and elaborated on the reasons from their own perspectives.

Procedure

On the first day of class, an informed consent form was signed by the students agreeing to participate in the study. After students signed the form, the instructors administered the pre-test. One class (control group) followed the traditional instruction (using a CD player and a pronunciation textbook, *Tree or Three?*, by Baker, 2006); another class (experimental group one) followed the traditional instruction that integrated the use of accent reduction software (Pronunciation Power I); and the final class (experimental group two) followed the traditional instruction that integrated the use of accent reduction and text-to-speech software (Text Aloud mp3 with NeoSpeech voices—Paul and Kate). The study lasted for 16 weeks and the instructor met the groups for three hours each week. With the results obtained from the pre-test, and by means of a one-way ANOVA test, it was possible to establish whether or not there were significant differences between two groups of participants at the 0.05 alpha levels (see Table 6.1).

Table 6.1 Pre-Test Results

Group	N	Mean	Std. Deviation	Std. Error
control	10	5.60	.516	.163
experimental 1	15	5.73	.458	.118
experimental 2	10	5.60	.516	.163
Total	35	5.66	.482	.081

	Sum of Squares	df	Mean Square	F	Sig.
Between Groups	.152	2	.076	.315	.732
Within Groups	7.733	32	.242		
Total	7.886	34			

As can be seen, the significance level was higher than 0.05, $F(2,32) =$ .315, which leads to the conclusion that there were no significant differences between the groups. Once this point became clear, the study was carried out with these three groups. On the last day of class, the instructor administered the post-test to all groups. In addition, experimental group two was interviewed regarding their views on accent reduction and text-to-speech software. The scores obtained in the pre- and post-tests were analyzed to see whether there was a statistically significant difference among the groups.

RESULTS

The post-test scores obtained by experimental and control groups were analyzed using the SPSS software package and the one-way ANOVA test to establish whether there were significant differences among the three groups of participants at the 0.05 alpha levels (see Table 6.2).

Table 6.2 shows that the significance level was higher than 0.05, $F(2,32)$ = 22.156, which leads to the conclusion that there were significant differences between the groups. The analysis used to address the first research question (Do accent reduction and text-to-speech technology result in better improvements in learners' pronunciation considering the scores on the tests given?) revealed significant practice effects on listening comprehension.

Considering the scores in the post-test, experimental group two, which was exposed to accent reduction and text-to-speech software, did better than the other groups. However, the study revealed that there were no statistically significant differences in the pronunciation of single words as all the groups did equally well. Nevertheless, there were statistically significant differences between the groups in the pronunciation of sentences, with experimental group two doing significantly better than the other groups.

Table 6.2   Post-Test Results

Group	N	Mean	Std. Deviation	Std. Error
control	10	32.50	4.859	1.537
experimental 1	15	70.33	6.651	1.717
experimental 2	10	78.10	2.283	.722
Total	35	70.31	7.851	1.327

	Sum of Squares	df	Mean Square	F	Sig.
Between Groups	1216.810	2	608.405	22.156	.000
Within Groups	878.733	32	27.460		
Total	2095.543	34			

During the semi-structured interview session, in order to answer the second research question (What are the learners' opinions regarding the use of accent reduction and text-to-speech technology?) the participants in experimental group two provided their opinions on accent reduction and the text-to-speech software. Their responses have been categorized as follows:

- **Addition of visual support.** The participants highly valued the visual activities provided by Pronunciation Power and the real-time visual illustrations of articulatory movements.
- **No stress or fear.** The participants enjoyed "playing" with the activities during sheltered practice sessions in which the participant could take risks without stress or fear of error.
- **Self-pacing.** The participants had the opportunity to study at their own pace, without having to try to keep up with the teacher or the classmates who were fast learners.
- **Immediate feedback.** The participants were provided with immediate feedback by the pronunciation software and the text-to-speech software.
- **Pronunciation of any word or sentence.** Text-to-speech software provided pronunciation of any words or any utterance entered by the participants. This provided a quick and efficient access without searching the words in their paper-based or CD/DVD dictionaries or any other resource.
- **Improved spelling and listening.** The participants also stated that they practiced spelling and writing while creating sentences and listening to these sentences created by TTS technology.
- **Lack of emotion and naturalness.** The participants, while listening to the longer sentences created by the TTS software, had the feeling that

the speaker lacked emotion or naturalness though his/her pronunciation was clear and understandable.

DISCUSSION

The integration of accent reduction and text-to-speech software into classrooms can help learners of English improve their pronunciation due to factors such as practice sessions in which the learner can take risks without stress and fear of error and can receive immediate feedback. However, this does not mean that only TTS technology and/or accent reduction software resulted in the participants' improved results in the tests reported in the study. By adding a variety of resources and enriching the classroom activities with audio and video materials, the classroom environment provided "optimal" conditions for learning, which can be noticed in the responses provided by the participants to the interview questions. The classroom atmosphere, teachers' guidance, and the somewhat relaxed state of mind facilitated the retention of material to its maximum potential. Thus, TTS technology and supplementary activities using appropriate software under the teachers' guidance seemed to be an invaluable resource not only in classroom activities but also beyond the classroom, exposing the learners to the language as much as possible. Although TTS technology is not designed for language teaching, it can be used for different purposes, as in the current study, in an EFL class, including:

1. **Practicing mispronounced words.** The teacher can note down the words generally mispronounced by the students and these words, with the help of TTS technology, can be listened to. This can be done by the students and/or the teacher. Instead of directly correcting the mistakes in the class, as it is probably more effective for students to correct their own mistakes, students can study on their own or in groups. Moreover, these words can be posted on blogs or wikis for later use.
2. **Listening to authentic materials/short stories/articles.** The Internet is an invaluable source for finding short stories, articles, authentic materials, and the materials designed for pedagogic purposes. Reading these materials can be accompanied by a listening activity, which will lead to longer retention of vocabulary and pronunciation of the words.
3. **Creating dialogues.** Using TTS, learners can create dialogues with different voices and accents, using their imagination. This will, hopefully, help them practice both writing and listening, and pronunciation.

Regarding the limitations of the study, it was carried out for two hours each week for 16 weeks, and with only a small number of participants due to the time constraint and the availability of the participants. It is suggested that similar experiments with a large number of participants through random assignment should be replicated.

CONCLUSION

In the past, sound and video materials were difficult to create and put into use in educational settings. However, with the fast development of technology, software, and equipment, it is now much easier to manage new audio and video materials because they are digital and offered in high quality. The quicker access to materials, and the use of these materials as learning and teaching objects, has made it possible to create a new learning and teaching experience in educational settings, especially in language classrooms. Considering the results in this study, the integration of accent reduction and text-to-speech software into classrooms has paved the way for helping learners of English improve their pronunciation, offering practice sessions in which the learner can take risks without stress and fear of error and providing the advantage of immediate feedback. TTS technology together with pronunciation practice software such as Pronunciation Power, with their potential for providing a valuable resource of pronunciation and enriching classroom activities, can greatly contribute to the field of language teaching and learning not only in the Turkish context but in others where the learner can go beyond the materials provided by course books. The combination of a human teacher together with opportunities for human–human interaction in the classroom or outside the classroom via text, and face-to-face or online communication supported by the technology, constitute the most desirable solution for both educators and students.

ACKNOWLEDGMENTS

I would like to gratefully and sincerely thank Dr. Françoise Blin for all her invaluable comments and suggestions.

REFERENCES

Azuma, J. (2008). Applying TTS technology to foreign language teaching. In F. Zhang & B. Barber (Eds.), *Handbook of research on computer-enhanced language acquisition and learning* (pp. 497–506). New York: Information Science Reference.

Baker, A. (2006). *Tree or three? An elementary pronunciation course* (2nd ed.). Cambridge: Cambridge University Press.

Celce-Murcia, M., Brinton, D., & Goodwin, J. (1996). *Teaching pronunciation.* Cambridge: Cambridge University Press.

Gilbert, J. (1995). Pronunciation practices as an aid to listening comprehension. In D. J. Mendelson & J. Rubin (Eds.), *A guide for the teaching of second language learning* (pp. 97–111). San Diego: Dominic Press.

Jenkins, J. (2005). Implementing an international approach to English pronunciation: The role of teacher attitudes and identity. *TESOL Quarterly, 39*(3), 535–543.

Kataoka, H. (2007, December). *Preparation for university entrance examinations: How to learn frequently-appearing English words with the TTS audios.* Paper presented at the Multimedia & Internet Seminar, Japan Association for Language Education and Technology (LET), Kansai Chapter, Osaka, Japan.

Kataoka, H., Funakoshi, Y., & Kitamura, Y. (2007). Utilizing text-to-speech synthesis for English education. In *Proceedings of the 23rd Annual Conference of Japan Society for Educational Technology* (pp. 429–430). Osaka: JSET.

Kenworthy, J. (1990). *Teaching English pronunciation.* New York: Longman.

Kiely, R. (2005). The role of television and televisual literacy in language teaching and learning. Retrieved from http://www.developingteachers.com/articles_tchtraining/tvpf_richard.htm

Kılıçkaya, F. (2006). Text-to-speech technology: What does it offer to foreign language learners? *CALL-EJ Online, 7*(2).

Levis, J. (2007). Computer technology in teaching and researching pronunciation. *Annual Review of Applied Linguistics, 27*(1), 184–202.

Ritchie, W. C., & Bhatia, T. K. (2008). Psycholinguistics. In B. Spolsky & F. M. Hult (Eds.), *The handbook of educational linguistics* (pp. 38–52). Singapore: Blackwell Publishing.

Seferoğlu, G. (2005). Improving students' pronunciation through accent reduction software. *British Journal of Educational Technology, 36*(2), 303–316.

Sha, G. (2009). Using TTS voices to develop audio materials for listening comprehension: A digital approach. *British Journal of Educational Technology, 41*(4), 632–641.

Tench, P. (1981). *Pronunciation skills.* London and Basingstoke: Macmillan.

7 Using Computer Keystroke Recording Software to Analyze Patterns of Revision in English Language Schools

Erifili Roubou

INTRODUCTION

Research on the potential of the word processor as a writing tool started in the early 1980s. However, the results produced have largely been inconsistent and even contradictory, suggesting that the effects of this medium are contingent on a number of parameters such as the design and the duration of a study, or the users and their prior computer and typing skills (Pennington, 1993; Roubou, 2008). To date, there has been almost no relevant research in the Greek context. However, the ubiquitous presence of computers and the introduction of computer-based versions of popular EFL exams make it a matter of urgency to investigate the effects of the word processor on the writing process. Contrary to expectation, Greek students do not use the word processor for extensive writing prior to entering higher education. Therefore, a better understanding of this tool will have practical applications as it will enable practitioners to consider the potential of this writing medium in general, as well as the investigation of whether or not students can benefit from this alternative mode of exam administration in particular. The present chapter focuses on one aspect of the writing process: the amount and types of revisions carried out by students composing on the computer.

WRITING RESEARCH BACKGROUND

The history of L2 writing research is a comparatively short one as its beginning can be traced back to the early 1960s (Matsuda, 2003). With respect to composition studies, very little published research on L2 writers appeared prior to the 1980s (Ferris & Hedgcock, 2005). This research gap can be attributed to the dominant audio-lingual approach to teaching, which emphasized the importance of spoken language over written forms (Fries, 1945). In that context, writing was not practiced as a skill per se but rather as a means of either reinforcing the oral patterns of language or testing knowledge of grammatical structures (Rivers, 1968). In addition, composing was viewed as simply linear and straightforward, while writing processes and subprocesses, which form an integral part of this demanding skill, were largely ignored. However, Flower and Hayes (1981), who emphasized the recursive nature of writing and the multiplicity of processes involved in composing, paved the way for substantial, in-depth research on writing, drawing on cognitive psychology and psycholinguistics. This interdisciplinary approach led to the emergence of a process approach to writing that, as the name suggests, shifted attention from *product* (i.e., the final piece of writing) to writers' *internal processes* as they compose.

At the same time, the microcomputer, used mainly by scientists, became available to a wider public, enabling more people to engage in CALL and L2 writing research (Levy, 1997). The introduction of the word processor in the writing class carried strong potential to reinforce the newly introduced process approach to writing. Indeed, its inherent features and commands can facilitate, and possibly encourage, the revising process, which forms part and parcel of the recursive nature of composing. Typically, text editors offer a wide range of editing and formatting options. The ease with which the text can be manipulated seems to alleviate some of the physical and cognitive constraints of writing, thus leading to writing of superior quality.

Research on word processing to date has focused mainly on its potential to improve writing quality, attitudes, amount and kinds of revisions, and planning. Bangert-Drowns (1993) conducted a meta-analysis review of 32 comparative studies that involved designs that employed two groups of students that received identical writing instruction but allowed only one group to use the word processor. The results showed that in two-thirds of the studies, word processing groups improved the quality of their writing. Similar findings were yielded by a meta-analytical review of studies dated from 1992 to 2002 (Goldberg, Russell, & Cook, 2003). The review included 26 studies and revealed significant mean effect sizes (effect size = .41) in favor of the word processor in relation to writing quality. With respect to attitudes, Cochran-Smith (1991) notes that the positive attitudes as a result of exposure to this tool are nearly universal in related studies. With regards to revising, although previous reviews did not arrive at unequivocal conclusions, Goldberg et al. claim that students composing on the computer tend to revise more than when writing by hand. In particular, it appears that the word processor tends to encourage mainly surface-level editing of texts. Yet, caution should be exercised when examining such generalized outcomes as the amount of revising and, more importantly, the kind of revisions carried out by students, is contingent on a number of factors such as language proficiency, previous computer writing experience, and the nature and length of the writing task (Pennington, 1993).

Readers familiar with word processing research might notice that most of the studies in the field were carried out in the 1980s. This issue was addressed back in 1998 by Susser, who argued that word processing as an instructional technology had by the early 1990s already disappeared from accounts of writing with computers (p. 347). In fact, many researchers claim that from about 1989, computer-assisted writing research abandoned word processing and moved to computer-mediated communication (CMC), the Internet, and other innovative technologies (Hawisher, LeBlanc, Moran, & Selfe, 1996). This was due to the word processor becoming "normalized," that is, reaching "the stage when technology becomes invisible, embedded in everyday practice" (Bax, 2003, p. 23), before being adequately investigated in a variety of contexts. In this light, research drawing on past studies, while avoiding previous pitfalls or parameters that skewed results, is essential to inform the use of the word processor, especially in an unresearched context like the Greek one where computer-based exams are gradually being introduced.

Nevertheless, computers do not only enhance and facilitate the writing process by offering text editing programs but can also contribute significantly to research in the field of L2 writing. The availability of computers has revolutionized the way in which writing processes, and in particular revising, are investigated as it allows for real-time studies. One of the most groundbreaking possibilities offered nowadays is the use of keystroke logging software.

Keystroke Logging Software

Due to the intricate nature of internalized writing processes, which were difficult to document, complex and sophisticated investigation techniques are required. Initially, cognitive theorists proposed think-aloud verbalizations as the main method for real-time studies (Newell & Simon, 1972), while direct observation and video recordings followed as more advanced techniques. However, the advent of the microcomputer made possible the use of keystroke logging software, an unobtrusive and reliable means of gathering such data. Keystroke logging software records all keystrokes executed by writers while they compose, and saves them in logs that can be subsequently coded and analyzed. As such software usually runs in the background, the process of recording does not interfere with the writing task.

Keystroke logging software has been used in many studies investigating self-assessment and autonomous learning (Sullivan & Lindgren, 2002), noticing and language awareness (Lindgren & Sullivan, 2006), discourse structure (Severinson Eklundh & Kollberg, 2003), composing processes (Levy & Ransdell, 1996; Spelman Miller, Lindgren, & Sullivan, 2008), pausing (Spelman Miller, 2000), and revising (Lindgren & Sullivan, 2006).

In early word processing studies, the examination and comparison between students' initial handwritten drafts and the final product served as a potential indicator and record of revising activity. This method, however, misses out a great amount of revising as it fails to document information on revisions that were made while actually composing a draft. In contrast, keystroke logging carries enormous potential for the recording of the actual, online process of writing, which constitutes a rich, detailed record of writers' revisions despite possible limitations that mainly involve errors in automatic analysis, if enabled, or the fact that we get no insight into the reasons behind specific revisions unless think-aloud protocols are used.

Justification

This chapter reports on a study that examined the potential of the word processor in the EFL writing class, with a particular focus on the revising behavior exhibited by learners. More specifically, it addresses the following research question: Does the writing tool (handwriting versus word processing) have any significant effect on the amount of revising activity? If so, what kinds of revision tend to be affected the most? This study is underpinned by two main contextual factors: computer familiarity and English-language status issues in the Greek context.

With regard to computer familiarity, although most Greek students attend computer classes for up to three years at their state junior high schools, they never use a word processor to write compositions. In some cases only, students are asked to type a brief report on various scientific issues but this is not typical of all schools. In fact, generally, the word processor is not used as a writing medium in educational contexts in Greece, with the exception of academic institutions. In effect, Greek students appear to lack computer literacy. According to a report by the Organisation for Economic Co-operation and Development published in 2006, Greek students at around the age of 15 use computers at a strikingly lower percentage than their peers in most member countries of the organization.[1] The same study revealed that these students' main preoccupation with computers was to play games and only to a lesser extent to learn new programs or to search the web for information.

On the other hand, English is widely recognized in Greece as an international language. Knowledge of the language is considered essential for entering the job market and for professional development in both the private and the public sector. In addition, language proficiency exams are required for entering university faculties such as English Language and Literature, Translation and Interpretation, and Tourism Studies. Given that Greece is a country that attracts a large number of tourists year-round, English is a prerequisite even for jobs requiring few other qualifications. As knowledge of the language is certified through official qualifications, international English proficiency examinations in Greece are so popular that the Greek context could be best characterized as exam oriented.

Because English classes at state schools do not provide adequate preparation for such exams, students very often resort to private language schools.

According to the last report published by the Greek Ministry of National Education and Religious affairs, in the academic year 2008–2009, there were 7,653 private language schools registered officially. According to the same report, 618,874 students attend such schools in order to learn English. In addition, many students receive private tutoring at home, especially in cases where the student is weak or in need of more intensive exam preparation. Stronger evidence is provided by a study conducted by Eurydice (2006) in Europe for the academic year 2005–2006. As reported, 87.4 percent of Greek children start learning a foreign language at the age of 8. Considering that foreign languages are introduced to schools for students at the age of 10, this implies that students turn to private schools or home tutoring much earlier.

METHODOLOGY

The present study took place during a whole academic year that spanned three terms (32 weeks). A comparative design was implemented, based on an experimental group to which the intervention was introduced, and a control group against which outcomes were measured.

Context

Research took place in a private language school with five branches spreading over adjacent neighborhoods. This school offers English lessons for all levels of competency and, typically, students attend classes for approximately eight years in order to reach the B2 level. The class investigated is in the seventh year of studies. This level involves six hours of instruction per week and at two branches these were broken down into three two-hour sessions. These classes cover all four language skills and try to build up students' competence in the language. According to the syllabus, students are taught the coursebook for four hours while the third session focuses on grammar. This teacher-researcher neither selected the materials nor introduced new methods regarding the teaching of the coursebook, besides the use of the word processor for writing.

Participants

The participants were 20 intermediate-level B2 students[2] (total N = 20) whose ages ranged from 13 to 15. Both the control group and the experimental group consisted of 10 students. Each group attended classes in a different branch of the same school. The groups were intact classes as students self-selected the branch they wanted to attend without any intervention from the school or the researcher. The selection of the branch that had the computer treatment was random. Both groups received identical instruction from the same teacher-researcher and were exposed to the same teaching materials in order to prevent extraneous, unrelated parameters from interfering with the outcomes of the intervention.

Data Collection Methods and Instruments

Taking into account students' limited familiarity with computers, the computer group received training in word processing skills prior to the study in order to ensure that lack of adequate skills would not present an obstacle to the effects of the word processor being materialized. In total, students completed 11 essay tasks in various genres. The first writing task was handwritten by both the experimental and the control group in order to keep a record of students' writing ability and revising behavior, and also to enable the comparison. The remaining 10 tasks were word processed by the computer group and handwritten by the control group. To facilitate the comparison of revising behavior, the handwriting group was asked to ensure that all the changes they made remained visible. Therefore, students were advised to simply cross out items they wanted to delete, or to use asterisks and arrows to add or move information in the text.

For the computer group, keystroke recording software, KGB Spy, was activated prior to the intervention. Students were able to use Microsoft Office Word, the software installed at students' Greek state schools and at the private school where the research took place, since it does not include a text editor. Once installed, KGB Spy ran at system boot and it operated in stealth mode in order not to interfere with the composing process. It logged all user activities into files that were later exported into HTML for analysis and it also provided information on the application name and the window caption. The software is easy to use, making it accessible to all language teachers even with limited computer skills. Another advantage of KGB Spy is that it has the ability to record language-specific characters. This is particularly useful because some Greek learners of English tend to write unknown words in Greek in their compositions expecting the teacher to translate them to English when they correct them.

Concerning the tasks, the word limit was 120 words per composition and students in both groups were given 50 minutes to complete each. All writing activity was carried out in the classroom for the handwriting group while the computer group moved to the lab. Writing partly paralleled exam situations due to the nature of the specific context. Therefore, students were not allowed to consult the coursebook, use dictionaries, or ask the teacher questions. In addition, in order not to give an advantage to the computer group, all proofing tools offered by the word processor, such as grammar and spelling checkers, were disabled prior to the study.

Although students completed 11 writing tasks throughout the year (i.e., 220 compositions in total), three tasks were selected for analysis purposes: (a) the first handwritten composition that constituted the baseline writing,

(b) another composition produced in the middle of the year, and (c) the very last writing task students completed at the end of the school year. The first and the last task belonged to the letter writing genre while the middle one consisted of a narrative.

Data Analysis

Once all writing and revising activity was exported into logs, the analysis of revisions was carried out by the researcher and a second coder, a public school English teacher with relevant research experience. All instances of revision were first quantified and categorized by the researcher and then by the second marker in order to establish the reliability of the analysis. Disagreements were resolved through discussion between the raters.

Following, an excerpt of a student's composition followed by its equivalent part as saved in the log is presented:

> "I would be greatful if you could teel me where is Queen's college located and if I can be reached there by public transport."
>
> [SHIFT]I would be greatful if you could teel me where is [SHIFT] Q[SHIFT]ueen's college located and if I can reashe there[LEFT] [LEFT][LEFT][LEFT][LEFT][LEFT]   [LEFT][LEFT][LEFT][LEFT] [LEFT][LEFT][LEFT] [BACKSPACE] be [RIGHT][RIGHT][RIGHT] [RIGHT][RIGHT][RIGHT][RIGHT][RIGHT]   [LEFT]d[DOWN] [LEFT][LEFT][LEFT][LEFT][LEFT][LEFT][LEFT]by public transport.   [UP][RIGHT][UP][RIGHT][UP][RIGHT][RIGHT][RIGHT] [RIGHT][RIGHT][RIGHT][RIGHT][RIGHT][RIGHT][RIGHT] [RIGHT][RIGHT][RIGHT][RIGHT][RIGHT][RIGHT][RIGHT] [RIGHT][RIGHT][RIGHT][RIGHT][RIGHT][RIGHT][RIGHT] [BACKSPACE]c[DOWN][DOWN][DOWN][LEFT][LEFT][LEFT] [LEFT][LEFT][LEFT][BACKSPACE][SHIFT]?[BACKSPACE]. [SHIFT]

Revision analysis was made according to Faigley and Witte's (1981) taxonomy (see Table 7.1). This taxonomy consists of two major categories, surface-level and text-base revisions. Surface-level revisions are further subdivided into formal changes (which involve mainly editing) and meaning-preserving changes (changes with minimal effects on meaning) while text-base revisions are further subdivided into microstructure (having an effect on meaning but not of overall consequence for the text) and macrostructure (affecting the whole body of the text).

A mixed ANOVA was used to examine whether there was an interaction effect of task/occasion and group on the amount of revisions, that is, if revising differed between occasions more in the computer group than in the control group. That was followed by tests of paired comparisons between occasions and also the trend test, which was used to detect any significant progression upwards or downwards in amount of revision across the three task/occasions in either group.[3]

RESULTS AND DISCUSSION

This being a comparative study, all discussion revolves around the comparison of the two groups and the three occasions which represent the three writing tasks students were asked to complete. Therefore, individual writing sessions were analyzed according to two criteria: (a) the total number of changes made, and (b) the types of revisions based on Faigley and Witte's (1981) taxonomy (see Table 7.1). Discussion starts with the overall number of revisions followed by an examination of all subcategories.

Overall Number of Revisions

Concerning the total number of revisions across all revision categories for the three tasks completed, the general pattern was that students increased the total number of changes they made on the second occasion but this was again decreased on the third occasion (see Table 7.2). The amount of revising differed between the two groups and a significant occasion by group interaction was produced only for students writing on the computer (F = 10.254, p < .000). This finding is supported by a significant trend (p = .001) for the experimental group resulting from significant differences between the first and second occasions (p = .000), and the first and third (p = .003).

The fact that students increased the amount of revising on the second occasion can be attributed to the genre of the second task, a narrative. Narratives present more difficulties for students as they involve using a wide range of tenses and reported speech. Therefore, students might have needed to make more revisions in order to cope with such demands.

Table 7.1   Faigley and Witte's Taxonomy

Surface-level changes		Text-base changes	
Formal	*Meaning-preserving*	*Microstructure*	*Macrostructure*
Spelling	Additions	Additions	Additions
Tense, Number & Modality	Deletions	Deletions	Deletions
Abbreviation	Substitutions	Substitutions	Substitutions
Punctuation	Consolidations	Consolidations	Consolidations
Format	Distributions	Distributions	Distributions
	Permutations	Permutations	Permutations

Table 7.2 Descriptive Statistics and ANOVA for the Total Number of Revisions

Task	Group	Mean	SD	N	Interaction	
					F	p
TN1	Computer	6.30	3.713	10	10.25	.000
	Handwriting	7.50	3.866	10		
	Total	6.90	3.740	20		
TN2	Computer	26.20	8.842	10		
	Handwriting	10.00	8.340	10		
	Total	18.10	11.792	20		
TN3	Computer	19.40	7.501	10		
	Handwriting	8.40	4.858	10		
	Total	13.90	8.347	20		

The findings here corroborate the outcomes reported by previous research (Li, 2006; Phinney & Khouri, 1993), which revealed that students writing with the word processor revised more extensively and produced a greater number of revisions compared to groups writing by hand. Overall, it seems that students writing on the computer took advantage of the text editing features offered by the word processor that allowed them to revise effortlessly while producing neat, well-presented papers.

Surface-Level Revisions

Surface-level changes refer to changes that involve editing of text features. Statistical analysis using mixed, two-way ANOVA showed that the interaction between the three occasions and the two groups was significant (F = 8.662, p = .001), suggesting that the word processor encouraged students writing on the computer to focus more on surface-level editing of their compositions. Table 7.3 presents the descriptive statistics for surface-level revisions and the two subcategories of formal and meaning-preserving changes. A post hoc pair comparison revealed that there were significant differences for the computer group between the first and the second occasion (p < .000) and the first and the third occasion (p = .004), but not between the second and the third (p = .544). In terms of progress of improvement, the trend test indicated that the linear trend was significant for the computer group only, showing a significant progression upwards. This implies that although the number of surface-level changes made by the computer group slightly decreased on the third occasion as compared to the second, the decrease was statistically nonsignificant. No significant differences were revealed for the handwriting group between any of the three occasions.

Table 7.3   Descriptive Statistics and ANOVA for Surface-Level Revisions and Subcategories

Task	Group	Mean	SD	N	Interaction	
					F	p
SF1	Computer	4.80	3.795	10	8.662	.001
	Handwriting	5.70	2.791	10		
	Total	5.25	3.275	20		
SF2	Computer	19.30	5.559	10		
	Handwriting	8.10	7.110	10		
	Total	13.70	8.461	20		
SF3	Computer	15.20	5.673	10		
	Handwriting	6.30	3.860	10		
	Total	10.75	6.569	20		
Fo1	Computer	3.50	2.635	10	19.600	.000
	Handwriting	4.20	2.440	10		
	Total	3.85	2.498	20		
Fo2	Computer	13.30	5.208	10		
	Handwriting	5.00	4.000	10		
	Total	9.15	6.209	20		
Fo3	Computer	14.40	4.881	10		
	Handwriting	4.70	4.029	10		
	Total	9.55	6.613	20		
Mng1	Computer	1.30	1.703	10	.829	.445
	Handwriting	1.50	.850	10		
	Total	1.40	1.314	20		
Mng2	Computer	1.90	1.792	10		
	Handwriting	1.30	1.252	10		
	Total	1.60	1.536	20		
Mng3	Computer	1.90	1.792	10		
	Handwriting	1.10	1.101	10		
	Total	1.50	1.504	20		

The decrease in revising activity by the end of the school year can be partly attributed to the novelty effects of the computer having considerably worn off. In addition, it seems that the effects of the word processor had already materialized by the time students completed the second task, although students appeared to reap some extra benefits by the time they completed the third task. Examining the handwriting group, although a similar pattern of revising behavior was produced (that is, students increased their number of revisions on the second occasion and this was followed by a slight decrease on the third occasion), there was not a significant linear trend either upwards or downwards. Similarly, examining the results of the post hoc comparison, no significant differences were observed between any of the three occasions.

Such findings support previous research which concluded that the word processor encourages surface-level editing (Li & Cumming, 2001; New, 1999), which is even more likely to occur when it involves inexperienced writers who tend to focus more on the word level because they lack the linguistic knowledge required for dealing with higher order concerns such as revisions at the phrase or discourse level.

Formal Changes

A very strong occasion-group interaction (F = 19.600, p < .000) was produced for this category. As denoted by the trend test, the computer group gradually increased the number of formal changes they made to their texts. More specifically, the post hoc comparison shows that there was a significant increase in the number of revisions between the first and the second writing task (p = .002), the first and the third writing task (p = .001), but not between the second and the third (p = 1). Yet, this is the only type of revision for which there was increasing revising activity from task to task for the computer group despite the lack of a significant difference between the second and the last writing task. This is also evident in the results of the trend test, which reveal a steady progression upwards for the experimental group. Among the further subtypes of revisions under formal changes, it was only spelling revisions for which the results showed significant occasion by group interaction for the experimental group (F = 11.206, p < .000), suggesting that students seemed mainly preoccupied with spelling. In a similar fashion, the handwriting group focused mainly on spelling changes despite the lack of significant differences from task to task.

Accounting for the large number of formal changes, a limited number of such changes might actually belong to the extra category of "computer changes,"[4] which was identified in the coding procedure for errors that could be attributed to typing skills or the keyboard. Yet, the principal explanatory factor for the strong focus on this type of revision on the part of students is the fact that spelling seems to be more amenable to revision and, in fact, is easier to perform by rather inexperienced writers. When in doubt about the spelling of a word, students very often experiment with different letters or combinations of letters in an already written word in order to decide which one seems to be the most likely version. This is common in handwritten essays as well, but it was to be expected that the nature of the word processor as a writing tool that encourages experimentation, and also the level of ability of the students, would accentuate such preference for this sort of revising.

Meaning-Preserving Changes

Considering meaning-preserving changes, both groups exhibited different revising patterns. The computer group increased the number of changes they made to their text on the second occasion and this number was exactly the same for the third occasion as well. By contrast, the handwriting group showed a steady decrease downwards in the number of changes carried out. Despite group differences, the interaction yielded was nonsignificant for both groups (F = .829, p = .445). In addition, a nonsignificant trend was produced. This implies that neither the control nor the experimental group showed any considerable increase in relation to this type of change. The examination of the subtypes of revisions within this category showed a significant interaction only for additions (F = 3.252, p = .050) for students writing on the computer.

Meaning-preserving changes might not be particularly popular among inexperienced writers, despite being easier to make than macrostructure revisions that affect larger segments of a text; novice writers are not usually eager and able to experiment freely with their evolving or finished texts. Therefore, they might avoid replacing segments with different ones that state more or less the same thing if they seem happy or simply satisfied with what they have already written.

Text-Base Revisions

The quantitative analysis of the total number of text-base revisions yielded similar findings to surface-level changes. A mixed, two-way ANOVA analysis revealed a significant occasion by group interaction favoring students writing on the computer (F = 5.259, p = .010) as well as a significant linear trend for this group (p = .026). Significant differences between only the first and the second occasion (p = .008) imply a steady progression upwards, which, however, did not dramatically continue after the second writing task. As far as the handwriting group was concerned, in line with surface level revising, students increased the number of revisions they performed but their progress did not yield significant results. Table 7.4 reports on the descriptive statistics for text-base revisions as well as microstructure and macrostructure revising.

Microstructure Changes

An examination of the two main categories of text-base changes, those of microstructure and macrostructure revising, yielded the following results: The occasion by group interaction for microstructure revising was significant (F = 5.344, p = .009) as the computer group outperformed the handwriting group in the number of this type of changes. There was also a significant linear trend (p = .040) for the same group due to the significant difference between the first and second occasion. Yet, with the exception of substitutions, no other subtype yielded significant differences between the two groups. Substituting can be greatly facilitated by the word processor since students can easily highlight and delete parts in order to overwrite something different. This sort of revision is more difficult to perform

Table 7.4 Descriptive Statistics and ANOVA for Text-Base Revisions and Subcategories

Task	Group	Mean	SD	N	Interaction	
					F	p
TB1	Computer	1.50	1.354	10	5.259	.010
	Handwriting	1.80	1.619	10		
	Total	1.65	1.461	20		
TB2	Computer	6.60	5.259	10		
	Handwriting	1.90	1.853	10		
	Total	4.40	4.616	20		
TB3	Computer	4.20	2.700	10		
	Handwriting	2.10	2.132	10		
	Total	3.15	2.601	20		
Micro1	Computer	1.40	1.265	10	5.344	.009
	Handwriting	1.80	1.619	10		
	Total	1.60	1.429	20		
Micro2	Computer	6.60	5.441	10		
	Handwriting	1.80	1.932	10		
	Total	4.20	4.675	20		
Micro3	Computer	3.60	2.221	10		
	Handwriting	1.50	2.014	10		
	Total	2.55	2.328	20		
Macro1	Computer	.10	.316	10	1.358	.270
	Handwriting	.00	.000	10		
	Total	.05	.224	20		
Macro2	Computer	.70	1.059	10		
	Handwriting	.20	.422	10		
	Total	.45	.826	20		
Macro3	Computer	.60	.966	10		
	Handwriting	.10	.316	10		
	Total	.35	.745	20		

on paper as it involves crossing out segments, making smudges, and using signs to indicate where the new part appears if there is no space to add it on the spot. This, however, not only ruins the appearance of a paper but also limits students in relation to the amount of changes they can make.

Macrostructure Changes

Interestingly, results differ when it comes to macrostructure changes as the groups failed to produce a significant interaction for this type of revision ($F = 1.358$, $p = .270$). In line with this finding, there was no significant trend for either of the two groups. Regarding macrostructure revising, it is noteworthy that the handwriting group gradually increased the total number of such changes from the first occasion to the third despite having made fewer overall changes than the computer group. The computer group exhibited a similar pattern to most of the other kinds of revisions, as participants made more revisions on the second occasion followed by a slight decrease on the third. Among the five subtypes of revisions, none proved to be significant for either of the two groups. In fact, students failed to produce any permutations, distributions, or consolidations whatsoever.

The word processor could have encouraged and facilitated macrostructure revising because of the relative ease of moving large segments in the text, and the fact that additions or deletions of whole chunks of text can be carried out effortlessly; yet, in this study, this kind of revision was limited to a very small number of changes. It is likely that the fact that the participants were novice writers contributed to this result. Moreover, as the writing tasks were limited to 120 words, it could be argued that the shorter the text, the more difficult it becomes to make extensive macrostructure changes.

The following arguments should also be discussed in an effort to account for the lack of a significantly higher number of macrostructure revisions by the computer group. Hyland (1993) argues that only instruction can play a major role in developing effective revision strategies. It is possible that students might have improved their writing skills further if, besides using the word processor, they had received explicit instruction on how to revise. However, it must be stressed that revising does not necessarily lead to improved quality.

It was deliberate that students in this study did not receive any instruction in revising as this would have introduced an extra parameter besides the intervention that could have influenced its outcomes. In other words, it would have been difficult to determine whether students made a greater number of and more varied revisions because of the instruction they received or due to the properties of the word processor as a writing tool. As research to date indicates, when there is no instruction in revising strategies, students tend to use the word processor to revise in ways they revise when writing by hand (Cochran-Smith, 1991). In reality, all they do is transfer the revising strategies they employ on paper to the word processor. Considering that these students are inexperienced writers, it was not surprising that the differences that appeared between the two groups were mainly related to a higher overall number of formal revisions, as these are typical of the revising behavior of students at this writing proficiency level (Van Gelderen & Oostdam, 2002). Yet, students in the computer group also exhibited a significantly greater increase in microstructure changes, that is, changes that have an effect on meaning. It could be argued that although these students may not be experienced enough to carry out extensive macrostructure revising, they used the word processor in order to make changes that affected the meaning of their texts even at the paragraph level.

CONCLUSION AND FURTHER RESEARCH

The contribution of this study is twofold. First, it researched a context that has been neglected in previous studies. The main contexts of investigation so far have been the Western European and American ones. However, the Greek context is more similar to Asian countries as it is highly exam oriented concerning ELT. Second, the specific age group has rarely been targeted before as studies so far have largely focused on elementary school children or academic writers.

The results suggest both qualitative and quantitative effects of the word processor on students' revising behavior. Quantitative effects have to do with the amount of revising in total. Statistical analysis showed that the computer group produced a significantly higher total number of revisions, suggesting that the word processor can facilitate or at least encourage greater revising compared to handwriting. On the other hand, from a qualitative perspective, students writing on the computer differed with respect to the types of revisions they made. Although both groups focused mainly on surface-level editing, the computer group carried out significantly more microstructure changes, that is, revisions that affect the meaning of the text. Considering that in the baseline writing task students in both groups produced similar types and amount of changes, the increase in microstructure revising is indicative of the qualitative effects of composition mode on revising. Finally, the noticeable lack of macrostructure changes across both groups possibly implies that students of this proficiency level were not linguistically ready to manipulate larger segments of text.

Based on the findings of this study, the following implications and recommendations for composition teaching in Greek private language schools and similar ELT contexts can be proposed:

1. It is imperative that students who write on the computer receive adequate training that will allow them to touch-type or at least to type quickly. Otherwise, it appears that the word processor slows down the writing process and interferes with the writing task.
2. In the light of the positive results of the present study, educators could also consider alternative technologies for promoting computer-assisted writing and for tracking revisions, such as wikis and other electronic encyclopedic webpages that allow for collaborative writing projects since pages can be easily created and edited by all users.
3. Future research could focus on L1 to L2 writing strategy transfer by means of a quantitative and qualitative comparison of revising in a

native and foreign language. Relating this information to composition mode could also be of interest to educators.

NOTES

1. For a complete list of the member countries visit http://www.oecd.org/count rieslist/0,3351,en_33873108_33844430_1_1_1_1_1,00.html.
2. Based on the Common European Framework (CEF).
3. The trend test is for multiple comparisons between ordered correlated variables and is used for reporting post hoc pair comparisons.
4. A typical computer change is to produce "1" instead of "!" as a result of not pressing the shift key properly.

REFERENCES

Bangert-Drowns, R. L. (1993). The word processor as an instructional tool: A meta-analysis of word processing in writing instruction. *Review of Educational Research, 63*, 69–93.

Bax, S. (2003). CALL-past, present and future. *System, 31*, 13–28.

Cochran-Smith, M. (1991). Word processing and writing in elementary classrooms: A critical review of the literature. *Review of Educational Research, 61*(1), 107–155.

Eurydice. (2005). *Key data on teaching languages at school in Europe*. Retrieved from http://eacea.ec.europa.eu/portal/page/portal/Eurydice/showPresentation? pubid=049EN

Faigley, L., & Witte, S. P. (1981). Analyzing revision. *College Composition and Communication, 32*, 400–414.

Ferris, D. R., & Hedgcock, J. S. (2005). *Teaching ESL composition: Purpose, process, and practice*. Mahwah, NJ: Lawrence Erlbaum.

Flower, L. S., & Hayes, J. R. (1981). A cognitive process theory of writing. *College Composition and Communication, 32*(4), 365–387.

Fries, C. C. (1945). *Teaching and learning English as a foreign language*. Ann Arbor: University of Michigan Press.

Goldberg, A., Russell, M., & Cook, A. (2003). The effect of computers on student writing: A meta-analysis of studies from 1992 to 2002. *Journal of Technology, Learning and Assessment, 2*(1), 1–52.

Hawisher, G., LeBlanc, P., Moran, C., & Selfe, C. (1996). *Computers and the teaching of writing in American higher education. 1979–1994: A history*. Norwood, NJ: Ablex.

Hyland, K. (1993). ESL computer writers: What can we do to help? *System, 21*(1), 21–30.

Levy, M. (1997). *Computer-assisted language learning: Context and conceptualisation*. Oxford: Oxford University Press.

Levy, M., & Ransdell, S. (1996). Writing signatures. In M. Levy & S. Ransdell (Eds.), *The science of writing* (pp. 149–161). Mahwah, NJ: Lawrence Erlbaum Associates.

Li, J. (2006). The mediation of technology in ESL writing and its implications for writing assessment. *Assessing Writing, 11*(1), 5–21.

Li, J., & Cumming, A. (2001). Word processing and second language writing: A longitudinal case study. *International Journal of English Studies, 1*(2), 127–152.

Lindgren, E., & Sullivan, K. P. H. (2006). Analysing online revision. In G. Rij-laarsdam (Series Ed.) & K. P. H. Sullivan & E. Lindgren (Vol. Eds.), *Studies in writing: Vol. 18. Computer keystroke logging: Methods and applications* (pp. 157–188). Oxford: Elsevier.

Matsuda, P. K. (2003). Second language writing in the twentieth century: A situated historical perspective. In B. Kroll (Ed.), *Exploring the dynamics of second language writing* (pp. 15–34). Cambridge: Cambridge University Press.

New, E. (1999). Computer-aided writing in French as a foreign language: A qualitative and quantitative look at the process of revision. *Modern Language Journal, 83*, 80–97.

Newell, A., & Simon, A. (1972). *Human problem solving.* Englewood Cliffs, NJ: Prentice Hall.

Organisation for Economic Co-operation and Development. (2006). *Are students ready for a technology-rich world? What PISA studies tell us.* Retrieved from http://www.oecd.org/home

Pennington, M. C. (1993). Exploring the potential of word processing for non-native writers. *Computers and the Humanities, 27*(3), 149–163.

Phinney, M., & Khouri, S. (1993). Computers, revision, and ESL writers: The role of experience. *Journal of Second Language Writing, 2*, 257–277.

Rivers, W. M. (1968). *Teaching foreign language skills.* Chicago: University of Chicago Press.

Roubou, E. (2008). Dealing with the inconsistency of previous word processing research: Solutions applied to a PhD project. *Essex Graduate Papers in Linguistics, 10*, 76–96.

Severinson Eklundh, K., & Kollberg, P. (2003). Emerging discourse structure: Computer-assisted episode analysis as a window to global revision in university students' writing. *Journal of Pragmatics, 35*, 869–891.

Spelman Miller, K. (2000). Academic writers on-line: Investigating pausing in the production of text. *Language Teaching Research, 4*, 123–148.

Spelman Miller, K., Lindgren, E., & Sullivan, K. P. H. (2008). The psycholinguistic dimension in second language writing: Opportunities for research and pedagogy. *TESOL Quarterly, 42*(3), 433–454.

Sullivan K. P. H., & Lindgren, E. (2002). Self-assessment in autonomous computer-aided L2 writing. *ELT Journal, 56*(3), 258–266.

Susser, B. (1998). The mysterious disappearance of word processing. *Computers and Composition, 15*, 347–371.

Van Gelderen, A., & Oostdam, R. (2002). Improving linguistic fluency for writing: effects of explicitness and focus of instruction. *L1 Educational Studies of Language and Literature, 2*(3), 239–270.

8 Modeling Language Learners' Knowledge

What Information Can Be Inferred from Learners' Free Written Texts?

Sylvie Thouësny and Françoise Blin

INTRODUCTION

Learner models store information about learners that enable intelligent tutoring systems to select the most appropriate pedagogical intervention for a particular student. Inferring a learner's knowledge of grammatical forms from free written texts is, however, a complex endeavor. In particular, it requires the use of instruments that can help distinguish between errors (competence-dependent) and mistakes (performance-related). In this chapter, we explicate how we constructed such an instrument.

A learner model is a core component of an intelligent tutoring system (Bernsen & Dybkjær, 2008), which typically stores information about the learner and can be called upon by the system to decide which pedagogical intervention is most suited to his/her current level of proficiency. In other words, learner models enable intelligent tutoring systems not only to assess students' performance, record their progress, and provide them with personalized feedback, but also to adapt tutoring strategies depending on their progress (Heift & Schulze, 2007). Different approaches to designing and maintaining learner models can be found in the literature (for a comprehensive overview, see Heift & Schulze, 2007). Most attempt to form a representation of a learner's knowledge from his/her performance. Adaptive student modeling systems may draw inferences about the student's knowledge using different methods, such as the knowledge tracing method (Beck & Sison, 2006), the probabilistic approach (Conati, Gertner, & VanLehn, 2002), or the overlay technique (Brusilovsky & Millán, 2007), to mention but a few. When integrated into Intelligent Computer-Assisted Language Learning (ICALL) applications, learner models enable the observation, recording, analysis, and even inference of reasons for an ill-formed word (Heift & Schulze, 2007).

Inferring the reasons for an ill-formed word in order to adapt the pedagogical intervention to the learner, be it in the form of corrective feedback or remediation activities, is a complex endeavor, especially when dealing with written compositions as opposed to discrete sentences or grammar-focused exercises. Whether computerized or human, tutors have to differentiate between incorrect forms due to the learner's physical or emotional states and incorrect forms due to a lack of underlying competence. Occasional lapses in a learner's performance are considered by some as mistakes, whereas gaps in a learner's competence are regarded as errors (Ellis, 1997). For Corder (1967), errors are systematic and affect the learner's knowledge or competence, whereas mistakes are unsystematic or occasional and affect his/her performance. From a sociocultural perspective, Aljaafreh and Lantolf (1994) claim that when learners rely on themselves to correct their own written texts without help or with minimum help, incorrect forms may be considered as genuine "slips of the pen." In this case, "whenever aberrant performance does arise [...] noticing and correcting errors do not require intervention from someone else" (p. 470). Distinguishing competence errors from performance mistakes in essay-type productions should therefore enhance the modeling of learner knowledge by providing reliable information about their linguistic strengths and weaknesses.

In this chapter, we posit that if a student is able to correct an ill-constructed form without explicit information on the error type, that is, with minimal assistance, the error is deemed to be a mistake. If, on the contrary, the student can only correct the erroneous form when additional information is provided, the incorrect form is deemed to be an error. Different levels of competence can then be inferred depending on the amount of assistance required to produce the correct form (e.g., errors highlighted only, error-type made explicit, metalinguistic explanations given, etc.). We thus propose and discuss a method to distinguish between errors and mistakes produced by intermediate learners of French in essay-type compositions so that variable performance can be taken into account and learner knowledge more reliably represented. More specifically, we investigate whether computing the ratio of incorrect to correct forms, which can help us represent language performance at a given time, provides enough information to model learner knowledge.

CREATION OF A TAGGED LEARNER LANGUAGE CORPUS

Thirteen university first-year students volunteered to contribute texts to the corpus. All participants were English native speakers and were studying French at an intermediate level. They were enrolled in a French module of 12-week duration, with three face-to-face sessions per week. The module adopted a project-based curriculum, which entailed students to organize a French film festival. The project involved presenting a movie to the class, writing a synopsis of the film, and finally reflecting on one's language learning experience and outcomes. In order to create our corpus, participants were asked to write a 200-word review of one of four given short films.

These short films were not well known to the general public, which prevented texts being copied and pasted from online blockbusters' reviews or from critics, and maintained a certain amount of authenticity and originality in learners' written productions.

Students were asked to submit their review via the university virtual learning environment (Moodle—http://moodle.org/) and subsequently requested to revise their initial text and to resubmit it in two successive stages. To do this, they were provided with web-based corrected copies of their initial text and were asked to self-edit their own work twice in succession during a controlled laboratory session. The purpose of the laboratory session was to ensure that students did not have access to external help, such as human assistance or online dictionaries. For the first self-editing exercise, students were provided with an electronic copy of their own text, where all incorrect forms were highlighted without any comments. Participants were asked to provide an appropriate alternative for each highlighted form. For the second self-editing exercise, students received additional information on the error type for each incorrect form. The error types were visible with a mouse rollover action on the incorrect forms. Each correction exercise was performed in a relatively restrained time period of 10 to 15 minutes. Two students, however, took more than the time allocated, up to 20 minutes for one exercise. Upon completion of the two self-editing exercises, all students received metalinguistic feedback about their written productions.

Learners' input was first error-encoded with the assistance of Markin (http://www.cict.co.uk/software/markin/index.htm)—a program enabling teachers to correct and annotate students' electronic submissions—and then tagged with *TreeTagger* (http://www.ims.uni-stuttgart.de/projekte/corplex/TreeTagger/), a part-of-speech (pos) tagger.

Error Encoding

Students' original texts were retrieved from Moodle and saved as plain text files. Incorrect forms were encoded according to a four-error type classification, based on Mackey, Gass, and McDonough's (2000) research on the nature of specific types of errors and corrective feedback. The four main error categories were defined as selection, syntactic, morpho-syntactic, and misspelling. Only one error per word or group of words was encoded according to the following level of precedence: (a) selection, (b) syntactic, (c) morpho-syntactic, and (d) spelling. Table 8.1 outlines the morpho-syntactic error types, which consist of incorrect, misplaced, or missing morphemes in a semantically correct word. In an error tag such as *mo_ag_dn*, the sequence *mo* stands for a morpho-syntactic error as main category, *ag* for an agreement error subcategory, and *dn* for an error occurring between a determinant and a noun.

Table 8.1   Error Types Considered: Morpho-Syntactic Error Category

Error category	Error sub-category	Error type	Error tag
		determinant/noun	mo_ag_dn
		noun/adjective	mo_ag_na
	agreement	pronoun/antecedent	mo_ag_pa
		past participle	mo_ag_pp
morpho-syntactic		subject/verb	mo_ag_sv
		plural	mo_fo_pl
	formation	conjugation	mo_fo_co
		partitive determinant	mo_fo_pd

Error tags were inserted using Markin, a Windows application enabling teachers to correct and comment on texts that have been electronically submitted by students. The reasons for using Markin were twofold. Firstly, the in-built error annotations were easily customized to match our error classification. Secondly, the annotated text, including teacher's comments, could be exported as rich text format (rtf) or hypertext markup language (html), both easily readable by students, as well as plain text files (.txt). Error statistics along with comments, grades, and other features could also be included in the feedback provided to students at the end of the laboratory session.

The error-encoded students' texts were exported as unformatted texts in order to computationally process the information on error types required for estimating the learners' performance. More specifically, error tags were used to count the incorrect forms in the students' free written productions.

Part-of-Speech Encoding

While incorrect forms were tagged with the assistance of Markin, correct forms remained to be automatically identified, marked, and counted. Thus the corpus of error-encoded texts had first to be pos tagged. TreeTagger was used to apply the most likely pos tag of each token (i.e., not only words but also punctuation marks, symbols, or abbreviations) in the learners' error-encoded texts.

TreeTagger is a probabilistic pos tagging tool using decision trees to obtain reliable pos estimates, which differentiates it from other taggers based on first-order or second-order Markov Models (Schmid, 1994, September). It had been tested on data from the Penn Treebank corpus (Marcus, Marcinkiewicz, & Santorini, 1993), and had achieved a tagging accuracy of 96.34 percent, which qualifies TreeTagger as a "high-quality tool for the annotation of corpora with part-of-speech information" (Schmid, 1994, para. 7).

Improving TreeTagger Reliability

The reliability of pos taggers trained on native input can be severely challenged depending mostly on the correctness of the text with regard to grammatical and lexical appropriateness. As observed by Díaz-Negrillo, Meurers, Valera, and Wunsch (in press), taggers perform less efficiently when processing text genres on which they were not trained. With language learners exhibiting misspellings, foreign and invented words, and incorrect syntactic constructions, the tagger accuracy did not reach the same expectation level of performance as the one obtained with texts generated by native speakers. For this reason, we increased the accuracy of the tagging process through a series of different steps.

Firstly, we added a set of handwritten rules based on the observation of inconsistencies during the tagging process. The replacement of erroneous pos tags is based on the analysis of lexicon and contextual information. In other words, the system applies replacement rules depending on the token itself, as well as prior and/or subsequent pos tags and lemma information already applied by TreeTagger. For instance, TreeTagger does not distinguish between a past participle ([VER:pper]) and a past participle employed as an adjective ([ADJ]). The rule allowing the replacement is written as follows:

VER:pper -> ADJ / NOM_

In this example the word tagged as past participle will become an adjective when occurring after a word tagged as a noun ([NOM]).

Secondly, each pos-tagged token is checked against the teacher's correction. If the token contains a lexical or grammatical error, the pos tag is compared to the error type tag. If a discrepancy occurs, the pos tag is updated in accordance with the error type. For example, the following extract includes a verbal group marked by the teacher as incorrect in terms of conjugation formation (<mo_fo_co>). TreeTagger incorrectly identified the past participle *du as a determinant ([DET] instead of [VER: pper]):

> **Student original text :** . . . l'article a *du être . . . (. . . *the article had to be* . . .)
> **Error encoded text (Markin):** . . . l'article <mo_fo_co>a *du</mo_fo_co> être . . .
> **Pos-tagged text (TreeTagger):** . . . l'[DET] article[Noun] <mo_fo_co>a[VER:conj] du[DET] </mo_fo_co> . . .

In the preceding example, the tokens *l'* and *article* were not marked as incorrect by the teacher. As a result, the pos tags are no further processed, the initial pos tag is left as such, and the word is marked as [correct]. Token *a* is enclosed with an error tag. Since the error type (<mo_fo_co>) and the pos-tag ([VER:conj]) are related (both refer to verb conjugation), the latter is not modified. On the other hand, the pos and error type of token *du* are not related ([DET] vs. <mo_fo_co>). The initial tag is therefore updated in accordance with the error type. In this particular case, the system replaced the pos tag "determinant" by "past participle." Each token is then stored in an XML file, along with its position in the input string, the pos, the lemma information, and the error type if marked as incorrect.

Evaluating TreeTagger Accuracy

Using the same tag set, the 13 participants' written texts were also manually pos tagged, resulting in a total of 2,462 tokens, with 303 incorrect forms over 2,083 words. The output produced by the tagger before and after improvements was compared with the manually tagged output. The hand-annotated pos corpus defined our "gold standard" and was not to be used as an objective to be achieved per se by TreeTagger, but rather as an indicative target. Given that, at best, the mean rate at which annotators disagree with one another in the context of a tagging task is 3.5 percent (Marcus et al., 1993), the target ceiling of the agreement between TreeTagger and human researchers was set at around 96–97 percent (Vanroose, 2001), as measured by the Kappa coefficient. The proportion of agreement between human and machine, after chance has been excluded, is displayed in Table 8.2.

The rate of human–machine agreement rose from 91.5 percent (Kappa = .915, $p < .0005$) before improvements to 96.6 percent (Kappa = .966, $p < .0005$) after improvement, thus reaching our target of 96–97 percent. The performance of TreeTagger, before and after improvement, was also

Table 8.2   Kappa Coefficient of Agreement between the Gold Standard Data and TreeTagger before and after Improvements

Gold Standard vs. TreeTagger		*Value*	*Asymp. Std. Error[a]*	*Approx. T[b]*	*Approx. Sig*
Measure of Agreement	Kappa (before improvements)	.915	.006	155.090	.000
	Kappa (after improvements)	.966	.004	159.740	.000
	N of Valid Cases	2462			

a. Not assuming the null hypothesis.
b. Using the asymptotic standard error assuming the null hypothesis.

Table 8.3   Overall F-Measure before and after Improvements of the Tagging Process

Improvements	F-measure Beta = 0.5
before	85.59%
after	95.32%

evaluated by means of recall and precision measures, which are widely used to estimate the effectiveness of a pos tagger (Voutilainen, 2003), where:

recall = number of correct constituents in TT/number of correct constituents in gold data
precision = number of correct constituents in TT/number of total constituents in TT.

High scores in recall and precision may only be considered as valuable if the recall and precision measures are evenly balanced. In the event of a big discrepancy between recall and precision measures, both figures may be combined together into the F-Measure (Hull & Gomez, 2002) in order to normalize the compromise between recall and precision:

F-Measure = $(\beta+1.0)(P)(R)/\beta(P)+(R)$
where β gives varying weights to recall (R) and precision (P).

While a beta value of 1 gives equal weights to recall and precision, a beta value of 0.5 emphasizes precision and a beta value of 2, recall. Table 8.3 displays the F-measure obtained (before: 85.59 percent, after: 95.32 percent, β = 0.5). This measure gives more weight to precision and therefore provides useful information about the tagging process accuracy. With an F-measure of 95.32 percent and a Kappa coefficient of 96.6 percent after improvements, the tagging process was considered robust and much improved, even if further refinement is still possible.

REPRESENTING LEARNER KNOWLEDGE

Computing the Incorrect to Correct Forms Ratio

To represent a learner's performance with respect to a particular form, the ratio of incorrect to correct forms (*IncF:CorF*) is computed by counting the number of pos tags that are accompanied by an error tag and the number of pos tags that are not. A score representing the percentage of success in producing the correct form is then calculated according to the formula *CorF / (CorF + IncF) x 100*.

Table 8.4   Details of Jane's Incorrect Entries for each Error Type

	error type	*incorrect entries*	*count*
mo_ag_dn	determinant/noun		0
mo_ag_na	noun/adjective	[chaud], [malheureux], [drole], [important], [longue]	5
mo_ag_pa	pronoun/antecedent		0
mo_ag_pp	past participle	[modifier]	1
mo_ag_sv	subject/verb	[est]	1
mo_fo_pl	plural		0
mo_fo_co	conjugation	[prends], [blessé], [brulé], [attendre], [as coincé]	5
mo_fo_pd	partitive determinant	[de le], [de le]	2

For example, if the learner wrote 1 instance of noun/adjective agreement incorrectly, whereas 10 other adjectives, not marked as incorrect, occur in the same text, then the learner had the opportunity to write 10 other occurrences of noun/adjective agreement correctly. The ratio in this case would be 1:10, which means that the percentage of success in writing correct noun/adjective agreements would be equal to 90.9 percent.

The computer counts the number of errors classified by type and the number of pos tags corresponding to the error type being analyzed. For illustration purposes, Table 8.4 lists all incorrect forms written by Jane (not her real name) and grouped by error type.

Jane did not produce any determinant/noun, pronoun/antecedent agreement errors, nor did she make any plural formation errors. All corresponding occurrences are therefore marked by the system as correct ([correct]). However, she produced five noun/adjective and one subject/verb agreements, one past participle, five conjugation formation, and two partitive determinants incorrectly. Each of these was marked using the corresponding error tag. When analyzing a particular pos tag (e.g., [ADJ] or adjectives), the computer sorts all pos entries according to the type of correction attached to the entry (e.g., [correct], [mo_ag_na], [sp_ac], etc.).

Jane wrote 16 adjectives in total, of which eight are marked as correct, five as noun/adjective agreement errors (mo_ag_na_), and three as misspelling (sp_ac_) due to missing accents. Since morpho-syntactic errors take precedence over misspellings, the three occurrences marked as missing accent are considered correct in terms of noun/adjective agreement. With respect to the latter, the ratio of incorrect to expected correct productions is therefore equal to 5:11. Consequently, Jane's percentage of success in producing correct noun/adjective agreements is 68.75 percent. A graphical representation of all results obtained for this student is displayed in Figure 8.1.

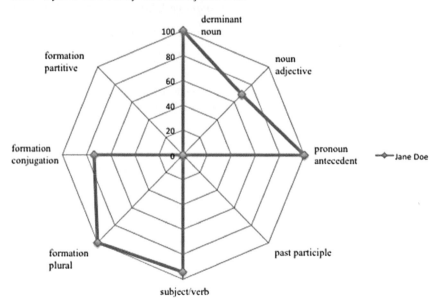

Figure 8.1   Graphical representation of Jane's performance in terms of morpho-syntactic errors.

Distinguishing between Errors and Mistakes

Interpreting the percentage of success in producing correct forms is, however, not straightforward. While Figure 8.1 gives us a snapshot of Jane's performance with regards to specific morpho-syntactic constructs at a given time, it does not tell us whether the incorrect forms can be deemed to be mistakes or errors. More generally, if a learner produces one incorrect form of a particular grammatical point, whereas hundreds of other forms of this same grammatical aspect occur correctly in the same text, one can safely assume that the learner has mastered the construct and the incorrect form may be deemed to be a mistake. But if the same learner produces only a small number of instances of the same form, whether correct or incorrect, the corresponding percentage of success does not provide any reliable information on the underlying knowledge of this particular form. To represent the latter, we need to identify whether the incorrect forms are mistakes or errors, and if the correct ones are merely guesses.

To determine whether the incorrect forms are errors or mistakes, the student's two attempts at revising his/her initial text are analyzed. As explicated earlier, minimal assistance is given to students in the form of highlighted incorrect forms in the first self-editing exercise, whereas error types are also made explicit in the second self-editing one. Looking back at Jane's production of noun/adjective agreements (*mo_ag_na*), it is useful to examine whether she was able to propose correct alternatives to the five incorrect forms detected in her original text. During the first self-editing exercise, Jane was unable to propose correct alternatives with respect to noun/adjective agreements. She left two blanks (*l'eau *chaud, le film n'est pas trop *longue*), corrected one misspelling (*les choses *drole → les choses *drôle*) but missed the required agreement (plural), tried another orthography but introduced a misspelling (*les choses *malheureux → les choses *malheureaux*), and replicated one item (*les choses *important → les choses *important*). During the second self-editing exercise, and although she was provided with the error type for each incorrect form, she still left one blank (*le film n'est pas trop *longue*), corrected the misspelling (missing accent) but still missed the agreement (*les choses *drôle*), again replicated one word (*les choses *important*), tried another word class (*les choses *malheur*), and finally provided one correct alternative (*les choses chaudes*).

Furthermore, four of the preceding five adjectives (*chaud, malheureux, drôle,* and *important*) are written in the masculine singular, that is, under the French dictionary entry for adjective, and do not take into account the gender and number of the nouns they qualify. Equally, the eight correct occurrences of noun/adjective agreement are also in the masculine singular form. This would suggest that Jane knows the masculine singular form of the 16 adjectives she produced, but either does not know how to construct their feminine and/or plural or has not mastered noun/adjective agreement in French. Since Jane is not able to notice the error type and correct herself without overt feedback from the teacher, we may assume that the correct noun/adjective agreements she wrote in her initial text may have occurred by chance. As a result, her knowledge of noun/adjective agreements in French cannot be easily inferred from the relatively high percentage of success (68.75 percent) she obtained in her first attempt at writing a short composition. Similarly, she obtained a high percentage (73.68 percent) of success in correctly forming verb conjugation (*mo_fo_co*). Yet, she could not offer correct alternatives to the erroneous verb forms whether without or with assistance. In both cases, we can safely assume that the incorrect forms are in fact errors. By contrast, her percentage of success in forming partitive determinants (*mo_fo_pd*) was 0 percent, thus indicating that all initial occurrences were incorrect. In this case, however, she was able to correct, without and with assistance. These incorrect forms can therefore be deemed to be mistakes.

Distinguishing Similar Levels of Initial Performance

The preceding discussion suggests that modeling observable learners' performance to infer their language competence by merely counting error type and pos tags in order to compute the incorrect to correct forms ratio and the percentage of success is not sufficient. Neither initial high nor low percentages of success adequately reflect the student's underlying knowledge of a particular form or construct. Similarly, when students take computer-based language tests, "the score itself does not prove with all certainty that the examinee's [. . .] level is low" (Chapelle & Douglas, 2006, p. 97).

To arrive at a better representation of learners' knowledge, our system computes the ratio of correct to incorrect forms in the original text and compares it to the ratios obtained after each self-editing exercise. If the percentage of success with regard to a particular form increases after the first self-editing exercise (i.e., with minimal assistance), it can be inferred that learners rely on their own resources to correct the incorrect form. The latter can then be deemed to be a mistake. If the percentage of success only increases after the second self-editing exercise, where the error types are made explicit to the learner, it can be inferred that, although s/he knows the grammatical rules, these have not yet been fully internalized. The learner may thus require further assistance to produce the correct form. Finally, if no significant increase in the percentage of success is observed after both self-editing exercises, the incorrect form can be deemed to be an error due to a lack of underlying knowledge. The learner is likely to require overt feedback in order to produce the correct form.

This method is also useful in personalizing the level of intervention or feedback to individual students exhibiting a similar level of initial performance. Indeed, the interpretation of a practically identical representation of two learners' performance may convey a different appreciation in terms of their respective underlying knowledge. While one incorrect form may be deemed to be an error for one particular student, the same incorrect form may be regarded as a mistake in another student's text. To illustrate these differences, we looked at the performance of two students, Louis and Marie, who both performed relatively well with respect to morpho-syntactic errors in their initial essay (see Figure 8.2).

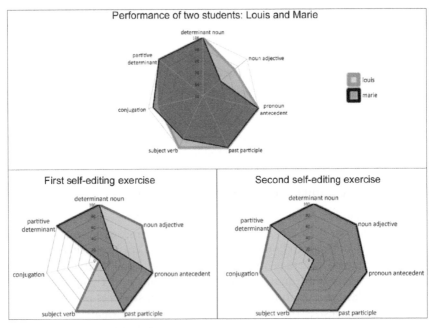

Figure 8.2   Performance of two students: Louis and Marie.

Taking the example of the formation of conjugated verbs, both Louis and Marie achieved a rather excellent score of over 90 percent. However, neither student was able to propose correct alternatives to their incorrect forms without assistance, which suggests that even with a result of more than 90 percent success in one specific form-focused feature, the 10 percent of incorrect forms cannot be considered as mere mistakes. The alternatives submitted during the second self-editing exercises show that while Louis was able to propose a correct replacement to his incorrect forms with the error type provided, Marie, on the contrary, was unable to do so. This suggests that she is likely to require more explicit feedback from the teacher or the tutoring system in order to resolve this issue. Figure 8.2 illustrates the extent to which both students could correct their incorrect ill-formed words when the error type was provided. In the case of conjugated verbs, Marie's incorrect forms reveal a different underlying knowledge from Louis's. She is thus likely to require further intervention and more overt feedback from the system or her teacher.

CONCLUSION

In this chapter, we have presented and discussed a method to distinguish between errors and mistakes in language learners' written texts, so that more robust learner models can be developed. More specifically, we were interested in investigating whether computing the ratio of incorrect to correct forms, which can help us represent language performance at a given time, provides enough information to model learner knowledge. The findings of our preliminary analysis focusing on morpho-syntactic errors have shown that, on its own, the incorrect to correct forms ratio is often inadequate to help us distinguish between errors and mistakes. As a result, the accompanying "success" score cannot be reliably used to represent a student's underlying knowledge. Indeed, while a high score in relation to a particular form may suggest that the student performed rather well in this respect, it would be wrong to assume that the remaining incorrect forms are the result of mistakes. Conversely, a low score does not necessarily mean that the incorrect forms are an indication of errors as opposed to mistakes. However, the amount and type of assistance required by learners to successfully correct their written production provides valuable information on their actual language knowledge. For example, we have demonstrated that students achieving very similar scores in relation to specific morpho-syntactic errors may in fact present a very different underlying knowledge.

The implications of these preliminary findings are twofold. Firstly, they call into question correcting practices that focus more or less exclusively on incorrect forms produced by language learners in free written productions, while ignoring correct ones. In doing so, a language tutor, whether human or machine, may not be in a position to identify areas where pedagogical intervention is most required. By extension, it also raises questions on the nature and quantity of feedback that should be provided to a learner at a given time. While many researchers have investigated the efficacy of written corrective feedback provided to language learners, and this without reaching a definite consensus, enabling performance-related errors to be ruled out from the scope of the error correction task would offer new perspectives to practitioners and researchers alike. From a practical point of view, language teachers would be able to save time when correcting their students' essays, an activity often referred to as stressful and unrewarding. In turn, learners may be less overwhelmed by too many annotations that may be irrelevant to them depending on their actual level of language development.

Secondly, the design and implementation of learner models in intelligent language tutoring applications could be enhanced through the integration of a refined module adopting our approach thus far. Few ICALL systems go beyond the idea that learner knowledge can be inferred from surface descriptions, and fewer again attempt to distinguish between errors and mistakes. Furthermore, the creation of a large corpus of learners' texts, where performance-related and competence-dependent errors would be clearly flagged, may offer a new angle for the study of learners' interlanguage. We continue to refine the approach presented in this chapter so that learner knowledge, as opposed to learner performance alone, can be adequately integrated into robust learner models, which will enable further investigations of learner interlanguage variability.

REFERENCES

Aljaafreh, A., & Lantolf, J. P. (1994). Negative feedback as regulation and second language learning in the zone of proximal development. *Modern Language Journal, 78*(4), 465–483.

Beck, J. E., & Sison, J. (2006). Using knowledge tracing in a noisy environment to measure student reading proficiencies. *International Journal of Artificial Intelligence in Education, 16*(2), 129–143.

Bernsen, N. O., & Dybkjær, L. D. (2008). Modelling spoken multimodal instructional systems. In R. Luppicini (Ed.), *Handbook of conversation design for instructional applications* (pp. 363–387). New York: Information Science Reference.

Brusilovsky, P., & Millán, E. (2007). User models for adaptive hypermedia and adaptive educational systems. In A. Bunt, G. Carenini, & C. Conati (Eds.), *The adaptive Web: Methods and strategies of Web personalization* (pp. 3–53). Berlin: Springer.

Chapelle, C. A., & Douglas, D. (2006). *Assessing language through computer technology*. Cambridge: Cambridge University Press.

Conati, C., Gertner, A., & VanLehn, K. (2002). Using Bayesian networks to manage uncertainty in student modeling. *User Modeling and User-Adapted Interaction, 12*(4), 371–417.

Corder, S. P. (1967). The significance of learner's errors. *IRAL—International Review of Applied Linguistics in Language Teaching, 5*(4), 161–170.

Díaz-Negrillo, A., Meurers, D., Valera, S., & Wunsch, H. (in press). Towards inter-language POS annotation for effective learner corpora in SLA and FLT. *Ms. Universidad de Jaén/Universität Tübingen.* Retrieved from <http://arbuckle.sfs. uni-tuebingen.de/~dm/papers/diaz-negrillo-et-al-09.pdf>

Ellis, R. (1997). *Second language acquisition.* Oxford: Oxford University Press.

Heift, T., & Schulze, M. (2007). *Errors and intelligence in computer-assisted language learning; parsers and pedagogues.* New York: Routledge.

Hull, R., & Gomez, F. (2002). Automatic acquisition of biographic knowledge from encyclopedic texts. In A. Kent & J. G. Williams (Eds.), *Encyclopedia of microcomputers: Volume 28* (pp. 1–16). New York: Marcel Dekker.

Mackey, A., Gass, S., & McDonough, K. (2000). How do learners perceive inter-actional feedback? *Studies in Second Language Acquisition, 22*(4), 471–497.

Marcus, M. P., Marcinkiewicz, M. A., & Santorini, B. (1993). Building a large annotated corpus of English: The Penn Treebank. *Computational Linguistics, 19*(2), 313–330.

Schmid, H. (1994, September). *Probabilistic part-of-speech tagging using decision trees.* Paper presented at the International Conference on New Methods in Language Processing, Manchester, UK.

Vanroose, P. (2001). *Part-of-speech tagging from an information-theoretic point of view.* Paper presented at the 22nd Symposium on Information Theory in the Benelux.

Voutilainen, A. (2003). Part-of-speech tagging. In R. Mitkov (Ed.), *The Oxford handbook of computational linguistics* (pp. 219–232). Oxford: Oxford University Press.

9 Automatic Online Writing Support for L2 Learners of German through Output Monitoring by a Natural-Language Paraphrase Generator

Karin Harbusch and Gerard Kempen

INTRODUCTION

Many foreign language learners, especially students at the level of secondary or tertiary education who are learning to write in the target language, want feedback on the grammatical quality of the sentences they produce. This raises the question how Intelligent Computer-Assisted Language Learning (ICALL) systems can provide feedback on the grammatical structure of their L2 sentences—for instance, in essay writing exercises. The usual Natural-Language Processing (NLP) approach to this problem is based on *parsing*. After the student has typed a sentence, the parser evaluates it and provides feedback on the grammatical quality. However, the more errors a sentence contains, the less accurate the feedback tends to be: A parser working with a large lexicon and a rich grammar usually finds many correction options but has no criteria to select the option that fits the message the student wishes to express. A related problem is caused by ambiguity. Hardly any sentence can be parsed unambiguously (cf. the proverbial *Time flies like an arrow*, for which Wikipedia lists no less than seven different interpretations). Hence, it is notoriously difficult to produce highly reliable feedback based on the parsing results.

We propose a *generation*-based approach aiming at the *prevention* of errors (*scaffolding*). Students construct sentences incrementally, and the ICALL system intervenes immediately when they try to build an ill-formed structure. We use a natural-language sentence and paraphrase generator—briefly called *paraphraser*—with a graphical drag and drop user interface. In our system, the student drags words into a workspace where their grammatical properties are displayed in the form of syntactic "treelets" as defined in the lexicalized Performance Grammar (PG) formalism (Harbusch & Kempen, 2002; Kempen & Harbusch, 2002, 2003). The treelet(s) associated with a word express(es) conditions on the syntactic environment(s) in which the word can occur (subcategorization restrictions). In the workspace, the student can combine treelets by moving the root of one treelet to a foot (i.e., a nonlexical leaf) of another treelet. In the generator, this triggers a unification process that evaluates the quality of the intended structure. If the latter is licensed by the generator's syntax, the tree grows and a larger tree is displayed. In case of licensing failure, the generator informs the student about the reason(s). This feedback follows directly from the unification requirements. The level of detail of the feedback can be parameterized with respect to the assumed proficiency level of the student. At any point in time, the student can issue a request for grammatical information—not only about syntactic rules, but also about the structure under assembly: *informative feedback on demand.*

The system presented here monitors the process of combining words and word groups into clauses and sentences (including coordinate and subordinate structures). The current prototype focuses on constituent order in German as L2 and checks correctness of attempted orderings. Feedback is based on the correctly applied L2 ordering rules. The paraphrase generator can provide the student with the correct ordering(s) on demand. Additionally, typical errors due to intrusions from L1 (currently English) are handled by *malrules.*

The chapter is organized as follows. First, we outline the state of the art in ICALL systems for essay writing based on NLP techniques. In subsequent sections, we sketch the PG formalism, illustrate how it represents contrasts between well-formed and ill-formed structures, and describe the prototype of our generation-based L2–learning system called COMPASS-II,[1] the generator that monitors the sentence construction process, the user interface, and various types of feedback. In the final section, we take stock and discuss desiderata for future work.

ICALL WRITING TOOLS: STATE OF THE ART

Computer-supported learning of how to write grammatically correctly in L1 and L2 figures prominently in the ICALL literature. Here, we cursorily review systems based on NLP techniques that provide students with online support in writing novel sentences that are grammatically well formed.

Virtually the entire literature on NLP applications to the syntactic aspects of first- and second-language teaching is based on parsing technology (Heift & Schulze, 2003). A *parser* computes the syntactic structure of input sentences, possibly in combination with their semantic content (provided that all words in the sentence are in the vocabulary, that the grammar available to the system covers all constructions mastered by the student, and that the input does not contain any errors). However, as indicated earlier, these systems struggle with ungrammatical input and need special measures preventing the parsing quality from becoming unacceptably poor. For example, in the FreeText system (L'haire & Vandeventer Faltin, 2003), the syntactic–semantic analysis is supplemented with *constraint relaxation* and *sentence comparison*. Other systems invoke matches with corpus texts (Granger, 2004). Yet another option is the addition of malrules to cover frequent errors (Fortmann & Forst, 2004).

Probably the first *generator*-based[2] software tool capable of evaluating the grammatical quality of student output was developed by Zamorano Mansilla (2004), who applied a sentence generator (Bateman, 1997) to the recognition and diagnosis of writing errors ("fill-in-the-blank" exercises). Zock and Quint (2004) converted an electronic dictionary into a drill tutor. Exercises were produced by a goal-driven, template-based sentence generator, with Japanese as the target language. More recently, Harbusch, Itsova, Koch, and Kühner (2008, 2009) developed the "Sentence Fairy"— an interactive tutoring system for German-speaking elementary schoolers who are about 10 years old, which supports writing little stories in L1. The pupils perform limited tasks such as combining simple clauses into compound or complex sentences. A sentence generator (described in Harbusch, Kempen, van Breugel, & Koch, 2006; see also next section) calculates all correct paraphrases, and an avatar (the Sentence Fairy) provides feedback.

Both the Sentence Fairy and the COMPASS-II system presuppose a minimum level of explicit grammatical knowledge in the student. Without it, the feedback information provided by the systems would be incomprehensible. Hence, systems of this type—but also parsing-based systems that are able to elucidate the parse trees they deliver—can only be used in the context of courses where the necessary grammatical concepts, structures, and rules have been, or are being, explained. Although this requirement entails a restriction on the range of potential users, in view of the increasing *grammatical awareness* in present-day language instruction (cf. Levy, 1997; Roehr, 2007), we believe this drawback is a minor one.

PERFORMANCE GRAMMAR

The PG formalism distinguishes three aspects of the structure of sentences: *dependency* relations, *constituent* structure, and *linear* order. The dependency relations and the constituent structure together form the *hierarchical* (or *dominance*) structure. The dependency relations include functional relations (subject, direct and indirect object, head, complement, determiner, modifier, etc.). The constituent structure comprises word categories (parts of speech) and word groups (the various types of phrases and clauses). As (a subset of) these concepts and structures are taught in many grammar courses, PG structures are relatively easy to apprehend—easier than the structures defined in many other formalisms. This advantage is enhanced by the fact that PG does not make use of movement transformations. Where certain other formalisms invoke such transformations, PG uses word order rules that assign constituents to their final positions in one go. PG's hierarchical structures can be visualized as rather flat unordered trees. The application of linear order rules may give rise to structures that can be depicted as ordered trees with crossing branches (graphs). Taken together, given the fact that PG's theoretical apparatus is rather close to what the students learn in pedagogical grammars, and that the structures it generates can be visualized in a transparent manner, we believe that PG is attractive as an ICALL formalism.

We now turn to some key technical aspects. PG's key operation is *Typed Feature Unification*—widely used in theoretical and computational linguistics (e.g., in Sag, Wasow, & Bender, 2003). Moreover, PG is *lexicalized*, that is, every constituency rule is associated with a *lexical anchor* consisting of at least one word (form).

Figure 9.1 (a) illustrates an *elementary treelet* (also called *lexical frame)* for the German word form *Junge* (boy). The rightmost branch specifies the lexical anchor of the treelet: *Junge* is a n[oun] functioning as the h[ea]d of a N[oun]P[hrase]. The second layer of nodes represents grammatical functions: det[erminer], q[uantifier], mod[ifier], etc. The third layer consists of phrasal nodes that specify which types of constituents are allowed to fulfill the function above them (the slash '/' separates alternative options). For example, the modifier role can be played by a P[repositional]P[hrase], an A[djectival]P[hrase], or a S[entence] (more precisely, a relative clause). One node in the third layer specifies the word category of the head, that is, the lexical anchor (here n[oun]).

Every node of a lexical treelet has associated with it a set of morpho-syntactic features. They are specified in the lexicon of word forms.[3] A feature is a combination of a property and a value specification. The latter may be a single term (which holds for the features of the noun *Junge*, with the feature-value pairs: wordform = Junge, lemma = Junge, gender = masculine, person = 3rd, case = nominative, and number = singular) but it may also be a disjunctive set of alternative value options. For instance, the word form *Jungen* (for "boy" or "boys") has the same treelet associated with it, except for the leaf node *Jungen*. However, the feature structure for the noun *Jungen* expresses the fact that *Jungen* can have *genitive* or *dative* or *accusative case* if, and only if, its *number* is *singular,* whereas it can have *nominative, genitive, dative,* or *accusative case* if, and only if, its *number* is *plural.* In disjunctive feature structures, the alternative value options are enumerated within curly brackets (the logical inclusive OR), and square brackets enclose an AND enumeration. The feature specification for the word form *Jungen* at node n[oun] now looks as follows:

[wordform=Jungen AND
lemma=Junge AND
gender=masculine AND
person=3rd AND
{[case={gen OR dat OR acc} AND number=singular] OR
[case={nom OR gen OR dat OR acc} AND number=plural]}]

Phrasal leaf nodes (*foot nodes*) can be expanded by an appropriate treelet whose root node carries the same label, thus forming more complex phrases. This operation (technically called *unification*) merges a foot node of one treelet with the root node of another treelet. In Figure 9.1 (b), the D[eterminer]P[hrase] foot node has been expanded by the DP root node dominating the appropriate masculine definite article *der*, and the ADJ[ective]P[hrase] root node dominating the word form *kleine* (small) expands the foot node of a mod[ifier][4] branch. Whether a root and a foot node can be merged ("unified") or not, depends not only on their label but also on the associated features. The feature specifications are used by the unification operation to select legal expansions. For instance, the fact that S-type modifiers within NPs should be relative clauses (rather than, say, main clauses) is controlled by features. Similarly, other features control the selection of the inflected word form *kleine* instead of the uninflected *klein*. For details of the unification process, in particular on how it deals with phenomena of grammatical agreement, we refer to the papers cited earlier.

Associated with every treelet is a *topology*. Topologies serve to assign a linear order to the branches of lexical frames. Here, we only illustrate the topologies associated with lexical frames for verbs ("clausal treelets"). A topology is a left-to-right sequence of slots that can be occupied by one or more constituents. In the current PG grammar for German, clausal topologies comprise nine slots, grouped into three "fields": one slot in the Forefield (slot F1), six slots in the Midfield (slots M1 through M6), and two Endfield slots (E1 and E2). The terminology derives from the *Topologische Felder* in German structural linguistics. Every grammatical function (subject, head, direct object, complement, etc.) has a small number of placement options (slots) in the topology associated with its "own" clause, that is, within the verb's lexical frame. Here are some of the slot fillers:[5]

F1:   Subject, topic, or focus in a declarative main clause (one constituent only); a wh-constituent (a phrase including an interrogative pronoun) in an interrogative main clause; a wh-constituent in a complement clause.

M1:   Finite verb in a main clause; the complementizer *dass* "that" of a complement clause.

M2–M5:   Non-wh subject, direct object, indirect object, non-finite complement clause.

M6:   Finite verb, possibly preceded by particle and pre-infinitival *zu* "to," in a subordinate clause.

E1–E2:   Nonfinite complement preceding finite complement.

Example Sentence 1 shows PG's linear order system at work. The hierarchical structure is depicted in Figure 9.1 (c). The root S-node of the verb treelet associated with the word form *sage* (say) in the complement clause has been unified with the complement (cmp) S-node of the word form *will* (wants) of the verb in the main clause:

> (1) Was will der kleine Junge dass ich sage?
>   what wants the little boy that I say
>   'What does the little boy want me to say?'

Each of the verbs instantiates its own topology. Constituents fulfilling a "major" grammatical function (i.e., a function immediately dominated by an S-node) receive a position in accordance with the preceding slot assignment rules (cf. Figure 9.1 [d]). In the main clause, the subject (which is neither a focused nor a wh-constituent) goes to M2; the verb is assigned M1; and the entire complement clause ends up in E1–E2. At the subordinate clause level, the direct object—a wh-constituent—goes to F1, the subordinating conjunction *dass* (that) goes to M1, the subject to M2, and the verb to M6, as prescribed by the rule for subordinate clauses.

How is the direct object NP *was* (what) "extracted" from the complement clause and "promoted" into the main clause? "Movement" of phrases between clauses is due to *lateral topology sharing*. If a sentence contains more than one verb, each lexical frame instantiates its own topology. In certain syntactic configurations (not to be defined here; but see Harbusch & Kempen, 2002), the topologies of two verbs are allowed to *share* one or more identically labeled lateral (i.e., left- and/or right-peripheral) slots. Sentence 1 embodies such a configuration. *After two slots have been shared, they are no longer distinct; in fact, they are unified and become token-identical.* In Sentence 1, the embedded topology shares its F1 slot with the F1 slot of the matrix clause. This is indicated by the dashed borders of the lower F1 slot of Figure 9.1 (d). Sharing the F1 slots effectively causes the embedded direct object *was* to be *preposed* into the main clause (black dot in F1 above the single arrow in Figure 9.1 [d]). The dot in slot E1–E2 in the main clause topology above the double arrow marks the position selected by the remainders of the finite complement clause.

Figure 9.1 (e) shows the linearly ordered structure after slot assignment. It also includes details concerning the linear order assignment to nodes within nonclausal constituents. For, not only clauses but in fact all constituents have—usually very simple—topologies associated with them. For instance, NP topologies have five slots, labeled NP1 through NP5, for determiner, quantifier, prenominal modifier, head, and postnominal modifier, respectively. The line connecting the S-node below "E2:cmp" and the node labeled "F1:dobj" represents the promotion of the wh-constituent *was* (what) from the subordinate clause into the main clause (see also the F1 slots in Figure 9.1 [d]): The promoted element fulfills a function in the subordinate clause but surfaces in the main clause.

134   *Karin Harbusch and Gerard Kempen*

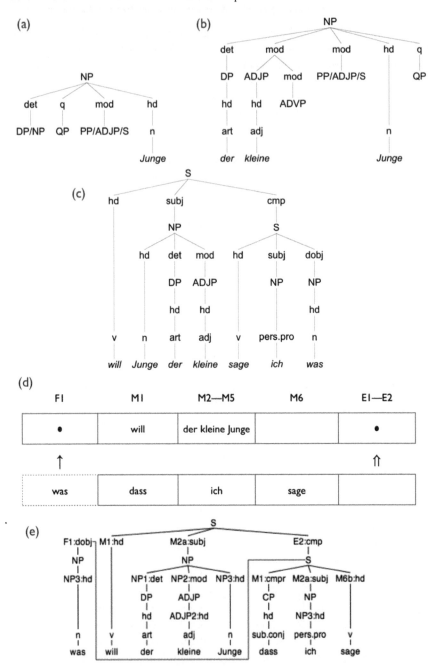

Figure 9.1
(a) Elementary treelet for the noun *Junge*.
(b) *Junge* treelet unified with a determiner and an adjective.
(c) Hierarchical structure of example (1), with arbitrary word order.
(d) Topology slot assignments of the major constituents of main and subordinate clause of sentence (1).
(e) Linearly ordered tree spelling out the final topological slot positions of the major constituents of sentence (1).

"SCAFFOLDED" SENTENCE CONSTRUCTION
BASED ON NATURAL-LANGUAGE GENERATION

In this section, we describe how COMPASS-II lets students compose sentences in PG format while the generator is monitoring this process and providing online feedback. This is followed by a sketch of the user interface and its parameterization options.

Student Actions and Feedback by the System

The student drags word forms one by one from an online lexicon into a *workspace*. The dragging actions are continually monitored by the generator. Each time a word form is entered into the workspace, the system reacts by depicting the lexical treelet associated with that word. As soon as the workspace is populated by more than one word, the student can combine them by dragging the root of one treelet over one foot of another treelet.[6] The system then checks whether root and foot node can be unified, and if so, pretty-prints the resulting larger tree (hierarchical structure) in the workspace. Furthermore, it provides a *positive feedback* message. If unification fails, *negative feedback* is provided (see next subsection). By pressing a button at the bottom of the workspace, the student can undo any action even after the system has accepted them (unrestricted undo). No constraints are imposed on the order in which the student performs the actions. For instance, all noun phrases can be built prior to selecting a verb; and all NPs can be assigned a grammatical function without spelling out their linear order. Clauses can be combined into more complex sentences by linking them via coordinating or subordinating conjunctions. We call this way of composing sentences *scaffolded writing* as it prevents the students from constructing incorrect sentences. At any point in time during the sentence composition process, the student can *query* the system by clicking on any node of a tree(let) in the workspace. In response, the system provides *informative feedback* by displaying the morpho-syntactic features of that node (or a subset thereof).

   The student actions described so far lead to the construction of *hierarchical* structures for partial or complete sentences. In order to specify a possible linear order for the branches of a hierarchical structure, the student can drag nodes (and the subtrees they dominate) to a position left or right of one of its siblings. When the node is released, the workspace is updated and the system pretty-prints the branches in the new left-to-right order. Because several drag and drop actions may be needed before the student is satisfied with the tentative linear order of constituents, the systems checks well-formedness of the current order only when explicitly requested to do so. When during a linear order check the generator notices that an obligatory constituent is missing (e.g., the subject of a finite verb or the direct object of a transitive verb), the system asks the student to expand the obligatory node before word order checking takes place. This is necessary because the generator needs the focus and wh-features of that constituent in order to determine its slot position.

Importantly, the positive or negative feedback supplied by the system in response to composition actions is not just a "correct" or "incorrect" signal. Positive feedback is accompanied by a summary of the linguistic action just performed, and its effect. Negative feedback includes a statement of the reason(s) why the unification or ordering attempt failed. Notice that the content of such feedback is conceived by the generator itself, in response to concrete unification or ordering attempts by the student.

The User Interface and its Parameterization Options

When starting up, COMPASS-II initializes four windows: to the left a window where the lexicon is displayed; to the right a window for feedback messages; in the upper central region of the screen a window for linear order manipulations on word strings; and in the lower central region a large window serving as workspace. Special push buttons at the bottom of the workspace enable the following system actions: get word order in selected tree, erase optional branches in selected tree, delete selected tree, and undo last tree manipulation, respectively. The upper central region includes a button labeled "Check word order."

All windows allow manipulation by the student, except for the right-hand window, which is reserved for system feedback. The student can select word forms from the left-hand window. The upper central window can display the terminal leaves of a tree selected in the workspace; to this purpose, the student can push the button labeled "Get word order in selected tree" (see next section).[7]

The user interface of COMPASS-II can be *parameterized* in the following respects:

1. Size of the lexicon
2. Level of detail concerning the visible hierarchical structure and associated features
3. Level of detail concerning the feedback
4. L1-specific malrules.

Ad (1) The size of the lexicon can be tailored to a specific task, that is, to the limited vocabulary addressed in a lesson. However, the full range of CELEX word forms (Baayen, Piepenbrock, & Gulikers, 1995) is available to the paraphraser; hence, in another parameterization, advanced students can freely formulate and check the sentences they want to write in L2. New lemmas and their word forms can be added by hand.

Ad (2) The student drags words into the workspace in order to build a phrase or a sentence. This action is monitored online by the paraphraser. How many grammatical details known to the paraphraser become visible to the student is a matter of parameterization. Showing treelets and feature structures in PG notation is the default parameterization. The grammatical terminology used in the feedback messages can be tailored to the vocabulary the learner is familiar with (e.g., L1 terms for elementary school children versus international terms for advanced learners). However, the system requires a lower bound on the level of visualized grammatical detail. Selected word forms are often ambiguous, that is, they have several readings, of which the student might not be aware. By displaying all alternative readings, the system forces the student to select the reading to be used in the construction process. Such confrontations with syntactic facts can serve to raise the student's grammatical awareness.

Ad (3) The level of detail of the feedback messages is determined as follows. As outlined earlier, every system action is associated with a feedback message. Actually, this message has the form of a template with placeholders in PG terminology. The placeholders get automatically instantiated as terms in the student's grammatical vocabulary. Moreover, the set of templates can be adapted to teacher preferences (e.g., as was done in the Sentence Fairy system; see Harbusch, Kempen, & Vosse, 2008).

How often syntactic nodes are queried, is completely in the student's hands. Simply moving the mouse over a node of a tree in the workspace triggers the presentation of the morpho-syntactic features of that node. Thus, students can verify their guesses as regards the features of the selected word form, or simply learn which features characterize a word form they have not used before. In the example of NP *den kleinen Jungen*, they might be insecure about its number and case features (as mentioned earlier, *Jungen* can be singular or plural). By checking these features, they can predict whether a desired unification action will work properly (e.g., moving the treelet to the direct or indirect object NP foot node of a verb will yield a successful unification whereas the subject option causes unification failure). At any point in time, the student can query other nodes or resume the sentence construction task.

While performing the sentence construction task, every composition action is commented in terms of positive or negative feedback as indicated at the end of the previous section. When the student attempts to merge the root node of one treelet with a foot node of another treelet, this triggers a unification process that evaluates the well-formedness of the intended structure. If the unification is licensed by the paraphraser's syntax, the feedback window flashes in green and displays a text saying that the node labels and the feature structures match (the student need not pay attention to the text; the green color is a signal to go on).

In case of unification failure, the background of the feedback window turns red, informing the students that the intended unification is not executed, and inviting them to read the explanatory text. In addition to the reason(s) of unification failure, this text may provide small hints on how to continue, for example, a list of other word forms belonging to the same inflectional paradigm as the offending word.

Ad (4) The paraphraser can run *malrules* that derive from typical errors users make in L2, given their L1. For instance, the erroneous string *der kleiner Junge* is "accepted" by the system but triggers a negative feedback message (the correct string is *der kleine Junge*; the confusion may arise from the correct *ein kleiner Junge* [a little boy]). In COMPASS-II, the malrules can be parameterized for different L1s.

Constructing a Sentence in COMPASS-II

The following example illustrates how students can construct sentences in their personally preferred manner. Let us assume a student wants to compose Sentence 2.

> (2) *Heute baut Anja eine Rakete weil ihr Freund morgen zum Mond fliegen will*
> Today builds Anja a rocket because her friend tomorrow to-the moon fly wants-to
> 'Today Anja builds a rocket because tomorrow her friend wants to fly to the moon'

She is allowed to perform the various subtasks in any order. For instance, main and subordinate clauses may be constructed, inclusive of their internal linear order, before they get combined. Alternatively, she may first concentrate on the overall structure of the sentence as a whole. In any case, only during the final steps can she determine the ultimately correct word order based on her (implicit or explicit) knowledge of the L2 linear order rules.

Suppose the student moves the determiner *einen*$_{ACC,MASC}$ "a" to the foot node of the det[erminer] branch of the feminine noun *Rakete* (rocket). The feedback window now turns red and requires the student to pay attention to the gender mismatch. The two trees snap back to their original positions and the system refuses to perform the erroneous action. The student may now inspect the features in detail (by querying some nodes) in order to pick up ideas for further actions. Suppose the student now decides to erase the treelet for *einen* by pushing the "Erase selected tree" button and to select the word form *eine* (in response to a hint in the feedback window). Moving the determiner *eine* (a) to the foot of the det[erminer] branch of the *Rakete* (rocket) treelet elicits positive feedback. The feedback window turns green and the two treelets merge to form one overall dominance structure. The feedback text summarizes the individual steps taken by the paraphraser on its way to the tree structure displayed in the workspace.[8]

The remainder of the example illustrates how our student can determine word order. Orderings of lexical leaves of any hierarchical structure can be changed by dragging subtrees horizontally and releasing them to the left or right of sister subtrees, whereupon the resulting tree is prettyprinted. The paraphraser does not immediately check whether the resulting linear order of words (lexical leaves) is grammatically well-formed; instead, it waits until the student issues an "order check." This check is executed in two steps. A press on the "Get word order in selected tree" button below the workspace causes the system to copy the lexical leaves of a selected tree into the word order window above the workspace. Then, when the button "Check word order" is pressed, the paraphraser determines whether the copied leaf string (i.e., the word group or sentence) is in the list of well-formed linear orders, and provides feedback accordingly. Additionally, or alternatively, the student can reorder the words of the sentence in a cut-and-paste manner, followed by an order checking request. In case of positive feedback, the system shows the hierarchical structure with topology slot assignments (as illustrated in Figure 9.1 [e]). In case of negative feedback (e.g., caused by the ill-formed string *heute Anja baut eine Rakete.*), the system shows a list of correct orderings in the feedback panel. This list can be queried by selecting one of the alternative orders, whereupon the system shows the corresponding tree with slot assignments (informative feedback).

In order to demonstrate the effect of *malrules*, we show how COMPASS-II reacts to two typical word order errors by L2 learners of German whose L1 is English. In German subordinate clauses, the finite verb goes to a clause-final position whereas in main clauses it is "verb-second." Let us assume that our student has violated both rules and has already produced Sentence 3.

(3) *Heute Anja baut eine Rakete weil morgen ihr Freund will zum Mond fliegen*

A malrule is a special grammar rule that "allows" the paraphraser to build ungrammatical structures but simultaneously triggers an error message. When analyzing the main clause of Sentence 3, where the finite verb is verb-third rather than verb-second, the paraphraser "accepts" the substring *heute Anja baut* but immediately provides negative feedback and prints the content of the malrule. Another malrule reacts to the incorrect verb-second position of the finite verb *will* (wants) in the subordinate clause introduced by the subordinating conjunction *weil* (because); here, the finite verb should occupy a position at the end of the midfield (cf. the aforementioned topology rules). Additionally, the system lists all correct orderings in the default feedback mode. They can be queried as yet another piece of informative feedback.

DISCUSSION

We view the current version of the COMPASS-II as the prototype of an "engine" that can drive the automatic evaluation and diagnosis of sentences produced by L2 students of German. The system is far from complete and not yet usable in the classroom. Several software aspects are in need of improvement, in particular the robustness of the system and the way feedback information is couched in nontechnical terms. We hope, however, that the foregoing description rouses the interest of the ICALL community in the great potential of generator-based systems as providers of online L2 writing support to students whose knowledge and understanding of sentence grammar is at high school or beginning-university level.

Profitable deployment of a COMPASS-II-type tool in the classroom requires embedding it in a tutoring system tailored to the requirements imposed by specific student populations and by specific L2 courses and exercise types. The resulting system should be evaluated with real students under realistic conditions. Of particular interest will be empirical studies that pit a generator-based writing support tool like COMPASS-II against a parser-based or a traditional (template-based) tool.

In the absence of pertinent supporting empirical data, we speculate that an important asset of systems like COMPASS-II is the fact that they do not impose upon the student any specific learning strategy (exploration, trial and error, drill and practice). Via the embedding tutoring system, they can be adapted to the strategy preferred by student or teacher. Another advantage—emphasized in the preceding sections—is the prospect of enabling effective feedback: feedback that, in line with the notion of scaffolding, is immediate, reactive, and assistive.

We are keenly aware that COMPASS-II makes heavier demands on the student's explicit grammatical knowledge than many other writing support tools. However, in quite a few languages, rules for spelling and other aspects of writing presuppose that the writer is able to explicitly recognize detailed syntactic properties of the sentence under construction. Well-known examples are morpho-syntactic distinctions that got lost in pronunciation but are maintained in spelling—for example, the distinction between *dass* (subordinating conjunction) and *das* (determiner or pronoun) in German, and numerous inflectional suffixes in French and Dutch. We suggest that COMPASS-II-type tools can be employed fruitfully in integrated writing and grammar courses.

A particularly useful approach to teaching grammar and writing in an integrated fashion—one that is relatively easy to implement in COMPASS-II—is to focus on an interrelated set of syntactic constructions and the rules controlling their shape. An example concerns coordinate structures and their elliptical forms: *forward conjunction reduction, gapping, right node raising*, and so on. Recently, we have laid the PG-oriented linguistic and computational groundwork for these constructions, which have very high usage frequencies (Harbusch & Kempen, 2006, 2007; Kempen, 2009). One of the topics we might address in the near future is to build a COMPASS-II application based on this groundwork.

ACKNOWLEDGMENTS

We are indebted to Theo Vosse for his collaboration in general, and in particular for making available his C++ software for word order checking.

NOTES

1. COMPASS-II (see also Harbusch, Kempen, & Vosse, 2008) is an acronym for <u>COM</u>binatorial and <u>P</u>araphrastic <u>A</u>ssembly of <u>S</u>entence <u>S</u>tructure, version II. It is an improved version, implemented in JAVA and C++, of the COMPASS system described by Harbusch, Kempen, van Breugel, & Koch (2006).
2. A *generator* produces a sentence or a set of paraphrases from an abstract representation of the content, often called *logical form* (see Reiter & Dale, 2000, for an authoritative overview of sentence and text generation technology). In the case of *paraphrase generation*, the generator delivers all possible ways of linguistically realizing the input logical form, given the lexicon and the grammar rules. Virtually all recent natural-language generation systems work in a *best-first* manner, i.e., produce only one output sentence rather than the set of all paraphrases. As it is not easy to change the control structure of such a system, the choice of generators is very limited. The paraphrase generator deployed in COMPASS-II does not take logical forms as input but a set of "lexical treelets" as defined in PG, which are connected via dependency links. It delivers all possible sentences licensed by the grammar (see next section).
3. Word forms are members of an inflectional paradigm. For instance, *Junge* and *Jungen* both belong to the same paradigm: the paradigm of the "lemma" *Junge*. Lemmas are referred to by one member of the paradigm—here the word form *Junge*.
4. Except for modifiers, every grammatical function in an elementary treelet occurs there once at most. Some of them are *obligatory*, like subjects of finite verbs and direct objects of transitive verbs, whereas others are *optional* (e.g., many indirect objects). To allow more than one modifier, when a branch of this type is expanded by a unification partner, another exemplar is added immediately.
5. The description in this chapter conflates the individual slot positions M2–M5 and E1–E2, respectively. The more differentiated PG rules allow simple but fine-grained word order specifications. For instance, an indirect object in the form of a personal pronoun is allowed to precede a full (i.e., nonpersonal-pronoun) subject NP.
6. The mouse handling need not be very precise. The root of a tree(let) gets selected by a mouse click anywhere within the tree(let). In order to connect the root node of the currently selected tree to a foot node of another tree(let), the student only needs to drag the former tree toward the targeted foot node of the latter. The nearest foot node calculated by the system is highlighted. Releasing the mouse triggers a unification attempt for the root

and foot nodes involved. If the student made a mistake and initiates an undo action, the system returns to the previous state of the workspace.

7. For a guided tour through the system, see http://www.uni-koblenz.de/~harbusch/COMPASSII-guided-tour.html.

8. Furthermore, the PG specifies which branches are optional or obligatory in terms of a feature on grammatical function nodes. The student can remove any optional branch by selecting a tree, and then pressing the button labeled "Remove optional branches in selected tree" at the bottom of the workspace.

REFERENCES

Baayen, R. H., Piepenbrock, R., & Gulikers, L. (1995). *The CELEX lexical database (release 2.5, CD-ROM)*. Philadelphia, PA: Linguistic Data Consortium.

Bateman, J. A. (1997). Enabling technology for multilingual natural language generation. *Natural Language Engineering, 3*, 5–55.

Fortmann, C., & Forst, M. (2004). An LFG grammar checker for CALL. In R. Delmonte, P. Delcloque, & S. Tonelli (Eds.), *Proceedings of the InSTIL/ICALL2004 Symposium* (pp. 59–61). Padova: Unipress.

Granger, S. (2004). Computer learner corpus research: Current status and future prospects. In U. Connor & T. Upton (Eds.), *Applied corpus linguistics: A multidimensional perspective* (pp. 123–145). Amsterdam: Rodopi.

Harbusch, K., Itsova, G., Koch, U., & Kühner, C. (2008). The Sentence Fairy: A natural-language generation system to support children's essay writing. *Computer Assisted Language Learning, 21*, 339–352.

Harbusch, K., Itsova, G., Koch, U., & Kühner, C. (2009). Computing accurate grammatical feedback in a virtual writing conference for German-speaking elementary-school children: An approach based on natural language generation. *CALICO Journal, 20*, 626–643.

Harbusch, K., & Kempen, G. (2002). A quantitative model of word order and movement in English, Dutch and German complement constructions. In S.-C. Tseng (Ed.), *Proceedings of the 19th COLING, Taipei, ROC* (pp. 328–334). San Francisco, CA: Morgan Kaufmann. Retrieved from http://www.aclweb.org/anthology/C/C02

Harbusch, K., & Kempen, G. (2006). ELLEIPO: A module that computes coordinative ellipsis for language generators that don't. In *Proceedings of the 11th EACL, Trento, Italy* (pp. 115–118). East Stroudsburg, PA: ACL. Retrieved from http://www.aclweb.org/anthology/E/E06/#2000

Harbusch, K., & Kempen, G. (2007). Clausal coordinate ellipsis in German: The TIGER treebank as a source of evidence. In J. Nivre, H.-J. Kaalep, K. Muischnek, & M. Koit (Eds.), *Proceedings of the 16th NODALIDA*, (pp. 81–88). Tartu: University of Tartu. Retrieved from http://dspace.utlib.ee/dspace/handle/10062/2683

Harbusch, K., Kempen, G., van Breugel, C., & Koch, U. (2006). A generation-oriented workbench for Performance Grammar. In N. Colineau, C. Paris, P. Wan, & R. Dale (Eds.), *Proceedings of the 4th INGL, Sydney, Australia* (pp. 9–11). Morristown, NJ: Association for Computational Linguistics. Retrieved from http://www.aclweb.org/anthology/W/W06/W06-14.pdf

Harbusch, K., Kempen, G., & Vosse, T. (2008). A natural-language paraphrase generator for on-line monitoring and commenting incremental sentence construction by L2 learners of German. In T. Koyama, J. Noguchi, Y. Yoshinari, & A. Iwasaki (Eds.), *Proceedings of WORLDCALL, Fukuoka, Japan* (pp.

190–193). Fukuoka: The Japan Association for Language Education and Technology (LET). Retrieved from http://www.j-let.org/~wcf/proceedings/proceedings.pdf

Heift, T., & Schulze, M. (Eds.). (2003). Error diagnosis and error correction in CALL. *CALICO Journal, 20*(3), 433–436.

Kempen, G. (2009). Clausal coordination and coordinate ellipsis in a model of the speaker. *Linguistics, 47,* 653–696.

Kempen, G., & Harbusch, K. (2002). Performance Grammar: A declarative definition. In M. Theune, A. Nijholt, & H. Hondorp (Eds.), *Computational linguistics in the Netherlands 2001* (pp. 146–162). Amsterdam: Rodopi.

Kempen, G., & Harbusch, K. (2003). Dutch and German verb constructions in Performance Grammar. In P. A. M. Seuren & G. Kempen (Eds.), *Verb constructions in German and Dutch* (pp. 185–222). Amsterdam: Benjamins.

Levy, M. (1997). *CALL: Context and conceptualization.* Oxford: Oxford University Press.

L'haire, S., & Vandeventer Faltin, M. (2003). Error diagnosis in the FreeText project. *CALICO Journal, 20*(3), 481–496.

Reiter, E., & Dale, R. (2000). *Building applied natural language generation systems.* New York: Cambridge University Press.

Roehr, K. (2007). Metalinguistic knowledge and language ability in university-level L2 learners. *Applied Linguistics, 29,* 173–199.

Sag, I. A., Wasow, T., & Bender, E. (2003). *Syntactic theory: A formal introduction* (2nd ed.). Stanford, CA: CSLI Publications.

Zamorano Mansilla, J. R. (2004). Text generators, error analysis and feedback. In R. Delmonte, P. Delcloque, & S. Tonelli (Eds.), *Proceedings of the InSTIL/ICALL2004 Symposium* (pp. 87–90). Padova: Unipress.

Zock, M., & Quint, J. (2004). Converting an electronic dictionary into a drill tutor. In R. Delmonte, P. Delcloque, & S. Tonelli (Eds.), *Proceedings of the InSTIL/ICALL2004 Symposium* (pp. 41–44). Padova: Unipress.

10 EFL Acquisition of English Causative Alternation with Integrated Concordances

Yuxia Wang and Suen Caesar Lun

INTRODUCTION

In the field of second language acquisition, English causative alternation has been identified as a consistent challenge for learners of English as a foreign/second language. To promote the acquisition of the target form in the classroom, our research investigated the effects of integrating concordances in two different learning conditions (inductive and deductive). As an example, consider the English causative alternation.

The English Causative Alternation

(1) a. The boy opened the door.
    b. The door opened.
    c. The boy made the door open.
    d. The door was opened.
(2) a. *The magician appeared a bunch of roses in his hand.
    b. A bunch of roses appeared in his hand.
    c. The magician made a bunch of roses appear in his hand.
    d. *A bunch of roses was appeared in his hand.

English verbs, as shown in the preceding examples, present varied syntactic properties. Some verbs, such as *open*, can be used in transitive form as in sentence (1a) to express a causative event[1] and in intransitive form as in (1b) to denote an inchoative event.[2] Without any overt morphological change, verbs such as *open* can participate in the so-called English causative/inchoative alternation; these are called alternating verbs. Unlike alternating ones, verbs like *appear* can only be used in intransitive forms to express inchoative meaning and not in transitive forms to show causative meaning (as in 2a). These two types of verbs also perform differently in periphrastic causative forms[3] and passive voices, as illustrated in sentences 1(c, d) and 2 (c, d) respectively. Alternating and nonalternating verbs were selected as the target verb types.

This study borrows heavily from Levin and Rappaport Hovav (1995), who claimed that verb syntactic usage is closely associated with verb semantic meaning. To enable learners of English as a foreign language (EFL) to assimilate a pedagogical rule and to make that rule applicable in classroom teaching, alternating verbs in this study express that something changes its physical state either internally or caused by an external agent. On the other hand, nonalternating verbs describe that something comes into existence or sight due to its inherent properties. The pedagogical rule is a simplification of the full range of linguistic facts determining causative alternation.

Given that these verbs exhibit complicated syntactic patterns and minute semantic differences, it is particularly difficult for EFL learners to acquire native-like knowledge of which verbs alternate and which ones do not. Montrul (2005) found that the target form was problematic for learners with a different first language background. This is also true with Chinese learners. For example, Yip (1995) reported that Chinese learners had a tendency to add the lexical predicate "make" for causative events and to use passive voices for inchoative events. Although the literature has documented a substantial amount of evidence in this problematic area, few studies have been conducted from the perspective of pedagogical second language acquisition (SLA), that is, how to facilitate acquisition through instructional treatment. Therefore, it is theoretically and practically important to investigate whether the target form is teachable and to determine the extent to which this can be done.

THE INTEGRATION OF CORPORA AND
CONCORDANCES IN LANGUAGE TEACHING

The rapid development of corpus technology has brought new perspectives to the field of SLA. The integration of corpora and concordances promises a wide application in language acquisition and hence may influence language learning in a number of fundamental ways (Chambers, 2007; Vannestål & Lindquist, 2007). The literature has provided an increasing, albeit limited, number of empirical studies, suggesting that the use of corpora and concordances appears to be beneficial in the acquisition of lexical and grammatical features. For example, Cobb (1999) observed a facilitative role of using concordance and database software to resolve the breadth–depth dichotomy in lexical learning. Horst, Cobb, and Nicolae (2005) argued that concordances played a positive role in the expansion of learners' academic vocabulary. Vannestål and Lindquist (2007) found the effectiveness of teaching English grammar with concordance in a college grammar course. Despite these results, however, more studies are needed to explore whether the integration of concordances in language instruction is effective in acquiring other linguistic features. To the best of the researchers' knowledge, no research has yet focused on using concordances to promote the acquisition of an accurate understanding of transitivity properties of English verbs.

INDUCTIVE VERSUS DEDUCTIVE LANGUAGE LEARNING

Integrating corpora in language learning increases the accessibility of an enormous amount of input in authentic contexts. The provision of rich exposure creates further inductive and deductive learning opportunities that are not available in traditional pedagogical grammar (Aston, 2001; Hunston, 2002). Induction is defined as a thinking process moving from the general to the specific, while deduction is an opposite process from the specific to the general. In inductive learning, EFL learners observe language usages in concordance data, and then discover and generalize usage patterns and rules. In deductive learning, learners test the rules or patterns they have already learned against corpora data. Although many empirical studies were conducted to compare the different effects of inductive learning versus deductive learning, no consensus has been reached (Erlam, 2003). Of the few empirical studies that incorporated concordances as instructional treatments and investigated a direct comparison between inductive and deductive learning, the studies mentioned in the following are of particular interest for the current study.

Sprang (2003) employed a concordance-like program as an intervention to introduce enhanced input in acquiring German verbs with inseparable prefixes (*be-* and *er-*). She designed three instruction groups: a control group wherein participants received reading comprehension tasks, a meaning group wherein participants had access to the concordance-like program (inductive learning), and an instructed group wherein learners received explicit rule explanation before they were involved in the program (deductive learning). Her results revealed that learners in all groups showed gains over time. Moreover, the instructed group outperformed the meaning group and also the control group. The researcher attributed the superiority of the deductive learning group to explicit rule explanation which allowed participants to understand the meaning of the concordance activity and made them more engaged in the learning activity.

Liu and Jiang (2009) investigated the effects of using corpora in lexico-grammar learning and reported several positive effects of the approach, such as better command of lexico-grammar rules and patterns, and enhanced skills of learning through discovery. More importantly, they suggested that the greatest challenge lay in analyzing concordance data to identify language rules and patterns. The majority of participants in their study stated that they were overwhelmed with an extremely large number of examples generated by their concordance searches and with the limited time accorded to them to process and analyze the data. Therefore, the researchers suggested that in actual classroom learning, it might be useful to provide students with rules and patterns before engaging them in inductive activities because testing a taught rule against concordances is much easier than formulating a rule out of concordances.

This chapter presents an empirical study on the effectiveness of a learning program with the integration of concordances in adult Chinese learners' acquisition of English causative alternation. It also addresses which instruction type (inductive versus deductive) is more compatible with the provision of concordances. The following research questions are investigated and the detailed methodological description is given in the next section.

1. Will participants in both concordance groups outperform the control group as measured in the production and grammaticality judgment tests?
2. Will the inductive concordance group outperform the deductive concordance group as measured in both the production and grammaticality judgment tests?

METHOD

Participants

Participants for this study were 75 adult Chinese learners of English, aged between 18 and 22 years. All the participants were freshmen students from the Department of Information Technology at a university in Guangdong Province, People's Republic of China. They were registered in the same English course but were divided into three classes as subgroups that were taught by one instructor. To test their English proficiency level, they all took the Oxford Placement Test (grammar section). The results reported that they were low intermediate learners (*mean* = 72.40, *standard deviation* = 6.234). No significant proficiency differences were observed among the three classes. In addition, 25 native speakers were recruited to take the pre-test, including grammaticality judgment (GJ) and production tasks. Their performances were taken as the reference points.

The three intact classes were randomly assigned as a control group, an inductive group, and a deductive group, with each group engaged in different learning conditions. The control group participated in a reading comprehension task in which target verbs were embedded implicitly. The inductive group engaged in a computerized learning program with integrated concordances, and the deductive group received both explicit rule instruction and the program containing concordances used in the inductive group.

Instructional Materials

The goal of teaching the English causative alternation was to help participants differentiate alternating verbs from nonalternating ones as well as acquire their semantic syntactic properties. For this study, three verbs from each class were selected as the instructed verbs. They were *break*, *burn*, and *open* from the alternating type, and *appear*, *die*, *and happen* from the non-alternating type. These six verbs were basic, typical verbs in each class and appeared early in learners' English courses. These verbs are often discussed in the literature. Furthermore, it might be easier for learners to understand English causative alternation by learning these basic verbs, which might perform a prototypic effect in applying what they have learned to future recognition and production of new verb items.

The control group participants were engaged in a reading comprehension task. The purpose of this task was to implicitly present target verbs and their transitivity properties (i.e., transitive, intransitive, passive, or "make ... do" structures) through meaningful input. Therefore, selecting reading paragraphs became important. This study used a learners' corpus, the 1.7-million-word New Horizontal College English Corpus, which covered a series of college English textbooks from the beginner to advanced levels. With the aid of the popular concordance program WordSmith, target verbs were searched, a concordance for each verb was produced, and all occurrences of that verb were studied and referred back to the original context. Eighty paragraphs were selected to present those verbs and their syntactic properties concerning the causative alternation. Most paragraphs contained one target verb, which was embedded and highlighted in red. The end of each paragraph had a multiple-choice question to check learners' comprehension.

The selection process can be further illustrated with the example of the verb *break*. The corpus produced 771 lines about the verb *break* and its participle forms (i.e., *breaks*, *breaking*, *broke*, *broken*), which made it neither possible nor necessary for learners to analyze all searched sentences in the classroom. A review of the search results suggested that *break* was used in causative, inchoative, and passive forms in the corpus. Then, five or six examples of each syntactic usage were selected in their original context, and presented through reading comprehension. A typical paragraph looks like this:

> If you often feel angry and overwhelmed, like the stress in your life is spinning out of control, then you may be hurting your heart. If you don't want to <u>break</u> your own heart, you need to learn to take charge of your life where you can—and recognize there are many things beyond your control.
> Q: If you often feel angry, _____.
> a) you may be hurting your heart. b).you may not hurt your heart.

Participants in the inductive group and the deductive group were asked to examine the English causative alternation in a computerized learning program that was created in two steps: (a) production of concordances of target verbs with the aid of WordSmith, and (b) integration of concordances in a computerized learning program, Verb Explorer (VE). In the first step, to control the amount of language input among groups, all reading paragraphs in the control group were encoded into a text file and used as the source data in WordSmith. The researchers produced concordances of target verbs, which had the following advantages. First, the sorted concordances suited participants' English proficiency levels. Second, the target form was presented in a sufficient yet not overwhelming amount of input. Third, irrelevant verb usage (e.g., phrasal verbs) was eliminated from these concordances. Fourth, unlike traditional English learning activities where learners fumble for verb usage in a piecemeal manner, the concordances gathered, analyzed, and provided target verbs with their complete syntactic properties regarding transitivity. Figure 10.1 illustrates the concordance result of *break*. The verb *break* was used in causative forms for the first six sentences, in inchoative forms for the next five, and in passive forms for the last six.

In the second step, all concordances were integrated into the learning program VE, which was designed using PowerPoint 2007. The program began with the activity instruction:

> In this activity, you will have a chance to study verb usage with concordances. Please try to understand the meaning and usage of the highlighted verbs in each line. Read through them quickly and answer the related questions. You can choose any one of the following six verbs to start with.

After learners clicked on one verb, the program moved on to the concordances of the chosen verbs on a new page. While studying concordances, participants could click on a concordance line to produce the source text if they needed more contextual information. After their completion of a target verb, they were asked, "ready to take questions?" Clicking "yes," they were brought to a new page on verb usage questions. They were asked whether or not the target verb could be used in causative, inchoative, passive, or periphrastic structures. During this exercise, they could return to the previous concordance page and go over example sentences. For example, learners were asked yes-or-no questions on whether the verb *break* could be used in *i) you broke your ankle, ii) you made your ankle break, iii) the cable broke,* and *iv) the cable was broken.* After they made their judgment, the program provided instant corrective feedback. Participants were requested to finish the six target verbs. The learning program created an intentional learning condition by starting with activity instruction and ending with follow-up questions.

Although both groups received the same learning program VE, the inductive group differed from the deductive group in the following respects. First, the deductive group received an explicit rule instruction before working on concordances while the inductive group got no explicit explanation of the target rule throughout the treatment session. Second, for the corrective feedback, the inductive group members received correct answers while those from the deductive group had correct answers together with

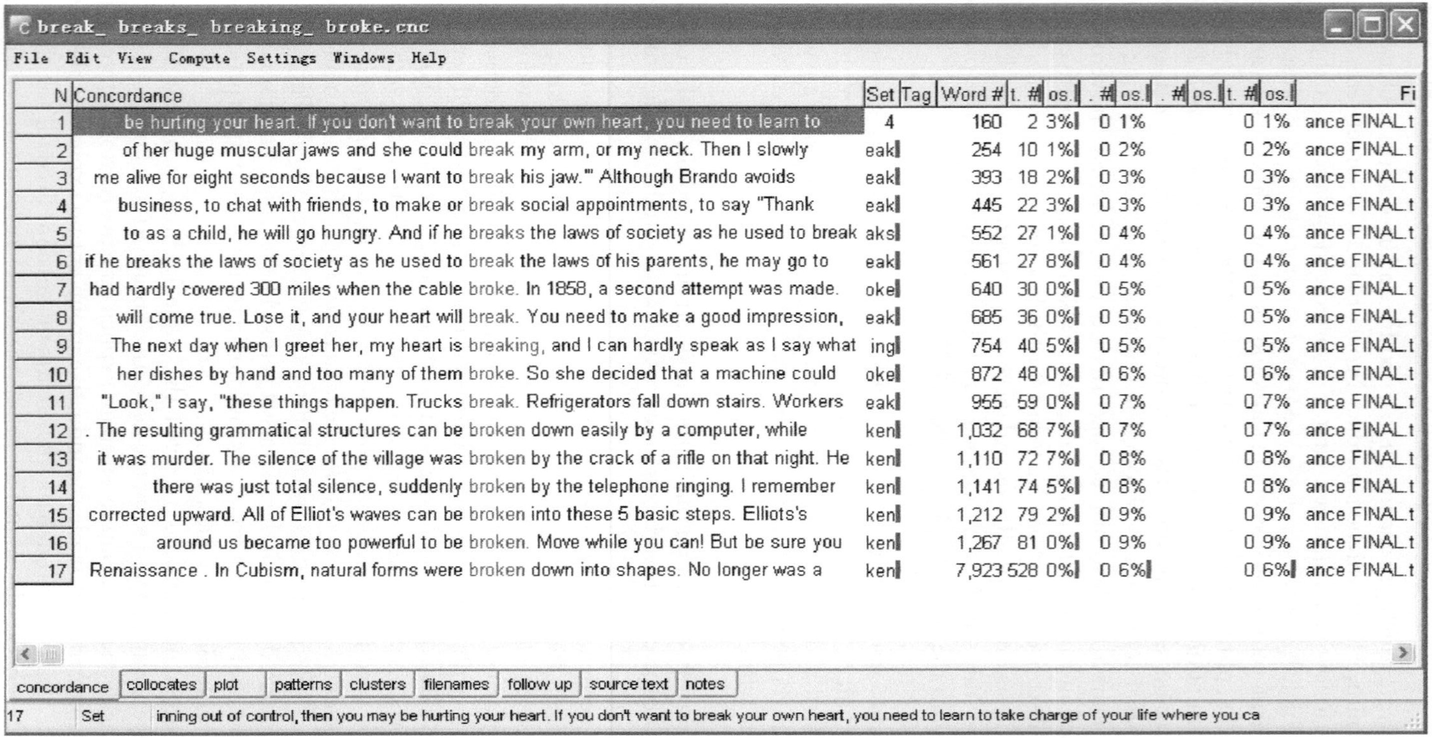

C break_ breaks_ breaking_ broke.cnc

File   Edit   View   Compute   Settings   Windows   Help

N	Concordance	Set	Tag	Word #	#t. #os.	. #os.	#os.	t. #os.	Fi
1	be hurting your heart. If you don't want to break your own heart, you need to learn to	4	eak	160	2 3%	0 1%	0 1%	ance FINAL t	
2	of her huge muscular jaws and she could break my arm, or my neck. Then I slowly		eak	254	10 1%	0 2%	0 2%	ance FINAL t	
3	me alive for eight seconds because I want to break his jaw." Although Brando avoids		eak	393	18 2%	0 3%	0 3%	ance FINAL t	
4	business, to chat with friends, to make or break social appointments, to say "Thank		eak	445	22 3%	0 3%	0 3%	ance FINAL t	
5	to as a child, he will go hungry. And if he breaks the laws of society as he is used to break		aks	552	27 1%	0 4%	0 4%	ance FINAL t	
6	if he breaks the laws of society as he is used to break the laws of his parents, he may go to		eak	561	27 8%	0 4%	0 4%	ance FINAL t	
7	had hardly covered 300 miles when the cable broke. In 1858, a second attempt was made.		oke	640	30 0%	0 5%	0 5%	ance FINAL t	
8	will come true. Lose it, and your heart will break. You need to make a good impression,		eak	685	36 0%	0 5%	0 5%	ance FINAL t	
9	The next day when I greet her, my heart is breaking, and I can hardly speak as I say what		ing	754	40 5%	0 5%	0 5%	ance FINAL t	
10	her dishes by hand and too many of them broke. So she decided that a machine could		oke	872	48 0%	0 6%	0 6%	ance FINAL t	
11	"Look," I say, "these things happen. Trucks break. Refrigerators fall down stairs. Workers		eak	955	59 0%	0 7%	0 7%	ance FINAL t	
12	. The resulting grammatical structures can be broken down easily by a computer, while		ken	1,032	68 7%	0 7%	0 7%	ance FINAL t	
13	it was murder. The silence of the village was broken by the crack of a rifle on that night. He		ken	1,110	72 7%	0 8%	0 8%	ance FINAL t	
14	there was just total silence, suddenly broken by the telephone ringing. I remember		ken	1,141	74 5%	0 8%	0 8%	ance FINAL t	
15	corrected upward. All of Elliot's waves can be broken into these 5 basic steps. Elliot's		ken	1,212	79 2%	0 9%	0 9%	ance FINAL t	
16	around us became too powerful to be broken. Move while you can! But be sure you		ken	1,267	81 0%	0 9%	0 9%	ance FINAL t	
17	Renaissance . In Cubism, natural forms were broken down into shapes. No longer was a		ken	7,923 528 0%		0 6%	0 6%	ance FINAL t	

concordance | collocates | plot | patterns | clusters | filenames | follow up | source text | notes

17   Set   inning out of control, then you may be hurting your heart. If you don't want to break your own heart, you need to learn to take charge of your life where you ca

Figure 10.1   Concordance for the verb *break*.

metalinguistic information. To summarize, participants in the control group were exposed to an implicit learning condition, in which attention was not guided to the target form. In contrast, learners in the inductive group were involved in an implicit, intentional learning condition where learners were guided to the subject matter, and learners in the deductive group were engaged in an explicit, intentional environment, where participants received explicit rule instruction in addition.

Assessment Materials

To assess learners' ability in *producing* the target form, a picture-stimulated production task was conducted. To test learners' ability in *recognizing* the target form, a picture-stimulated GJ task was administered. The assessment was arranged for three times, as pre-/post-/delayed tests. In addition to the six instructed verbs, six uninstructed verbs were included to measure whether or not participants could apply the knowledge they had acquired to new verbs. The uninstructed verbs were *dissolve, freeze*, and *sink* in the alternating type, and *emerge, disappear*, and *occur* in the nonalternating type. Also, there were three verbs as distracters, namely, *build, create*, and *destroy*.

Each verb was tested through a set of two pictures: one in the intransitive form wherein only the theme was portrayed, and the other in the transitive form wherein both the agent and the theme were drawn. In the production task, participants were required to describe the event in the picture using a given verb, while in the GJ task, they were asked to judge a pair of sentences with similar structures in a given picture-stimulated context and to mark their judgment on a 5-point Likert scale. Therefore, the production and GJ tasks had a total of 30 and 60 items respectively. As both tasks used the same pictures, the production task was conducted before the GJ task to avoid test effects. An example of the GJ task is illustrated in Figure 10.2.

Procedure

Two weeks before the treatment (i.e., Day 1), the participants completed a background questionnaire and a pre-test containing production and GJ tasks to ensure that the sample was homogeneous in their knowledge of the target form. No significant differences were found among groups in the pre-test. Pedagogical treatment was conducted on Day 15, when different groups received different instructions. The inductive and deductive group had an additional 10-minute briefing session, during which learners were guided to use the learning program VE and concordances. One day after the treatment (Day 16), the participants completed an immediate post-test with the same tasks as the pre-test. Finally, two weeks after the treatment, the participants received a delayed post-test with the same tasks. Table 10.1 lists the treatment timeline and the overall procedure adopted for this study.

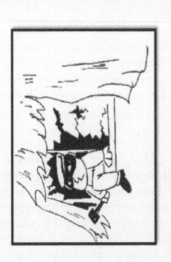

The robber came to the front of the house. And then,

- he broke the window.   [-2 -1 0 +1 +2]

- he made the window break.   [-2 -1 0 +1 +2]

(a). Transitive context (lexical causative form)

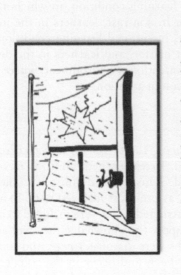

It was a very quiet night. And suddenly,

- my window broke.   [-2 -1 0 +1 +2]

- my window was broken.   [-2 -1 0 +1 +2]

(b). Intransitive context (inchoative form)

Figure 10.2   Examples of the picture-stimulated GJ task.

Table 10.1   Treatement Timeline and Overall Procedure Adopted for the Study

Stages	Timeline	Control Group	Inductive Group	Deductive group
Pre-treatment	Day 1	Oxford Placement Test, Background Test, Pre-test		
Briefing	Day 15	N/A	10 Minutes' Briefing	
Treatment	Day 15	Reading Comprehension	Integrated Concordance and Inductive Instruction	Metalinguistic Information Integrated Concordance and Deductive Instruction
Post-treatment	Day 16		Immediate Post-test	
	Day 30		Delayed Post-test	

RESULTS

Raw data in the production task were calculated using mean percentage, that is, at what percentage participants answered these questions correctly. As for the GJ task, mean scores were computed out of learners' responses to a 5-point Likert scale. The analysis of both tasks used the following statistical procedures: To address whether there were any statistical differences in learners' performance by instruction type (Group), and by test administered in three different times (Time), a 3x3 General Linear Model (GLM) repeated-measures ANOVA was conducted, with Group as the between-subjects variable, and Time as the within-subjects variable. If any main effect was found, further univariate ANOVAs were performed on the immediate and delayed post-tests, with Group as the between-subject factor and the pre-test scores as the covariate factor. For any significance found, Tukey's honest significant difference (HSD) post hoc test was performed to locate the exact source of differences.

The Picture-Stimulated Production Test

Table 10.2 presents mean percentages and standard deviations of learners' responses in the picture-stimulated test. The control group remained

Table 10.2   Mean Percentages and Standard Deviations of the Production Test

Group	Pre		Post		Delay	
	Mean	SD	Mean	SD	Mean	SD
Control group	.4544	.1707	.5025	.2148	.4896	.1615
Inductive group	.4944	.1187	.6412	.1177	.5924	.1798
Deductive group	.4924	.1136	.6676	.1799	.6592	.1855

at the same level throughout the learning period, while both the inductive and deductive groups improved their performance in the immediate post-test before losing a certain edge in the delayed post-test. Compared with their respective pre-tests, the inductive group increased by 14.68 percent in the post-test and 9.8 percent in the delayed test, while the deductive group improved by 17.52 percent in the post-test and 15.68 percent in the delayed test. It is important to point out, however, that instructed learners still lagged behind the native speakers who responded with 87.52 percent correctness.

To test whether participants in various learning conditions improved significantly in their post-test and delayed post-tests, a GLM repeated-measures ANOVA was run, with mean percentages in the pre-, post-, and delayed tests (Time) as the within-subjects variable and treatment groups (Group) as the between-subjects factor. Statistically main effects were found with Time—$F (2, 144) = 14.165, p < .000$; Group—$F (2, 72) = 8.967, p < .000$; and the combined effects of Time and Group—$F (4, 144) = 4.641, p < .05$.

Univariate ANOVAs were performed on the post-test and delayed post-tests, with Group as the between-subjects factor and pre-test scores as the covariate factor. Results revealed that main effects were found in the post-test—$F(2, 71) = 5.87, p < .01$, and also in the delayed test—$F (2, 71) = 5.26, p < .01$. The Tukey's HSD post hoc tests reported that honest significant differences existed between the control group and deductive group in both the post-test ($p < .01$) and the delayed test ($p < .01$). Comparing the control group and the inductive group, main differences were found in the immediate post-test ($p < .05$), but not in the delayed post-test ($p = .104$). Reliable differences were not found between the inductive group and deductive group in either immediate or delayed post-tests. The results suggested that instruction types played a significant role in learners' performance over the time of tests administered: Significantly greater performance was found with both concordance groups over the control group, while no significant differences were reported between the two concordance groups.

The Picture-Stimulated GJ Test

Table 10.3 reports means and standard deviations of learners' responses on a 5-point Likert scale. The descriptive data clearly show that the deductive group improved most, scoring at 0.933 and 0.677 in the immediate and delayed post-tests respectively; the inductive group gained progress by increasing 0.192 in the immediate post-test; and the control group remained roughly the same. Given that the maximum score was 2, and the native speakers scored at 1.7258 (standard deviation = 0.089), the participants still faced a difficult challenge.

Similar procedures were administered on the GJ test. The results of a GLM 3x3 repeated-measures ANOVA revealed that there were statistically significant effects in Time—$F(2, 144) = 29.732, p < .000$; Group—F(2,

Table 10.3 Means and Standard Deviations of the GJ Test

Group	Pre		Post		Delay	
	Mean	*SD*	*Mean*	*SD*	*Mean*	*SD*
Control Group	.2552	.3509	.3728	.3911	.3359	.4226
Inductive Group	.2585	.4671	.7508	.2964	.4133	.3358
Deductive Group	.3292	.4899	.9331	.2828	.6771	.3286

72) = 12.818, $p < .000$; and their combined effects Time x Group—$F(4, 144) = 4.359$, $p < .01$. Further univariate ANOVAs were conducted on the immediate and delayed post-tests, using the participants' mean responses as the dependent variable. The results suggested that reliable differences were found with the immediate post-test—$F(2, 71) = 22.414$, $p < .000$, and the delayed post-test—$F(2, 71) = 6.871$, $p < .01$. Detailed post hoc Tukey's HSD tests reported that for the immediate post-test, both concordance groups outperformed the control group at the alpha level $p < .000$, but reliable differences were not found between the inductive group and the deductive group. For the delayed post-test, the deductive group performed significantly better than the control group ($p < .01$) and the inductive group ($p < .05$), but no statistical differences were observed between the control group and the inductive group.

DISCUSSION

To address the first research question concerning whether both concordance groups outperformed the control group, the statistical analyses on the production and GJ tasks suggested the following: (a) in the immediate post-test, both concordance groups performed significantly better than the control group; and (b) in the delayed post-test, the deductive group yielded higher retention of learning gains and outperformed the control group, but the inductive group retained fewer gains and failed to perform better than the control group. Generally, this study reports a positive answer: Both experimental groups facilitated the acquisition and understanding of English causative alternation.

Given the fact that the three groups spent an equivalent amount of time processing the same amount of enhanced input (yet with different instruction types), the question arises: Why did the control group fail to progress and why did both concordance groups perform significantly better? One possible explanation is that in the control group, learners were involved in a meaning-focused activity where their primary purpose was comprehension. In such a communicative activity, the syntactic property of verb lexicon is not necessarily focused or analyzed. This means that learners in the control group might avoid attending to the formal aspects of lexical items but still manage to achieve a satisfactory level of comprehension. Comprehensible input might not require the processing of accurate syntactic frames, as argued by Swain (1995). And incidental vocabulary acquisition might not be effective in helping learners notice the syntactic aspects of a lexical item, as insightfully pointed out by Gass (1999). This may also partly reveal why the target form poses a big challenge with EFL learners even at their advanced proficiency levels.

As for the superiority reported with both concordance groups, the result could be attributed to the integration of concordances into the intentional, high-demanding learning program employed in the inductive and deductive groups. It is possible that target verbs in concordance lines are presented in the most salient position as they are placed in an isolated and central column, making it easier for learners to focus on these verbs and their syntactic usage. At the same time, the combination of activity instruction, concordances of target verbs, follow-up questions, and correct feedback successfully introduces a more "engaged" learning condition that attracts learners' attention to the target form and pushes them to conduct deeper processing. This agrees with the argument that the deeper learners process a word, the greater the chance of learning different aspects of that word (Hulstijn & Laufer, 2001). In this study, the activity instruction explains the purpose of the learning activity, which helps make the learning intentional; concordances provide enhanced input and present the target form in a salient, systematic manner; follow-up questions ensure that learners analyze and discover the target form; and corrective feedback functions as a hypothesis checker on learners' understanding formulated in a former stage.

Although the integration of concordances makes a major contribution to the overall learning effects brought by the learning program, it is dangerous to attribute the advantage found with both experimental groups solely to the use of concordances. This study actually suggests that concordances have a unique data presentation format, and if integrated organically to proper learning activities, they might bring optimal results in verb lexical-syntactic aspects, such as the English causative alternation in this study.

As for the second research question regarding the differential effects between the inductive group and the deductive group, statistical results suggested that there were no reliable differences between the groups as measured on both tests, except that the deductive group exhibited a certain edge. This suggests that the instruction of an explicit, metalinguistic rule does not bring significantly better effects, which argues against Liu and Jiang (2009) and Sprang (2003), who both found advantages with deductive learning. A possible explanation might be that the rule is not teachable because it could be too abstract to be understood by all participants.

There also appears to be an interactive effect between instruction types and assessment tasks. A close examination of learners' performance on the two assessment tests suggests that the GJ is more difficult. Comparing learners' performance with that of native speakers, a narrower gap was found in the production test, while a wider gap was found in the GJ test. The results also suggest that deductive learning is more compatible with the GJ test, because the deductive group outperformed not only the control group but also the inductive group in the delayed post-test. The reason might be that as learners are required to complete the GJ task, they are required to make fine-grained decisions on similar structures, making the task a bigger challenge. During the process, it is believed that explicit knowledge might play a certain role (Bialystok, 1979). Therefore, explicitly explaining a rule might help the deductive learning group perform better in the GJ test.

CONCLUSION

This chapter has shown that a learning activity with an integration of concordances could effectively promote EFL learners' ability to acquire English causative alternation. Its effectiveness might be attributed to the more "engaged" learning environment created through the combined features of activity instruction, concordances of target verbs, follow-up questions, and correct feedback in the program. Meanwhile, explicit rule instruction exhibits no major effects on learning. This chapter presented empirical evidence supporting the contention that integrating concordances in language teaching may play a beneficial role in acquiring a better understanding of verb lexical-syntactic properties. The technology of corpus and concordance, if integrated with appropriate pedagogical intervention, might have a promising future in facilitating the acquisition of a wide range of linguistic forms.

As this is one of the pioneer attempts to teach English causative alternation in the classroom, there are certain limitations with the current work. First, although all participants were registered in the same English course, they could still be engaged in other learning activities outside the experimental tasks that could have influenced their performance on the immediate and delayed post-tests. Better control of this aspect is desired in further studies. Second, the two-week interval between the two post-tests might be relatively short for fully assessing the long-term effects of the learning program and for investigating the issues of explicitness. Future studies are needed to examine the learning effects over a longer period of time. Third, to tap learners' knowledge, two types of assessment test (controlled written production and GJ) were employed. Further studies need to investigate whether the observed learning effects for learners in the three instruction types would be the same in different assessment tasks, for example, a free production task. Fourth, this study compared the effects of incidental learning without the integration of concordances versus intentional learning with integrated concordances, and reported the superiority of the latter. A logical expansion would be to compare the effectiveness of intentional learning without concordances (such as asking learners to pay attention to the target form in a reading comprehension task) versus incidental learning with concordances (such as presenting concordances without intentional guidance to the target form), in order to understand the effects of concordances and instruction types in a more detailed manner.

NOTES

1. A *causative event* refers to a verb event that involves one entity causing another entity to perform an action or to change its state.
2. An *inchoative event* refers to a verb event that involves one entity undergoing a change of state.
3. *Periphrastic causative form* refers to the structure of adding periphrastic verbs like *make* or *have* to express causative event, as in the sentence "*he made me laugh.*"

REFERENCES

Aston, G. (2001). Learning with corpora: An overview. In G. Aston (Ed.), *Learning with corpora* (pp. 6–45). Houston, TX: Athelstan.

Bialystok, E. (1979). Explicit and implicit judgements of L2 grammaticality. *Language Learning, 29,* 81–103.

Chambers, A. (2007). Integrating corpora in language learning and teaching. *ReCALL, 19,* 249–251.

Cobb, T. (1999). Breadth and depth of lexical acquisition with hands-on concordancing. *Computer Assisted Language Learning, 12,* 345–360.

Erlam, R. (2003). The effects of deductive and inductive instruction on the acquisition of direct object pronouns in French as a second language. *Modern Language Journal, 87,* 242–260.

Gass, S. M. (1999). Discussion: Incidental vocabulary learning. *Studies in Second Language Acquisition, 21,* 319–333.

Horst, M., Cobb, T., & Nicolae, I. (2005). Expanding academic vocabulary with an interactive on-line database. *Language Learning and Technology, 9,* 90–110.

Hulstijn, J., & Laufer, B. (2001). Some empirical evidence for the Involvement Load Hypothesis in vocabulary acquisition. *Language Learning, 51,* 539–558.

Hunston, S. (2002). *Corpora in applied linguistics.* Cambridge: Cambridge University Press.

Levin, B., & Rappaport Hovav, M. (1995). *Unaccusativity: At the syntax-lexical semantics interface.* Cambridge, MA: MIT Press.

Liu, D., & Jiang, P. (2009). Using a corpus-based lexicogrammatical approach to grammar instruction in EFL and ESL contexts. *Modern Language Journal, 93,* 61–78.

Montrul, S. (2005). On knowledge and development of unaccusativity in Spanish L2 acquisition. *Linguistics, 43,* 1153–1190.

Sprang, K. (2003). *Vocabulary acquisition and advanced learners: The role of grammaticization and conceptual organization in the acquisition of German verbs with inseparable prefixes.* Unpublished doctoral dissertation, Georgetown University.

Swain, M. (1995). The output hypothesis: Just speaking and writing aren't enough. *Canadian Modern Language Review, 50,* 158–164.

Vannestål, M., & Lindquist, H. (2007). Learning English grammar with a corpus: Experimenting with concordancing in a university grammar course. *ReCALL, 19*(3), 329–350.

Yip, V. (1995). *Interlanguage and learnability: From Chinese to English.* Amsterdam: John Benjamins.

Part III

Materials Design and Development

11 Blended Learning, Empowerment, and World Languages in Higher Education

The Flexi-Pack Project for "Languages of the Wider World"

Nathalie Ticheler and Itesh Sachdev

INTRODUCTION

In *A New Landscape for Languages* (2003), Kelly and Jones presented how the language landscape might look in the United Kingdom in 2007. Using the most recent statistics, the report was revisited by Canning (2008) in *Five Years On: The Language Landscape in 2007*, in which the actual landscape was compared with the one that was envisaged seven years ago. Kelly (2008, p. iv) explained in the foreword that "languages remain vulnerable, despite being strategically important for the future of the country. But there are signs that government initiatives and the efforts of language educators are beginning to have an effect, at least in slowing the decline."

Several organizations such as the National Centre for Languages (CILT) and the Higher Education Funding Council for England (HEFCE) report on the precarious situation of modern foreign languages in the United Kingdom as evidenced by the decreasing number of students on specialist language degree courses and the closure of university departments. Data from the Higher Education Statistics Agency (HESA), based on annual enrolment figures, reveal a decline of 5.3 percent overall on first degree language students in higher education between 2002 and 2003 and 2006 and 2007 (CILT, 2008). More recently, in a national review of modern foreign language learning in UK higher education (HE), Worton (2009, p. 3) reported:

> The consultation revealed a community which feels itself to be vulnerable and indeed beleaguered. There is a strong sense that the importance and the value of languages are not properly understood and recognised either by government or by potential students.

Worton mentioned a variety of research-oriented and training initiatives including the creation of five Language Based Area Studies Centres in the UK (funded by HEFCE and Research Councils) as well as funding by government departments to facilitate outreach and collaborative activities, such as "Routes into Languages" (http://www.routesintolanguages.ac.uk/index.html).

An important recent development in the field of language learning and teaching has been the increasing use of new technologies. In 2005, HEFCE funded and launched its 10-year strategy about e-learning (HEFCE, 2005). The strategy was revised in March 2009 and now focuses on enhancing learning, teaching, and assessment through the use of technology. In addition, following the publication of the HEFCE strategy, the Higher Education Academy was invited to lead an E-Learning and Benchmarking Programme (2005–2008) in partnership with the Joint Information Systems Committee (JISC; see JISC/HEA, 2008). The benchmarking exercise was intended to help institutions establish where they were in regard to embedding e-learning. The Pathfinder program, by contrast, was specifically designed to help selected institutions, on behalf of the sector, identify, implement, and evaluate different approaches to the embedding of technology-enhanced learning in ways that result in positive institutional change. Without going into greater detail, it suffices to say that UK HE now makes extensive use of virtual learning environments (VLEs) and related multimedia technology to support blended learning solutions in a range of degree and nondegree courses.

In another supportive development for languages, HEFCE in 2005 funded a Centre of Excellence for Teaching and Learning (CETL) in "Languages of the Wider World" (LWW CETL; http://www.lww-cetl.ac.uk) based at the School of Oriental and African Studies (SOAS) and University College London (UCL). The aim of this center is to promote excellence in the teaching and learning of languages that do not have a large presence in higher education in the United Kingdom but that are of increasing strategic importance locally and globally. The specific languages promoted include those of Africa, the Middle East, Asia, Eastern Europe, Scandinavia, and the Netherlands. A key objective of the CETL is to support blended language learning, which MacDonald (2006, p. 2) defines as "associated with the introduction of online media into a course or programme whilst recognising merit in retaining face-to-face contact." As one response to this, the LWW CETL launched the Flexi-Packs project to create a whole range of blended learning materials in Bengali, Nepali, Romanian, and Turkish (materials in other languages are also being developed). Flexi-Packs are sets of online language materials that are flexible in the way they can be used (either directly from a VLE, or "on the go" by downloading them) and also in terms of the variety of activities from which students can freely choose, complete, and assess themselves, giving them a greater say in their learning experience. Flexi-Packs complement language lessons by providing students with online materials tailored to their needs, both in terms of contents and level of difficulty. This chapter presents the pedagogical rationale behind the Flexi-Packs, together with results of a preliminary evaluation of the project, and also makes recommendations for appropriate use and future developments, with a view to enhancing the language learning experience. It is suggested that the current Flexi-Packs project, which combines e-learning and second language acquisition, presents a motivating learning experience for students and one practical way to promote blended language learning.

BRIEF CONCEPTUAL RATIONALE FOR THE FLEXI-PACK PROJECT

Students learn a language for a variety of reasons (Agnihotri, Khanna, & Sachdev, 1998; Dörnyei, 2001; Gardner, 1985). They frequently come from diverse educational backgrounds and their experience of second language acquisition will be different. Their learning styles and individual learning preferences may vary. Students make sense of the various influences that surround them and will act in their own personal ways. Therefore, what motivates one person to learn a foreign language and keeps that person going will differ from individual to individual. No two people will learn precisely the same thing from any particular learning situation. In this context, learning a foreign language is an essentially personal and individual experience, albeit with important societal and contextual underpinnings (Clément & Gardner, 2001).

Dörnyei (1994) proposes a three-level categorization of motivation. In Dörnyei's model, the language level encompasses various orientations and motives related to aspects of the second language, such as the culture and the usefulness of the language. These will influence learners and the goals they set themselves. Dörnyei's learner level involves individual characteristics that the learner brings to the learning task. Key features of this level are self-confidence and the need for achievement. Finally, the situation level includes components related to the course, the teacher, and the group dynamics. Dörnyei's formulation is helpful as it highlights the fact that motivation is multifaceted and likely to be affected by situation factors.

In addition, the significance of learners' control over their learning experience is highlighted by Williams and Burden (1997, p. 127):

> A number of researchers investigating cognitive approaches to motivation have proposed that the sense people have of whether they cause and are in control of their actions, or whether they perceive that what happens to them is controlled by other people is an important determinant in motivation. These factors are a part of what is known as a sense of agency.

Flexi-Packs take this issue into consideration and offer built-in flexibility so that students can choose where and how to use the materials, either directly from VLEs, or by downloading them. The objective is to empower students to have more control over their learning. Flexi-Packs also contain reference sections with key grammar points and essential vocabulary, together with learning tips, which learners are free to use as they wish. Extension sections including web links allow for a great variety of activities. A more detailed description of the Flexi-Packs project follows.

DESCRIPTION OF THE FLEXI-PACK PROJECT

Each language course unit or module offered at the SOAS and UCL comprises a series of lessons focusing on a variety of topics and language skills. Flexi-Packs complement these lessons by providing materials specially tailored to the students' needs.

Flexi-Packs aim to take into account the diversity of students' needs, the importance of communication between staff and students, and also the empowerment of teaching staff by providing resources that are easy to use, update, and improve. All these aims are in line with HEFCE's e-learning strategy outlined in 2005.

A typical Flexi-Pack, which is composed of a downloadable text file (pdf) and related audio (mp3) and/or video files, normally contains the following sections, although allowances can be made regarding authors' preferences and individual language requirements: learning objectives, various tasks based on the contents of the previous lesson (together with keys and transcripts to allow for student self-assessment), learning tips and cultural tips, and reference sections (vocabulary, grammar, and published materials available in libraries and other resource areas such as language resources rooms).

The SOAS-UCL LWW CETL commissioned the creation of Flexi-Packs as follows:

- Bengali: 30 Flexi-Packs in the form of pdfs and mp3s, uploaded on the institution's VLE (Blackboard), for complete beginners. These are supplemented with additional video clips from a previous project funded by CETL.
- Nepali: 20 Flexi-Packs (two terms of 10 weeks each), in the form of pdfs and mp3 files, uploaded on the institution's VLE for complete beginners on degree courses; with another 30 (three terms of 10 weeks each) in the same format for the Language Centre based at SOAS (which provides accredited and nonaccredited modules to internal students and members of the general public who enroll for self-standing language classes).
- Romanian: 20 Flexi-Packs, here again, in the form of pdfs and mp3 files, uploaded on Moodle, for lower intermediate and intermediate students based at UCL.
- Turkish: 10 Flexi-Packs for complete beginners, in the form of pdfs, mp3 files, and video clips, which correspond to one term's study in the SOAS Language Centre.

Flexi-Packs require only a limited level of computer expertise from their authors and users (teaching staff and students), and are easy to modify and update. In addition, they offer built-in flexibility so that students can choose where and how to use the materials, either directly from any VLE that may be in use at their institution (e.g., Blackboard, Moodle, etc.), or on the go by simply downloading the required files. Flexi-Packs provide independent self-learning online materials fully tailored to student needs. At the same time, independent learning does not mean learning in isolation: Flexi-Packs also have potential in enhancing collaborative learning by making use of built-in communication tools available on the VLE (like blogs and message boards), and by fostering a greater integration between taught classes and self-study or homework, with activities such as the writing-up of dialogues in preparation for the next class or extra pieces of written work to submit to their teacher.

One of the key aspects of Flexi-Packs is that they have been produced by teaching staff who have experience with the courses where materials will be used. The Flexi-Packs are tailored to the students' needs and students can complete or use them in a learning context where Flexi-Packs are linked as a follow-up to lessons. Moreover, Flexi-Packs contain transcripts to all the listening tasks, which are a useful source of help for users, as well as keys to all the activities. This means that students can assess themselves in an unobtrusive manner, check on how well they do, repeat activities when necessary, or prepare for their next class.

LEARNER AND TEACHER DATA FROM
PRELIMINARY EVALUATION

Data obtained from our preliminary evaluation, which included student self-completion questionnaires and interviews of teaching staff, indicate that an overwhelming majority of stakeholders view them favorably and would like to develop them further. The stakeholders included teachers and students at SOAS, UCL, and University of Manchester, as well as learners taught off-site (including commercial clients).

Learners

The preliminary evaluation yielded data concerning flexibility and empowerment that was consistent with the aims of Flexi-Packs. Feedback from students suggested that this was a clear benefit experienced by learners: "It is great to be able to do these at home and fit around my timetable" (intermediate Romanian student); "Flexi-Packs are a fantastic resource. It is great to be able to use them at home" (intermediate Romanian student).

It is important to note that students who participated in our evaluation repeatedly reported their satisfaction with the integrated nature of the Flexi-Packs and the fact that these materials were a good follow-up to their lessons: "Flexi-Packs really help. I can revise on my own what we have covered in class" (beginning Turkish student).

These aspects of the Flexi-Packs contribute to students' self-confidence and sense of achievement. Clearly the empowerment, flexibility, self-confidence, and sense of achievement offered by the Flexi-Packs are a great source of motivation. Other relevant aspects of the Flexi-Packs that can contribute to students' motivation range from realistic contents in terms of authentic audio and video files in the particular languages, to websites as gateways to many aspects of cultures and languages. Data from regular users underlined this point: "It is good to be able to use authentic dialogues. Flexi-Packs also structure your self-study" (intermediate Romanian student); "I like the visual layout. Topics are also well covered" (beginning Nepali student).

Feedback from learners also pointed to the role of Flexi-Packs in helping create a positive learning experience. For instance: "Flexi-Packs have formed the foundation of my Bengali learning. They have made Bengali as easy and fun to learn as possible" (beginning Bengali student). And: "Flexi-Packs are helpful and fun. I like the learning tips" (beginning Turkish student).

Interestingly, favorable comments concerning the use of Flexi-Packs for those studying languages where the range of suitable published materials may be fairly limited were also obtained. For instance, students of Romanian reported that Flexi-Packs were perceived as a good method to use for self-study when they were unable to find taught classes at the level they needed, while a Beginners Turkish student reported: "I think that Flexi-Packs are very useful and helpful, as there is not a great deal of study materials available to Turkish learners."

Overall, from the learners' perspectives, and in the words of an intermediate student of Romanian: "Flexi-Packs are an excellent learning tool." Furthermore, a student of Bengali for beginners, who had also learnt other languages, said: "Flexi-Packs are a great idea. It would be great if such a resource was available for other languages."

Teachers

The teaching staff involved in the study also commented on the motivating nature of the Flexi-Packs—not only for students but also for themselves. They reported feeling pleased about producing materials specially tailored to the needs of students and appreciated the blended learning approach presented to them. They also added that Flexi-Packs actually reduced their regular homework load once the production phase was over, as they only had to direct students to the materials. In addition, various staff, such as the Nepali and Romanian staff, indicated that they liked the fact that the Flexi-Pack project was introduced to them by a peer, with a similar professional background, who had previously gone through the same experience in terms of materials development. Authors of Flexi-Packs intended to make use of them whenever feasible and to expand their dissemination to other institutions and courses. Flexi-Packs vary according to the different languages and levels to ensure that the end product will correspond to the preferences expressed by relevant teaching staff and will meet the students' needs. (A range of sample materials can be seen by going to http://www. lww-cetl.ac.uk/part_3/part_3_flexipack.htm.)

In addition, in our preliminary evaluation, teaching staff reported on the great value of the extension tasks to be submitted by students and saw them as a valuable way to maximize the integration of the taught provision and the Flexi-Packs. Interviews with some of the teaching staff indicated that they sought feedback from the students and updated the Flexi-Packs when necessary (Nepali), and generally provided tips and guidance on how to use the materials as part of the normal routine of the lessons (Romanian). Finally, staff (in particular the Nepali teachers) described the websites listed in the Flexi-Packs as an ideal gateway towards Nepal, not only in terms of language through the use of authentic materials, but also in terms of access to culture.

As indicated in earlier sections, results of our preliminary evaluation show that Flexi-Packs are viewed positively both by students and staff, in terms of user-friendliness, contents, layout, and links between materials and lessons, creating a fully integrated package in line with a blended learning approach supported by MacDonald (2006). Interviews of staff reinforced the blended learning aspect of the project, as they explained what course of action they regularly took in order to maximize students' use of the materials. In addition, it is worth reminding readers that authors of Flexi-Packs were all teaching staff who had considerable experience with relevant modules, and used the materials with their own students. This clearly places teachers at the heart of the project, in the position of facilitators.

> The challenge is not to establish new pedagogies for e-learning in the simple sense of coming up with new things to do with learners. Instead, this more complicated picture requires a more conservative approach: finding out what teachers do and why, and then working out how technology can best be used to support that. (Oliver, 2006, p. 134)

In this context, we take the view that the tutor should play a central role in the creation and implementation of the Flexi-Packs, playing the part of a facilitator and working in tandem with students. This may constitute a shift from their more traditional position of source and transmitter of knowledge: "there should be no doubt of the essential role teaching presence plays in integrating the various elements of an educational experience made ever more challenging by the responsibilities of e-learning" (Garrison & Anderson, 2003, p. 66). Regular updates of materials by teaching staff following students' feedback are likely to assist in maintaining students' motivation and satisfaction. Indeed, students who are active participants of their own learning, in terms of what, when, and how they learn, are more likely to remain motivated.

Ideally, tutors who have previously taught or currently teach relevant modules should be regular authors of materials—including updates—to ensure greater integration between lessons. We also believe that the more tutors are involved in the production, the more likely they are to promote and share materials with others, including students, in line with principles of teacher empowerment and theories of collaborative learning. Clearly, teaching staff need to guide and motivate students to make regular use of resources and materials presented to them. For instance, tutors could give students a demonstration of Flexi-Packs early in the course, together with regular learning tips in class and the addition of materials and information to be consulted both in and out of class. In short, the key is to embed e-learning in regular learning and teaching activities, to seek feedback from stakeholders at regular intervals, and to ensure flexibility of the provision, in hand with careful training. Indeed, there is a need for teachers to adapt their pedagogy to make the best use of technologies available to them, in a context where digital learning design should facilitate the shift towards learner-focused activities (Laurillard, 2009).

CONCLUSION

This chapter promotes the use of Flexi-Pack e-learning materials as part of a blended learning approach. Findings from our preliminary evaluation indicate that Flexi-Packs are viewed positively by language learning students as well as by teaching staff, with both groups reportedly welcoming an expansion of such materials. Apart from the tremendously motivating role that such materials play in language learning, which includes important empowering aspects, the role of teaching staff is central: It is not limited to that of knowledge transmitter but is also more of a facilitator in areas such as e-learning skills and language study skills.

The overall findings of this project reinforce socio-constructivist approaches to learning. Such approaches promote the important notion that individuals learn together with other learners as a community, through mutual support and collective sharing of experience. Collaborative learning is generally perceived as being beneficial to learners, and further development of the Flexi-Packs for collaborative learning is therefore important (e.g., through the use of communication tools such as discussion boards in tandem). In conclusion, it is essential for teachers to fully understand and apply socio-constructivist approaches to ever-changing learning contexts, to review their pedagogical beliefs, and to redefine their role in order to boost the students' learning experience.

ACKNOWLEDGMENTS

We would like to express our thanks to all our colleagues who contributed to the Flexi-Pack project, in particular, Fotis Begklis, Arif Billah, Ramona Gönczöl-Davies, Nil Okan Paniguian, and Krishna Pradhan.

REFERENCES

Agnihotri, R., Khanna, A. L., & Sachdev, I. (1998). Introduction. In R. Agnihotri, A. L. Khanna, & I. Sachdev (Eds.), *Social psychological perspectives on second language learning* (pp. 1–10). New Delhi: Sage.

Canning, J. (2008). *Five years on: The language landscape in 2007.* Southampton: Subject Centre for Languages, Linguistics and Area Studies.

Clément, R., & Gardner, R. C. (2001). Second language mastery. In H. Giles & P. Robinson (Eds.), *The new handbook of language and social psychology* (pp. 489–504). London: Wiley.

Dörnyei, Z. (1994). Motivation and motivating in the foreign language classroom. *Modern Language Journal, 78,* 273–284.

Dörnyei, Z. (2001). *Teaching and researching motivation.* Harlow: Longman.

Gardner, R. (1985). *Social psychology and second language learning: The role of attitudes and motivation.* London: Arnold.

Garrison, D. R., & Anderson, T. (2003). E-learning in the 20th century. A framework for research and practice. London: RoutledgeFalmer.

Higher Education Funding Council for England. (2005). Strategy for e-learning. Retrieved from http://www.hefce.ac.uk/pubs/hefce/2005/05_12/05_12.pdf

Joint Information Systems Committee/Hither Education Academy. (2008). E-learning benchmarking and pathfinder programme. 2005/2008. An overview. Retrieved from http://elearning.heacademy.ac.uk/weblogs/ea/wpcontent/uploads/2009/03/bandpglossyfinal_update19mar09.pdf

Kelly, M. (2008). Foreword. In J. Canning (Ed.), *Five years on: The language landscape in 2007* (pp. i–iv). Southampton: Subject Centre for Languages, Linguistics and Area Studies.

Kelly, M., & Jones, D. (2003). *A new landscape for languages.* London: The Nuffield Foundation.

Laurillard, D. (2009). The pedagogical challenges to collaborative technologies. *International Journal of Computer-Supported Collaborative Learning, 4*(1), 5–20.

Macdonald, J. (2006). *Blended learning and online tutoring. A good practice guide.* Burlington, VT: Gower Publishing.

National Centre for Languages. (2008). Retrieved from http://www.cilt.org.uk/home.aspx

Oliver, M. (2006). Editorial. New pedagogies for e-learning? *Alt-J, Research in Learning Technology, 14*(2), 133–134.

Williams, M., & Burden, L. (1997). *Psychology for language teachers.* Cambridge: Cambridge University Press.

Worton, M. (2009). *Review of modern foreign languages provision in higher education in England.* London: HEFCE.

12 Intermediate Online English
An Example of Self-Access Courseware Development

Ana Gimeno-Sanz

INTRODUCTION

The increasing demand for high-quality innovative foreign language (FL) teaching and learning materials has no doubt influenced the fact that language teachers have had to develop new skills in Computer-Assisted Language Learning (CALL) materials design. Although many language specialists are still reluctant to develop their own materials using dedicated authoring tools, it is the changing understanding of methodological approaches to language learning that has driven the need to offer the FL teaching community a flexible and robust web-delivered authoring tool.

This was the goal underlying *Proyecto InGenio,* one of the research and development projects carried out by the CAMILLE[1] Research Group at the Universidad Politécnica de Valencia (UPV) in Spain: the creation of a web-delivered language-independent authoring tool capable of managing databases on a remote server and allowing teachers from around the world to design and publish materials to suit their students' particular needs. The implementation of materials is based on the template approach to software authoring (Gimeno, 2005), with predefined templates that integrate video, graphics, audio, and text. The system includes a "content manager" enabling subject specialists to create a database from which to share and select materials by organizing the multimedia components and materials (learning objects) according to a number of specifications (e.g., language, level, skill, target group, etc.), thus creating a pool of multimedia exercises and resources. The authoring tool automatically converts the contents into learner-ready materials in the form of an online course, delivered via the *InGenio* web-based Learning Environment. In addition, the system incorporates an online tutoring and student assessment utility that allows course tutors to supervise student scores, written input, and overall progress. Lastly, the *InGenio* system also includes a module allowing any of the courses designed with the authoring tool to be adapted into any number of source languages to comply with different learner L1 needs.

The use of Information and Communications Technologies (ICT) in the language curriculum has, to some extent, been responsible for the shift from focusing on the teacher to focusing on the learner when designing web-enhanced materials, and has led courseware designers to adopt a constructivist approach to learning, whereby the student is encouraged to actively construct knowledge and the teacher becomes a guide to support learners through the process of learning. In so doing, students must be equipped with all the necessary tools to become independent learners and take responsibility for their own learning. As pointed out by Blin (2005, p. 33), "Independent language learning environments present language learning opportunities that do not require the constant intervention of a teacher or that can be pursued outside the framework of an educational institution."

Thus, online learning resources such as the ones that can be developed using the *InGenio* system should ultimately encourage "active learning," that is, a context where the learner is encouraged to write, speak, actively participate, interact with fellow learners, and so on, in a resourceful and stimulating learning environment, yet not necessarily under the constant supervision of a teacher. This scenario naturally implies making use of currently available technologies such as video and audio conferencing tools, instant messaging tools, blogs, and wikis. The very nature of these tools provides learners with a fair amount of independence that nevertheless also requires guidance by a qualified tutor to help the learner orient his or her activity toward the learning process itself and avoid deviating their attention towards other possible distracting scenarios. Learner autonomy, understood as the capacity to self-manage learning, is also one of the key concepts that has rapidly evolved due to the integration of CALL into the language curriculum. As Littlewood (1997, p. 83) points out, "The autonomous learner takes responsibility for his or her own learning, has developed useful and effective learning strategies and is able to work independently." In CALL materials' design, most authors are aware of the fact that a variety of teaching strategies have to be implemented in the courseware in order to facilitate and encourage learners to take up the endeavor of second language acquisition. To this end, the *InGenio* authoring tool has been designed to include, in addition to a considerable number of exercise templates, reference materials such as grammar notes, cultural information, and multilingual sound-enhanced glossaries, in order to provide learners with all the necessary resources that contribute toward enriching comprehension and understanding of the target language. Another important factor to bear in mind is the need for the inclusion of meaningful corrective feedback on which the learner can rely to support the acquisition process.

In terms of methodology, *InGenio* can be adopted to suit a large number of teaching methodologies, ranging from structural methods to a more communicative approach to language learning. The exercise templates are particularly suitable for designing courses that attempt to acknowledge the fact that a true linguistic competence implies being able to use the language that is appropriate to a given social and cultural context in order to achieve a specific communicative goal. To do this, learners need knowledge of the linguistic forms, meanings, and functions for a given context. To achieve this end, *InGenio* provides a variety of goal-oriented learning strategies in a media-rich electronic environment that supports the study of the target language. The notion of supporting the study of the language is crucial here. Our objective was not so much the creation of software to "teach" a language, but the construction of learning resources in the shape of an environment that would provide the student with all the tools and information, short of a live teacher, that they might need to undertake a language course.

Because "there are strong arguments to support the notion that students will need higher levels of explicit and implicit assistance in computerised than in face-to-face environments" (Trinder, 2006, p. 97), online courseware must replace the absence of face-to-face interaction with techniques and strategies that give the student appropriate support and backing. To this end, the *InGenio* system has been designed to foster independent learning, and it ensures that the most recent Internet-based developments can be integrated into the online courses and, due to its versatility, can be constantly updated as the need may arise.

The following sections include a description of the *InGenio* system, illustrated with examples taken from one of the courses developed with the authoring tool, Intermediate Online English.

THE *INGENIO* SYSTEM

A recently published study on the impact of ICT and new media on language learning, conducted by European scholars, reveals that "about 70% of respondents 'strongly agreed' or 'agreed' that using technologies can **motivate** them more to learn a language" (Stevens & Shield, 2009, p. 30). It also shows that:

> overall, among the possible advantages offered as options, respondents most readily recognized that the use of technologies offers **flexibility and autonomy**, as well as opportunities for **self-improvement** in studies/work (more than 80% "strongly agreed" or "agreed"). There was a similar response, too, about the statement that "people learn languages differently when they use new technologies."

The survey, which was based on the findings of an online questionnaire answered by 2000 respondents from Europe and beyond, provided empirical proof of a number of facts that the CAMILLE Research and Development Group at the UPV had intuitively believed. The fact remains that, still today—and basically due to the wealth of media-rich online environments currently available—technology-enhanced language learning is seen to be appealing, as well as believed to provide flexibility (i.e., in terms of where and when one approaches learning) and autonomy (i.e., independence in terms of managing one's own learning needs and the pace at which it takes place). These factors were always present during the design process that led to the development of the *InGenio* system, a completely language-independent online authoring tool, content manager, and learning environment intended to foster independent learning by offering language specialists a robust tool to design attractive, motivating, and pedagogically sound language learning materials and/or courseware. But what is it that makes language learning materials efficient and motivating to the learner? It is obviously a combination of factors and these can, naturally, vary from learner to learner. Colpaert (2004) very appropriately points out that the efficiency of the development process will have an important impact on the quality of the software, its usability, and didactic efficiency. He defines these concepts thus (p. 40):

> **Software quality** includes aspects such as *performance* (connection capacity and execution speed), *flexibility* (the ease with which a system or component can be modified for use in applications or environments other than those for which it was specifically designed), *interoperability* (the ability of two systems or components to exchange information), *portability* (the ease with which a system or component can be "ported" to another platform or operating system), *reliability* (the ability of a system or component to perform its required functions under stated conditions for a specified period of time) and *scalability* (the ease with which a system or component can be modified according to changing circumstances such as the number of users, the amount of data etc.).
>
> **Usability** [. . .] Relevant for architecture design are *accessibility* and *cost*. Accessibility means the ease with which online systems can be installed and run on the user's computer. With a dial-in connection, being online costs money. [. . .] Broadband connections (ADSL-based or high-speed cable), in contrast, are kept open from computer start-up to shut-down. The user is no longer aware that his/her computer is connected. Broadband applications do not take connection time into account, but they must still take into account the number of service requests from servers; such demands can lead to more waiting time for the user.
>
> Efficiency of the development process should entail more **didactic efficiency** (Colpaert 1996a, Colpaert and Decoo 1997).[2] Courseware should be designed to make a significant contribution to learning, teaching, testing, and tracking activities in order to improve the language acquisition process and to match needs and expectations of both learners and teachers. The final goal is to increase *effectiveness* in terms of results.

These elements were all taken into account when designing the *InGenio* system. Its *quality* is endorsed by its capacity to comply with all the aspects mentioned above by Colpaert (2004), that is, optimized HTML programming, free of plug-ins or additional software requirements, to enhance performance speed; flexibility to be integrated into popular Learning Management Systems such as Moodle, Sakai, Blackboard, and so on; ability to perform reliably (without system failures) regardless of the number of users connected to the system at a given moment; and scalability in order to allow constant improvements and addition of contents (multimedia components).

Its *usability* in terms of accessibility and connectivity is founded on the grounds that any audio or video sequence integrated into the system can be accessed at three different transfer rates[3] in order to cater for slow or unreliable Internet connections such as those found in underdeveloped countries, or less powerful computers.

InGenio's didactic efficiency depends to a great extent on the language specialist's (materials writer's) skills in designing pedagogically meaningful activities with the 15 exercise templates that integrate the *InGenio* authoring tool. The templates have been designed to foster the development of a wide range of exercise typologies by means of combining different types of input to encourage multiple types of learner output (written or oral production, grammar, use of language, listening or reading comprehension, etc.).

The templates include a number of common features, such as enabling us to specify time limits or the number of attempts allowed to complete a given exercise, to facilitate the creation of assessment tests. Additionally, we can specify whether we wish any written learner input to be case-sensitive, a feature that may prove very useful when designing proficiency level materials or when creating exercises that focus more on meaning rather than form and where it may be relatively irrelevant whether punctuation is respected.

Provision of reference materials is also based on several specially designed templates. These can be designed as independent sources of information or linked into the exercises proper to ensure that the learner is not deprived of any element that may support acquisition of the target language, a feature that gains great importance when developing materials to serve autonomous learning. Such is the case also of supplying the user with appropriate glossaries, which can combine text (definitions or translations), audio (pronunciation), phonetic transcription, and image.

INTERMEDIATE ONLINE ENGLISH

Intermediate Online English was designed as a prototype to illustrate what could be done with the *InGenio* authoring tool and how it worked (see Figure 12.1). It has since been updated and is currently being used as the basis for a course delivered at UPV called Computer Assisted English. The online course is delivered through the *InGenio* Learning Environment

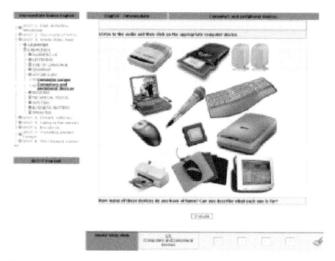

Figure 12.1 Sample vocabulary exercise from Intermediate Online English.

(LE), to which registered students have access. The online English course is intended for intermediate learners of English seeking to achieve level B2 of the Common European Framework of Reference for Languages (European Council, 2001).

Because one of the aims of the course was to reinforce technical English, Intermediate Online English was divided into two distinct parts: one devoted to semi-technical issues such as digital devices, ICT, electric vehicles, the WWW, and so on, which could be of general interest to our students; and another focusing on more general topics such as leisure activities, the Olympic games, theatergoing, film festivals, and the like. The aim of this division was to balance the intake of formal versus informal language and structures. The courseware aims to provide the conditions in which learners can develop communicative competences in their own way and in their own time. This is achieved, among other things, by presenting a default route to follow, offering diversity of activities (see Figure 12.2), and developing a progression that moves from receptive to productive skills. Various strategies have been included that are designed to encourage problem solving and resolution of specific tasks, aiming at developing the learner's ability to apply and adapt their knowledge of the target language to specific communicative scenarios. The problems and the tasks, therefore, have been designed to encourage learners to use the target language for a communicative purpose in order to achieve an outcome.

In Intermediate Online English, all eight units are preceded by a grammar section—aimed at revising grammatical notions that are relevant to the course contents—and are divided into the following subheadings: listening, use of language, grammar, vocabulary, reading, technical focus,

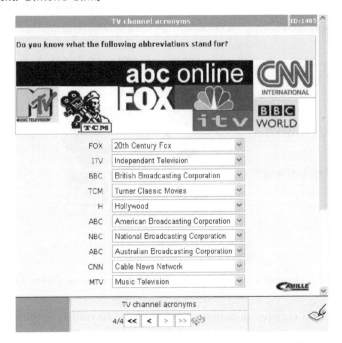

Figure 12.2   Sample multiple-choice exercise from Intermediate Online English.

writing, business matters, and speaking, which include a varied number of exercises relating to the section's prime focus. The course itself comprises over 300 exercises and activities designed to expose learners to the intricacies of the target language and generate a sound basis for acquisition and consolidation of knowledge.

Within this general course outline, the courseware also combines several interrelated teaching approaches; ranging from the more LSP-oriented[4] approaches such as the functional/notional approach, through the more traditional language form approach that primarily focuses on structures, to a more contextual approach. Among the approaches that were applied to determine the course design and structure, the functional/notional approach allowed us to specify the desired learning outcomes in terms of language functions (e.g., making a request, advising a colleague on how to proceed), general as well as specific notions (e.g., duration, location), and rhetorical skills (e.g., extracting information from a dialogue). The language form approach helped to shape the structures that were present in the language functions in order to achieve learner awareness as to the linguistic forms being used, and the contextual approach enabled us to determine the situations in which the functions, notions, and structures were embedded (Gimeno, 2009).

STUDENT ASSESSMENT AND FEEDBACK
IN *INTERMEDIATE ONLINE ENGLISH*

In terms of self-evaluation, progress reports can be called up at any point during the learning process since a link to the assessment function is permanently available on the screen. The data are automatically transferred to the server while the materials are in use, thus allowing students to monitor their progress during the course of their work. The results are presented in percentages, registering date and time, number of completed exercises, scores, and so on, as shown in Figure 12.3.

Since the system automatically registers and tracks student performance, tutors using the course materials with registered users may access progress reports, as well as the student's written production deriving from open input activities, in order for them to correct and mark these, and provide appropriate feedback. These marks will automatically be averaged by the system in order to give students a final mark or score. When specified in a template, learners may also upload any type of file (spreadsheets, audio, etc.) onto the server for their tutors to evaluate and assess together with any other course work.

Feedback is given to the learner in two distinct ways, either by providing automatically generated messages in response to the number of correct

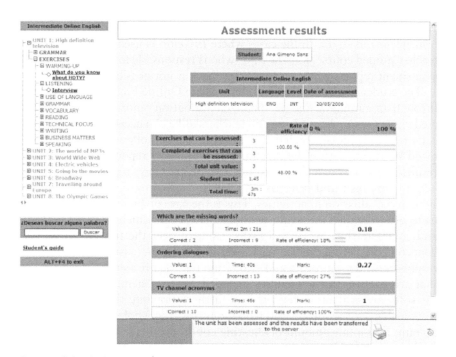

Figure 12.3   InGenio student assessment report.

or incorrect answers or by providing personalized feedback that has previously been introduced by the author of the exercise. In this last case, every element that a learner has to supply (i.e., by clicking on an item) to complete an exercise is susceptible to receiving personalized feedback. If, on the other hand, the exercise consists of writing open input, automatic correction is not provided and feedback depends on the tutor. "Tutorized" activities, therefore, are those that require human intervention in order to analyze responses more deeply and offer personalized assessment or corrective feedback. This is the case in some of the exercises focusing on oral and written production, where responses are generally more elaborate or cannot be limited or controlled in order to give students automatic feedback. The system, in this case, simplifies interaction between students and tutors in order to evaluate the completed activities; for self-assessment, students are encouraged to analyze their performance and progress by comparing with a model of the solution; for tutor assessment, the teacher is able to analyze, evaluate, and provide appropriate feedback.

Intermediate Online English was developed following several design principles in an attempt to offer the EFL community a useful and efficient educational tool. Since the requirements in designing self-access materials are completely different from designing face-to-face supplementary materials, great effort was put into providing learners with all the necessary tools and resources to support the autonomous learning process. These included the provision of self-explanatory reference materials, additional explanations to support theoretical concepts, links to external sources, student assessment principles, and so on. In the cases where *InGenio* is used to deliver a more teacher-guided course, it is the tutor who is responsible for offering detailed assessment reports when automatic feedback is not possible.

The students who undertake Intermediate Online English are evaluated through an automatic and personalized evaluation report that is also delivered via *InGenio*. As students and teachers alike can access the data, all the activities and contents included in the course must follow a clear and organized structure within the system. The evaluation reports show students' results and scores in a simplified but also precise way. Technology can also help in this task and offer useful tools for speeding up correction, revision, and evaluation of activities. This is the case of *InGenio*, which allows us to offer detailed information about the way in which students perform and complete their work and tasks. Control over the time spent by students on completing each activity, over their answers, visualization of their responses, and monitoring and evaluation reports are some of the solutions that are part of all the facilities included in the system. On carrying out the software evaluation reported on in the following, the tutor who was responsible for the subject and who monitored the whole process took into account that a fair amount of cheating could take place and that a student could be replaced by another at the moment of completing the course tasks, or that they could simply copy the answers and solutions from another partner in an attempt to improve their final results. This is the reason why the scoring system has been structured as follows: 70 percent of the final score results from the mark obtained when completing the online course and the remaining 30 percent is provided by a personal oral interview with the teacher in charge of the subject:

Subject mark = (7*Course mark + 3*Personal Interview)/10
Extra Activities > 5
Course mark <= 120 percent extra activities

The interview therefore aids in corroborating or adjusting possible deviations in relation to the results provided automatically by the system, as well as allowing us to carry out a more detailed and consistent evaluation of the students' oral production skills. This process also analyzes the communicative competence and verifies the authenticity of their online results, including their written compositions. Students must achieve at least 50 percent of the total score of the interview in order to pass the subject. If the mark obtained automatically when completing the online activities were 20 percent higher than the one provided by the evaluator according to the student's performance during the personal interview, the final grade would be reduced down to the 20 percent limit.

SOFTWARE EVALUATION RESULTS

During two consecutive years, all the learners who have taken Computer-Assisted English as a subject at UPV have been asked to complete an opinion questionnaire at the end of the semester. The results of these questionnaires have been analyzed and the results are discussed in the following. The 60 students who comprised the sample group were all students undertaking a technical degree at UPV and they had all completed the entire Intermediate Online English course.

Out of the 60 students who registered for the course, 35 of them responded to the opinion questionnaire, a sample of which can be found in Appendix 12.1. Generally speaking, the results were very positive in relation to the different aspects of the course analyzed and there was an overall high level of satisfaction among students.

The questionnaire consisted of 20 questions focusing on different aspects of the course, in which the students expressed their degree of agreement or disagreement for each of the items, as well as being able to include their personal comments. The questions were classified into five different categories including data regarding the following general topics:

- Usability of the course
- Quality of the exercises

- General opinion
- Objective achievement.

The first item, usability of the course, refers to the functional and technical features of the courseware. It is divided into six questions regarding different aspects of the interface: navigation, technical requirements, clarity, user-friendliness, vocabulary, and quality of the audio files.

Regarding the second item, quality of the exercises, we collected data specifically referring to the quality of the exercises and the activities, by means of five questions focusing on the characteristics of the audio files and of the reading comprehension texts, the usefulness of the exercises, their level of difficulty, and the extent to which the instructions in each exercise were appropriate.

In the item general opinion, we wished to know to what extent the students were satisfied and whether their expectations had been fulfilled or not. The data we collected from this section of the questionnaire were extremely valuable in terms of the students' general fulfillment of their expectations, and also to evaluate the use of the reference materials included in the course, such as grammar, functions of language, culture, and so on, as well as their degree of motivation in learning autonomously.

The last section of the questionnaire, objective achievement, queried about the characteristics of the goals to be achieved, an analysis of the time spent on completing the course, the vocabulary improvements, and the general achievements and benefits obtained by the students from this course.

The students' answers and the graph with the results are shown in Appendices 12.1 and 12.2. The results reveal that their overall level of satisfaction regarding the course was unanimously high, since they rated different aspects of the course and their improvement in terms of proficiency, motivation, and ability to work autonomously very positively.

As far as user-friendliness is concerned, almost all the students from our sample found the interface user-friendly, thought that navigation was intuitive, considered that it would not be hard for someone with minor computer skills to use this course, found the graphics and symbols clear, deemed the layout (use of colors, fonts, icons) to be good, considered that the input was meaningful and interesting, and were satisfied with the quality of the audio sequences.

As for the exercises, the students' opinions were positive in most of the aspects that were questioned, such as the clarity of the instructions or the usefulness of the reading and listening comprehension exercises, which most of the students found both of use and meaningful. There was less agreement amongst students concerning the level of difficulty of the exercises: Most of them considered the exercises were not easy to complete. This could obviously be taken as a positive aspect of the course, since it means that the activities were challenging and not too easy for them, but at the same time they could be completed by making an effort or referring to the reference materials.

With regard to the students' overall level of satisfaction, their answers to this question confirm that the students from our sample were generally satisfied. They also thought the content of the reference materials from the grammar section was sufficient and all the students referred to them before completing the exercises in each unit. All but one student considered that the course encouraged independent or autonomous learning (which is one of the basic aims of the online course).

As for the time the students from the sample spent in completing the course, most of them actually completed it in the 45 hours that were predicted. The students were under the impression that their general English vocabulary had improved and so had their technical vocabulary, and they had the feeling that their overall level of English had improved after completing the course. Over half of the students from our sample enjoyed lessons 5 to 8 the most—that is, the lessons focusing on topics dealing with leisure activities such as sports, theatergoing and cinema-going, and so on, and everyday vocabulary; while the rest of the students preferred lessons 1 to 4, which focused on semi-technical topics and technical vocabulary and made a more formal use of the language.

We would now like to highlight some of the comments made by the students in the last section of the questionnaire. In this section the students were given the chance to provide personal remarks. Their comments were very useful and enabled us to make improvements in the course materials, since both the strong and the weak points were commented upon by the students. The following are some of the more noteworthy comments that have had consequences on the future editions of the course:

- "In my opinion this kind of course is the future of the university."
- "It could be useful to introduce exercises about VRS (Voice Recognition Systems) in order to improve our pronunciation."
- "If the connection isn't very good as in my home, you can't complete the course as fast as if you complete it in the UPV, but you can complete the course with any Internet connection."

Although only one opinion on this matter has been quoted here, in the past two years several students have pointed out the fact that it would be very useful to include voice recognition exercises in the course. Although voice recognition systems (VRS) are commercially available, they are currently still underdeveloped for the Internet, which is the prime reason why they have not been implemented in Intermediate Online English. Nonetheless, a foreseeable rapid evolution and implementation of VRS on the Internet in the years to come will enable us to improve our course by integrating this technology in some of its exercises.

As we can see from the last comment, there is another drawback: Some of the registered students' Internet connections are not as fast or as reliable as we would expect, owing basically to differences in bandwidth. In fact, some students complain about their access from home to the course, which is much slower than it is from the university. As mentioned earlier, in order to reduce the negative consequences of this obstacle, all the courses created with the *InGenio* authoring tool integrate the option of transmitting the video files at three different transfer rates, in order to avoid problems caused by unreliable or slow Internet connections.

CONCLUDING REMARKS

The *InGenio* Intermediate Online English language course for engineering students, implemented in the Universidad Politécnica de Valencia since 2004, is one of the actions taken by the UPV in order to adapt to the European Higher Education Area (EHEA), by complying with EU recommendations regarding the Bologna process and the European Commission's "Action Plan for Language Learning and Linguistic Diversity."[5] This course adapts to the new trends and guidelines laid out in self-access and autonomous learning theories, and aids students in reaching a B2 level of proficiency in English while improving their technical vocabulary and their ability to learn autonomously. Its implementation is one of the ways in which the UPV follows the EU recommendation that European universities should put into practice a coherent language policy clarifying their role in promoting language learning and linguistic diversity. Furthermore, it can be considered as a step forward towards the achievement of the main goal of the said Action Plan, namely, to enable every citizen to communicate in at least two foreign or second languages.

The results obtained from evaluating the *InGenio* Intermediate Online English language course with UPV engineering students during two academic years show that the students' overall level of satisfaction is high, since different aspects of the course, such as user-friendliness, the quality of the exercises, the content and usefulness of the reference materials, and contribution to their overall improvement in terms of language proficiency, motivation, and ability to work autonomously, were rated very positively. These results have additionally led us to corroborate the belief revealed by respondents in the study on the impact of ICT and new media on language learning, stating that the use of technologies offers our students opportunities for self-improvement in their studies and in their preparation for their future work.

The CAMILLE Research Group continues to work and research into technology-enhanced language learning and testing, in order to conduct ongoing assessments of the courseware designed and published with the *InGenio* authoring system with a view to making future improvements and providing innovative solutions to autonomous and self-directed learning, as well as ameliorating existing courses in terms of quality, contents, user-friendliness, layout, efficiency, attractiveness, and functionality, while suiting the learner's level and individual needs and demands. At the same time, we aim to prepare our students for a society in which being able to communicate and interact fluently and spontaneously with speakers of other languages is becoming increasingly necessary.

NOTES

1. CAMILLE stands for Computer-Assisted Multimedia Interactive Language Learning Environment.
2. The articles referred to are Colpaert (1996) and Colpaert and Decoo (1997).
3. A choice of 56, 256, or 512 kbps is available in all the exercise templates.
4. Languages for Specific Purposes (LSP).
5. Available from http://ec.europa.eu/education/languages/archive/policy/index_en.html.

REFERENCES

Blin, F. (2005). *CALL and the development of learner autonomy—an activity theoretical study*. Unpublished doctoral thesis, Institute of Educational Technology, The Open University, UK. Retrieved from http://webpages.dcu.ie/~blinf/BlinThesis.pdf

Colpaert, J. (1996). Learning from the past, building new working hypotheses: The DIDASCALIA criteria framework for more added value in CALL. *CALL*, 9(4), 309–318.

Colpaert, J. (2004). *Design of online interactive language courseware: Conceptualization, specification and prototyping*. Antwerp: University of Antwerp.

Colpaert, J., & Decoo, W. (1997). More didactic efficiency through shared language contents for hard copy, electronic and interactive textbooks. *CALICO Proceedings of the 14th Annual Symposium "Content! Content! Content!"* CD-ROM.

European Council. (2001). *Common European framework of reference for languages: Learning, teaching, assessment*. Cambridge: Cambridge University Press.

Gimeno, A. (2005). New challenges in developing an online CALL authoring shell, content manager and courseware: The *INGENIO* model. *EUROCALL Review*, 7, 2–11. Retrieved from http://www.eurocall-languages.org/news/newsletter/7/index.html

Gimeno, A. (2009). Online courseware design and delivery: The *InGenio* authoring system. In I. González-Pueyo, C. Foz-Gil, M. Jaime Siso & M. J. Luzón Marco (Eds.), *Teaching Academic and Professional English Online* (pp. 83–105). Bern: Peter Lang.

Littlewood, W. (1997). Self-access: Why do we want it and what can it do? In P. Benson & P. Voller (Eds.), *Autonomy and independence in language learning* (pp. 79–91). Essex: Longman.

Stevens, A., & Shield, L. (Eds.). (2009). *Study on the impact of information and communications technologies (ICT) and new media on language learning*. (EACEA 2007/09 [Final Report]). Retrieved from http://eacea.ec.europa.eu/llp/studies/study_impact_ict_new_media_language_learning_en.php

Trinder, R. (2006). *Language learning with computers: The student's perspective*. Frankfurt: Peter Lang.

APPENDIX 12.1

LEARNER QUESTIONNAIRE
Tutor   Ana Gimeno
No. of students   35
Period   2007–2008 and 2008–2009
Subject   Computer-Assisted English (Intermediate Online English)

USABILITY		YES	NO	OTHER	N/A
Interface	Did you find the interface user-friendly?	33	1	0	1
Navigation	Is navigation intuitive?	34	0	0	1
Technical Requirements	Is it easy for someone with minor computer skills to use the online course?	33	0	1	1
Clarity	Are graphics/symbols clear to the user?	34	0	0	1
User-friendliness	Is the layout (use of colors, fonts, icons) appealing to you?	31	3	0	1
Vocabulary	Is the language input meaningful and interesting?	34	0	0	1
Quality of audio	Is the audio input clear and loud enough?	29	2	2	2
EXERCISES					
Listening	Did you find the listening comprehension exercises useful?	31	3	0	1
Reading	Did you find the reading comprehension exercises useful?	29	4	1	1
Usefulness of exercises	Did you find the exercises useful and meaningful?	31	2	1	1
Level of difficulty	Did you find the exercises easy to complete?	3	28	3	1
Instructions	Are the exercise instructions clear and precise?	30	1	3	1
OPINION					
Overall satisfaction	Are you satisfied with the variety of activities?	30	4	0	1
Content of reference materials	Did you find the reference materials (grammar section) sufficient?	29	4	1	1
Use of reference materials	Did you refer to the reference materials (grammar section) in each Unit before starting to do the exercises?	34	0	0	1
Motivation	In general, do you think that the online course encourages autonomous/independent learning?	28	1	5	1
ACHIEVEMENT OF OBJECTIVES					
Time	Did you complete the entire 8 Units of the online course in 45 hours?	30	2	1	2
Technical Vocabulary	Did Units 1–4 help you improve your technical English vocabulary?	33	0	1	1
General Vocabulary	Did Units 5–8 help you improve your general English vocabulary?	23	2	9	1
Overall improvement	In general, did your level of English improve after completing the online course?	31	0	3	1
Open input questions					
	Do you have any comments or suggestions to make in order to improve *Intermediate Online English?*				
	Which Units did you enjoy doing most? [1–4] [5–8]	9 [1–4]	20 [5–8]	0	6

APPENDIX 12.2

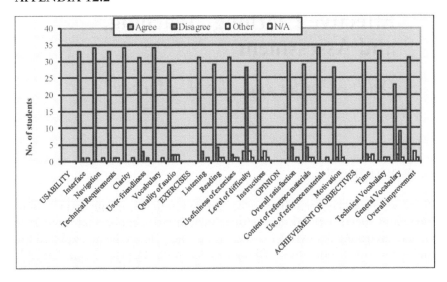

Graphic of Learner Overall Satisfaction

13 Integration of Technology for Effective Learning, Teaching, and Assessment

Debbie Corder and Alice U-Mackey

INTRODUCTION

Blogs, wikis, and e-portfolios are becoming familiar learning and teaching tools, and social networking websites including Facebook and multi-user virtual environments (MUVEs) such as Second Life are being explored for their educational potential for language learning (Deutschmann, Panichi, & Molka-Danielsen, 2009; Levy, 2009; Thorne, Black, & Sykes, 2009). These emerging technologies enable access to authentic materials and inter-action with native speakers for developing language and intercultural competence. They can also be used for development and assessment of learning competencies ("learning to learn"), including problem solving, critical analysis, reflection, and collaborative learning, central to lifelong autonomous learning (Levy, 2007; Murray, 2005).

However, to realize the affordances of technology, it must be integrated carefully into the curriculum and linked clearly to learning outcomes and learning, teaching, and assessment activities (Hoven, 1999; Levy, 2007; Stockwell, 2007); in other words, technology must be integrated to resolve pedagogical issues (Bax & Chambers, 2006; Boulton, 2008). Once technology is introduced, scaffolding of learners is essential to ensure understanding of technology as a tool in the learning process, both in terms of content knowledge and learning how to learn (Garrett, 2009; Stockwell, 2007). Use of tools such as blogs and e-portfolios requires the consideration of the "human element" (social dimensions). This involves the student being able to establish a social identity, ownership of content, and a feeling of belonging to a community, in order to ensure engagement (Dippold, 2009; Evans, Mulvi-hill, & Brooks, 2008; McLoughlin & Lee, 2008; Schneider & Evans, 2008).

The focus of this chapter is on two ongoing studies in BA programs at the Auckland University of Technology (AUT) that are evaluating the learning, teaching, and assessment approaches and activities into which technology has been strategically integrated. The courses are Japanese for Specific Purposes (JSP), a well-established course taught since 1995, and Introduction to Intercultural Competence (ICC), a new course with particularly complex learning outcomes, developed in 2007. The integration of

technology into the two courses was guided by the findings from two previous AUT studies: the evaluation of a kanji (Japanese characters) software
package (Corder & Waller, 2005, 2007), and the trialing of an e-portfolio
(Moffat, 2008), as well as the personal experience of one of the authors
(Corder, 2008). The studies showed that while technology could enhance
learning, teaching, and assessment, and provide the environment to foster
development of learning competencies especially through dialogue, there
were a number of key issues. The kanji software study showed the importance of scaffolding students, both to use the technology and to identify
learning needs. The e-portfolio study showed the need for the technology
to be integrated in such a way that both teachers and students saw its affordances as relevant and of value. Many students appeared to be familiar
with the emerging technologies such as Facebook, blogs, and wikis, and to
a lesser extent, portfolios. However, not many students appeared to make
the link that these technologies, especially the e-portfolio, could be used as
tools for their own learning. There was support for Jafari's belief that portfolios are not integrated into students' lives yet (Jafari, 2006). Additionally,
the design of the e-portfolio did not allow for student ownership, online
social networking, or development of online identity.

Finally, it was very evident that learning, teaching, and assessment
activities needed to facilitate the goals intended, particularly reflection and
critical thinking. In the case of the e-portfolio, the learning, teaching, and
assessment activities did not provide students with a learning experience on
which to reflect. As Prensky (2001, p. 5) says, "One of the most interesting
challenges and opportunities in teaching Digital Natives is to figure out and
invent ways to *include* reflection and critical thinking in the learning. . . .
We can and must do more in this area." However, students are not used
to reflecting on the learning process, or on themselves as language learners (Boulton, 2008; Sercu, 2004). In addition, as Garrett (2009, p. 730)
points out, although language teachers might espouse the concept of lifelong learning, "for the most part we have not yet integrated into language
programs explicit teaching of the tools and techniques students need to be
serious lifelong learners."

We now turn to a description of the JSP and ICC courses. The pedagogical rationale for integrating technology into learning, teaching, and
assessment activities will be discussed, together with the initial findings of
the evaluation of the integration, including the extent to which it became
"normalized" and used naturally by students (Bax & Chambers, 2006).
The approach in both courses is student centered, with a strong emphasis
on the development of learning competencies. However, each course has
specific aims and issues. For the purpose of this chapter, the term "technology" will be used, even though the tools have been mainly computer-
mediated Web 2.0 and 3D technology. In addition, the terms "intercultural
competence" and "intercultural communicative competence" will be used
interchangeably.

THE JSP COURSE

The JSP course, which is in the final year of the Japanese major, has business as a main component, and two smaller components, Japanese media and Japanese translation. The study described in this chapter is based on the translation component of 12 hours over six weeks. During the 15 years that the JSP course has been taught, there have been significant innovations in technology and the curriculum has needed to adjust accordingly. Changes have been most significant in the last three years, capitalizing on the increased university resourcing in technology and staff training and support, and the obligatory integration of the affordances of Blackboard, the Learning Management System (LMS). There have been five cohorts since the JSP study began (n = 79), and each cohort has consisted of a range of ethnicities and ages. The last two cohorts in particular were familiar with the university's LMS, many students owned electronic dictionaries, and every student had a mobile phone. The translation classes were held in the computer room so that students had ready access to technology as the need arose.

The aim of the translation component is to expose students to authentic material they might need to translate in the workplace. It is not intended to train them to be translators, but rather to develop self-assessment of their strengths and weaknesses in various genres, awareness of the role of culture in language, ethical issues, and technology as a translation resource. This is a new experience for our students because, as Garrett (2009, p. 729) observes, "Partly because language pedagogy still tends to proscribe using translation in elementary/intermediate language courses, we seldom teach our students explicitly how to use online translation tools and resources for real-life purposes after they leave the language classroom."

Students are introduced to online tools in the context of graded problem-solving exercises using authentic materials. These tools include online dictionaries and relevant websites. English as a second language (ESL) students have the opportunity to translate some material into their own language and to discuss this with other speakers of their language. There are ongoing discussions on the cultural differences influencing translations, along with the need to cross-check dictionary meanings and language style to ensure appropriateness for the context. Wikis in the LMS were introduced from the fourth cohort to facilitate collaborative learning by extending student–student and teacher–student dialogue beyond the classroom, to record work and reflection (learning to learn), and to manage group work. The use of wikis was justified by linking it to the concept of a community of translators.

Materials for the summative assessment had previously been selected by the teacher, but they had often been badly translated and poorly presented, which was probably a strong indication that students did not see the relevance of the tasks. Therefore, it was decided to give students more autonomy in designing their own assessment within clear guidelines of the requirements and learning outcomes. They could get help from any source they wished (technological or human), but they had to indicate the nature and extent of the help. Reflection on the experience was guided by trigger questions relating to language, intercultural perspectives, the translation process—including an analysis of any help received—and learning outcomes. Students had the option to work on their own, in pairs, or in groups of up to three.

THE ICC COURSE

When we first developed the ICC course in 2007, ICC was very new to language teaching in New Zealand. It was introduced as a first-year elective to complement language courses, to allow for development of the reflective and critical analysis that would be difficult to develop at the early stages of language learning (Garrett, 2009). As with the JSP study, there have been five cohorts since the study began (n = 97), with a range of ethnicities, and ages mainly ranging between 18 and 25. The course met for three hours a week, one of which was in a computer room. The students' experience with computers varied; most had used them to surf the Internet but not all were familiar with the LMS or with writing in blogs or wikis.

The daunting nature of the learning, teaching, and assessment needs, and the complexity of learning outcomes that did not lend themselves to traditional learning, teaching, and assessment approaches (Scarino, 2009), were the main reasons for our very strategic integration of technology into the course. ICC puts new demands on language teaching (Garrett, 2009) because in addition to cultural knowledge it includes cognitive, affective, and behavioral components. Rather than focusing just on content, importance is placed on the nature of learning (learning competencies) as a lifelong process, and the ability to notice, reflect, critically analyze, problem solve, and relate to others (Byram, 1997; Kohonen, 2005). For this type of learning to be achieved, dialogic interaction with others is essential, requiring a shift to a student-centered holistic experiential model of learning and teaching (Kohonen, 2005), and replacement of the traditional assessment methods such as essays or reports with alternative tools to measure changes in affective and behavioral dimensions over time (Scarino, 2009).

Our challenge was to translate this theory into practice, and we developed the following model (see Figure 13.1), based on Byram's (1997) savoirs and Kolb's (1984, p. 42) experiential learning model. It is an iterative process and technology has been integrated into all the learning, teaching, and assessment components shown on the periphery of the model, to achieve the learning outcomes shown in the center.

Activities such as discussions, role plays, critical incidents, and presentations provide the experiential learning, which is then conceptualized by

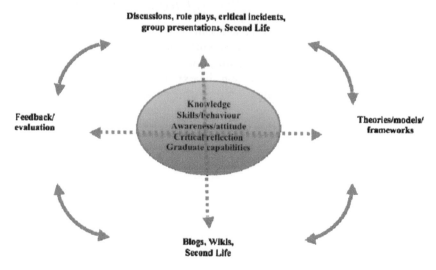

Figure 13.1   ICC Model for learning, teaching, and assessment.

theoretical frameworks. Students reflect on the experiences in class discussions and online, using blogs and wikis. Feedback is gained from debriefs and comments from peers and teachers in class and online, and the learning is then applied subsequently in new experiences. Formative assessment is primarily through the blogs and summative assessment is through the work done in wikis, a group presentation at the end of the course, and peer assessment. Although group work has inherent problems, for example, logistics of meeting times (Strauss & U, 2007), the necessity for peer interaction both face-to-face and online provides ideal opportunities to apply knowledge and skills of intercultural competence.

The most challenging aspect has been managing and assessing the development of the affective, behavioral, and meta-cognitive dimensions such as increase in awareness, changes in behavior, and development of critical analysis, reflection, and planning. This development is a longitudinal process. Managing the constant dialogue and collaboration needed for building, extending, and elaborating on concepts and processes is very difficult using paper-based methods, even without taking assessment into account. We did not have access to an e-portfolio that met our learning and teaching needs so we chose blogs and wikis within the LMS because of the affordances for social interaction, ease of use, and the fact that students had heard of them even if they had not used them. The possibilities for social networking are more limited than on open sites such as Blogspot.com; however, we believe that using the LMS has reduced possible technical barriers for students who are not "digital natives" (Prensky, 2001) and who are not so confident in the online environment.

The blogs were used initially to ease students into the online environment with self-introductions, and then to develop critical reflection with guidance from teachers (scaffolding) and peers. To enable collaboration and dialogue the blogs were open to the whole class and not just to the teachers, and it has been possible to map the longitudinal development of each student and their likelihood of meeting learning outcomes. The blogs have been a requirement because the e-portfolio findings showed that students tend not to engage if they do not think it counts towards their results.

Each group had a wiki for members to manage their learning and demonstrate reflection and critical analysis, responsibility for their own work, leadership, and collaborative learning. As with the blogs, the wikis were open to all the other groups in the class. Teachers could monitor the wikis providing scaffolding, and students could comment.

Some students had said they could not think of relevant life experiences on which to reflect, so we explored the use of Second Life to provide out-of-class intercultural experiences, particularly unpredictable situations that would push students out of their comfort zones without the real-life implications and embarrassments. Although there are very few studies on the use of 3D virtual worlds for language and culture learning, there is increasing interest in its potential (Deutschmann et al., 2009; Thorne et al., 2009). Research by Diehl and Prins (2008) indicates that Second Life provides the environment that could foster development of intercultural competence by providing opportunities for "cross-cultural encounters and friendships, greater awareness of insider cultural perspectives, and openness towards new viewpoints" (p. 102). Being placed in real-time intercultural encounters using avatars has real potential to enable students to link experiences and theory. For example, the limited body language of avatars such as nodding and shrugging highlights the role of nonverbal communication in social interactions.

Second Life was trialed with our third and fourth cohorts on the ICC course. Volunteer students from the third cohort took part in a series of five exchanges with engineering students in a Japanese university who were meeting people in Second Life for authentic experiences and then blogging in English about them. All the students in the fourth cohort of the ICC course were introduced to Second Life during class time over a few weeks, and one group based their group presentation on "Meeting people and making friends in Second Life."

Finally, with regard to assessment, and because of the complex learning outcomes in both courses, we have used performance indicators based on assessment criteria to assess the learning outcomes, combined with grade descriptors for final grades. We believe this allows for students to learn from mistakes during the course, and is a more reliable indicator of achievement by the end of the course than percentages and weightings.

METHODOLOGY

Both the translation section of the JSP course and the ICC course are ongo-ing action research studies. The authors teach in one or both of the courses, so all students in the courses were approached for consent after the final assessment, and the authors were informed about who had consented after the examination board had approved the final grades. To this end the data have been collected retrospectively, with minimum impact on students, and without compromising the research process. The data for initial findings for both studies have been based on course work and student evaluations, as well as online introspective methods, namely, blogs and wikis. This has been an iterative process with ongoing revisions depending on feedback and findings. A key research question is whether technology has been integrated so that it has enhanced learning, teaching, and assessment and whether it is used naturally and even spontaneously by students.

INITIAL FINDINGS AND DISCUSSION

The initial findings show that technology was naturally integrated into the translation section of the JSP course: Classes were in a computer room and many of the tools available were very relevant to the task of transla-tion. The results have shown increased engagement, evidence of deep learn-ing, and a much higher standard of work—even from the students who achieved a lower grade. The quality of student reflection and analysis has been beyond expectation, particularly from the higher-achieving students. Examples of student reflections included words such as "style," "expressive vocabulary," "written literally," "make it flow," "needed a simile," "great words that I'd like to remember," "literal translation," and "unnatural."

Increased engagement has extended to greater collaboration, with stu-dents sharing useful websites. The introduction of wikis to record reflection and manage group work has proved effective for collaboration and model-ing, as can be seen from the following comments:

> HI X. . . .
>   I read your Go Document {Yosuke is the staunchest but scrawniest actor, he's kind of hot though} Anyway I think you did a good transla-tion. Where is your steps and reflection though, I want to see how you translated it.
>   Have a look at mine if you have time
>   I did it on Proverbs
>   Y

> W, thanks for your comment. Its good to see that i wasn't the only one having trouble putting my words onto paper. If you ever do any

translation in the future a good site which I used to look up kanji reading s and meanings is www.popjisyo.com its not always right but it is
easy to use. ALso looking at your translation help me put mine into
better english so keep up those English grammar skills (^_^)

There is evidence of increased use of technology not just in terms of tools
to aid translation, but also for searching for materials to translate for the
assignment. Almost all the first cohort of students chose from hard copies
of magazines or newspapers and also used hard copies of dictionaries. In
the last cohort, all the students used online material. This might be because
it was easier to use the Internet to find something of interest, and convenient to read the online material using online pop-up dictionaries.

The translation section is reviewed annually to ensure its continued relevance to students, particularly the ESL students. To date not one student
has said that it is not relevant to their needs, nor has anyone commented
negatively about the technology. Instead, many have commented on how
useful the course has been, and a number have indicated interest in translating as a career. Students in practicum workplace placements have found
the knowledge and skills particularly relevant. They found the course challenging, especially the reflection and self-assessment, but enjoyed the freedom of choice and authenticity of tasks. We believe it was the combination
of authentic learning, teaching, and assessment activities, and integrated
relevant technology, that made it possible to enhance and extend the student experience and achieve the desired outcomes.

In the case of the ICC course, there is evidence that the integration of technology has been very effective for introducing content, and that the blogs
and wikis have become increasingly effective for learning to learn. However,
this has not happened without ongoing modifications to learning, teaching, and assessment activities, including greater clarity of requirements for
online elements and more effective scaffolding as the teachers became more
experienced. As Dippold (2009) found, confidence in scaffolding is important. An excessive number of online tools was found to be detrimental. The
interaction in the blogs increased following the removal of a complex online
reflective activity, with postings increasing from an average per student blog
of three postings (58 views, four comments) in the second cohort, to an average of ten (212 views, 19 comments) in the fifth cohort.

The following is an example of a blog entry by a mature student majoring in Chinese. He applied theory to critically analyze and reflect on the
Japanese way of complaining, and identified possible issues when interacting with Japanese people. The next step was to transfer this criticality to
reflect on social practices for making complaints in his own culture, as well
as in Chinese culture.

Today we talked about high vs low context cultures, and the ways in
which they differ with respect to making apologies, complaints and

requests. The contrast between them was pretty interesting. I liked the example of the Japanese women engaging in circumlocutionary back-flips to avoid giving offence when one was complaining about the oth-er's inconsiderate cleaning times. If someone was complaining to me in that manner, I'd get pretty annoyed—just tell me I'm keeping you awake and I'll do what I can. That's just another example of how I'd have trouble adjusting to Japanese society.

There was an increase in the interaction in the wikis with each cohort, the greatest increase being in the fourth and fifth cohorts. Compared to the first cohort, the fifth cohort showed an increase of 300 percent in the average number of views (517) per group and an increase of 218 percent in average edits. The greatest number of views and edits for a wiki was for the Second Life group in the fourth cohort (1,077 views, 205 edits).

Although not all students contributed actively in either the blogs or the wikis, their passive involvement (viewing only) was seen in the number of views. There was also evidence that students learned from their peers, for example, using other students' work as models. However, having to move to the computer room to work on blogs and wikis presented a barrier in terms of natural use of technology.

Not all the students engaged with Second Life, and this might have been for a number of reasons, including its use being voluntary and student per-ceptions that it was not useful or was too technological. However, when students did engage, the results were outstanding. Students were strongly motivated to engage in the learning process and there was marked collab-orative learning and enjoyment. The following is an example of the wiki belonging to the group in the fourth cohort who used Second Life as the medium for their project. It shows the group cohesiveness (social dimen-sions), the extent to which the students collaborated, and how they had integrated technology into their learning. One member (Z), who had ini-tially been anxious about computers, recorded the highest number of blog posts of any of the cohorts and used the wiki extensively.

> Hi X and Y—Hope you are not in holiday mode and are doing lots of stuff for next week's presentation. I think we need more communica-tion so we are prepared. I'll send you emails as well in case you are not coming onto the site. I've been chatting to W [in] SL about the project. Z, 21 Apr 2009.

> MEETING MEETING How does a meeting on Saturday afternoon at 1pm sound? I think Sat is best so it gives plenty of time to sort every-thing out. We probably need access to computer. Happy to host it at my place only i'm 10 minutes drive from town i will even provide biscuits!, no parking problems., or if thats inconvenient anywhere else is fine for me Im totally mobile, providing there is computer access. Happy

to do pickups in central city or west.Need to discuss: finalisation of "initial presentation" and whether we stick with "contentious foods" or change to "Second Life." Cheers W 23 April 2009

Hi X—W, Y and I had a good session [in] SL tonight and I am sure you would have enjoyed the exploring we did. I hope you will be able to join us here sometime to look at the different sites and meeting people en route. See you Saturday at W's. Z 23 April 2009.

I'll print out the wiki and bring a copy for each of us to the meeting tomorrow so we can see where we are at. X—I am meeting Y [in] SL tonight around 8.30 so if you are free please come and join us. Z 24 April 2009.

Hey guys, hope you had fun [in] SL. I just read that article "unintended outcomes in Second life"—WOW inspiring!. Discuss it tommorrow, hope you have time to read it too before our meeting.
See you, W

The learning demonstrated by the students in both Second Life trials far exceeded the authors' expectations in terms of development of intercultural competence. The following are examples of student reflections demonstrating use of theory and ability to notice and analyze:

- The people I have met on Second Life are very interesting and very friendly but it is hard to communicate . . . without the benefit of seeing them face to face [sic]. Part of this is because non-verbal communication is a huge part of speech, we take clues from the other persons [sic] face as to decipher some of the meaning eg [sic]: if it is meant to be humourous [sic] or not
- . . . real-world cultures don't really dominate in SL. SL cultures dominate in SL, with variations for each country.
- People interacting in SL have developed norms regarding how they act in the world.
- . . . body language . . . assumptions . . . politeness strategies . . .
- . . . a system that models (to an extent) human interaction, while providing interesting differences . . .
- . . . how people view themselves in cyberspace and the relation between that and the real world.
- I found it interesting how much more natural (for me, anyway) it was talking to strangers in Second Life, (where there is some sort of physical appearance that you can link them to) versus chatting to strangers on, say, MSN—which is totally impersonal.

With respect to learning style and preferences, in formal and informal feedback on the course, students' negative comments have focused on the activities and not on the technology. Positive feedback has identified the technology, as can be seen from the following comments:

- I'm finding wiki is useful for presentation. Also blog is another useful and helpful median between lecturers and students. It's abridge and way to know about each other for classmates.
- I enjoy the blog exercises as they allow us to interact with people from other cultures.
- Blogs very useful because we learnt from comments and other groups and become clear about what we should do later.
- I like the blogs. Made me think.

Learner Differences

The findings show correlations between the level of meeting the learning outcomes and the extent and quality of student engagement in the learning, teaching, and assessment activities, whether in class or using technology. Student engagement was linked to learner autonomy, involving self-motivation, intrinsic motivation, and learning strategies, rather than disadvantages arising from cultural background, first language, or feelings of discomfort with using technology. Students who did not blog regularly, or who did not respond to the scaffolding and continued to make irrelevant (albeit amusing) comments, did not achieve the learning outcomes or were low achievers.

INTEGRATION OF TECHNOLOGY AND IMPLICATIONS FOR TEACHING

There were many advantages of integrating blogs and wikis, particularly the ability to monitor student learning and provide timely intervention and the ability to assess the complex learning outcomes more effectively than by using traditional assessments methods and paper-based reflective tools. The main disadvantage was the increased demand on time. Giving regular and appropriate feedback was time-consuming, and, with the absence of RSS (Really Simple Syndication) feeds on the LMS, time was wasted checking blogs and wikis for late entries.

The learning achieved using Second Life was significant and the optional approach worked, because students who engaged with Second Life were motivated, learned quickly, and taught each other. If this aspect had been compulsory, then developing basic competency would have been more demanding on staff and students in terms of time. Depending on an individual's computer experience and the nature of the activities, basic competency development can take from 5 to 10 hours (Atkins & Caukill, 2009). As far as the technology issues were concerned, permission to go through an institution's firewall was necessary, and although there were no bandwidth issues within the university, bandwidth was a problem for some students at home. In addition, we needed to be prepared for the dark side of Second Life and be aware of the protocols for dealing with harassment or the occasional intrusion by unknown avatars.

CONCLUSION

The initial findings of the purposeful integration of technology into the JSP and ICC courses are promising, especially for developing and assessing learning competencies and complex learning outcomes. Blogs and wikis have provided an environment for student collaboration and dialogue, necessary for the development of skills in reflection and critical analysis. They have also enabled the monitoring and scaffolding of students over time in a way that would not have been possible with traditional approaches.

In both the JSP and the ICC courses, some of the technology tools were clearly relevant and engaging for students (YouTube, search engines, websites) and if students were familiar with them, they did not need much persuasion to use them. Others, such as the wikis and blogs, used as tools for learning to learn, might have been considered less functional or relevant, as some students needed encouragement from teachers to use them. Second Life showed strong potential for providing synchronous out-of-class experiential learning and for facilitating the social dimensions that foster collaboration, although mastering the technology demanded time.

It has been a learning curve for us. The most important lesson has been that integration of technology alone does not produce the promising results, and that it depends on what Stockwell (2007) calls the "symbiotic" relationship between pedagogy and technology. It is clear that technology must be easy to access and use without much training so that the focus is on the learning and not the technology. The choice of technology tools also needs to be evaluated: Workloads for staff and students engaged in online interaction need to be managed carefully, and being too zealous with the number of online tools can confuse students and increase workloads unnecessarily. Ultimately, the extent of student engagement in the learning process will depend on individual learner differences and motivation. However, as Garret (2009) points out, although technology will not address all the problems, we cannot begin to address problems without it.

REFERENCES

Atkins, C., & Caukill, M. (2009). Serious fun and serious learning: The challenge of Second Life. In J. Molka-Danielsen & M. Deutschmann (Eds.), *Learning and teaching in the virtual world of Second Life* (pp. 78–79). Trondheim: Tapir Academic Press.

200   *Debbie Corder and Alice U-Mackey*

Bax, S., & Chambers A. (2006). Making CALL work: Towards normalization. *System, 34*(4), 465–479.

Boulton, A. (2008). Learning to learn languages with ICT—But how? *CALL-EJ Online, 9*(2). Retrieved from http://www.tell.is.ritsumei.ac.jp/callejonline/

Byram, M. (1997). *Teaching and assessing intercultural communicative competence.* Clevedon: Multilingual Matters.

Corder, D. (2008). *Debbie's blog.* Retrieved from http://debbiecor.blogspot.com/2008/02/reflection-on-course-assignment-1.html

Corder, D., & Waller, G. (2005). An analysis of the effectiveness of an in-house CALL software package for the learning and teaching of kanji (Japanese characters) and the development of autonomous language learning skills. *CALL-EJ Online, 7*(1). Retrieved from http://www.tell.is.ritsumei.ac.jp/callejonline/

Corder, D., & Waller, G. (2007). Using a CALL package as a platform to develop effective language learning strategies and facilitate autonomous learning. In L. Miller (Ed.), *Learner autonomy: Autonomy in the classroom* (pp.7–26). Dublin: Authentik Language Learning Resources Ltd.

Deutschmann, M., Panichi, L., & Molka-Danielsen, J. (2009). Designing oral participation in Second Life—A comparative study of two language proficiency courses. *ReCALL, 21*(2), 206–226.

Diehl, W. C., & Prins, E. (2008). Unintended outcomes in Second Life: Intercultural literacy and cultural identity in a virtual world. *Language and Intercultural Communication, 8*(2), 101–118.

Dippold, D. (2009). Peer feedback through blogs: Student and teacher perceptions in an advanced German class. *ReCALL, 21*(1), 18–36.

Evans, N., Mulvihill, M., & Brooks, N, J. (2008). Mediating the tensions of online learning with Second Life. *Innovate, 4*(6). Retrieved from http://innovateonline.info/index.php?view=issue&id=27

Garrett, N. (2009). Computer-assisted language learning trends and issues revisited: Integrating innovation. *Modern Language Journal, 93*(S1), 719–740.

Hoven, D. (1999). CALL-ing the learner into focus. In R. Debski & M. Levy (Eds.), *World call: Global perspectives on computer-assisted language learning* (pp. 149–196). Lisse: Swets and Zeitlinger.

Jafari, A. (2006). Preface. In A. Jafari & K. Kaufman (Eds.), *Handbook of research on e-portfolios* (pp. xxxiii–xxxvi). Hershey, PA, and London: Idea Group Reference.

Kohonen, V. (2005). Experiential learning, intercultural learning and teacher development in foreign language education. In J. Smeds, K. Sarmavuori, E. Laakkonen, & R. de Cillia (Eds.), *Multicultural communities, multilingual practice* (pp. 123–135). Turku: Annales Universitatis Turkuensis B 285.

Kolb, D. (1984). *Experiential learning.* Englewood Cliffs, NJ: Prentice Hall.

Levy, M. (2007). Culture, culture learning and new technologies: towards a pedagogical framework. *Language Learning and Technology, 11*(2), 104–127.

Levy, M. (2009). Technologies in use for second language learning. *Modern Language Journal, 93*(S1), 769–782.

McLoughlin, C., & Lee, M. J. (2008). Future learning landscapes: Transforming pedagogy through social software. *Innovate, 4*(5). Retrieved from http://www.innovateonline.info/index.php?view=article&id=539

Moffat, S. (2008). *Student attitudes towards and perceptions of e-portfolios in a first year Japanese language programme.* Unpublished master's thesis, Auckland University of Technology, Auckland, New Zealand.

Murray, D. (2005). Technologies for second language literacy. *Annual Review of Applied Linguistics, 28*, 188–201.

Prensky, M. (2001). Digital natives, digital immigrants, Part II: Do they really think differently? *On the Horizon (NCB University Press), 9*(6). Retrieved from http://www.twitchspeed.com/site/prensky20 percent-20 percentdigital

Scarino, A. (2009). Assessing intercultural capability in learning languages: Some issues and considerations. *Language Teaching, 42*(1), 67–80.

Schneider, S. B., & Evans, M. A. (2008). Transforming e-learning into e-learning: The centrality of sociocultural participation. *Innovate, 5*(1). Retrieved from http://www.innovateonline.info/index.php?view=article&id=511

Sercu, L. (2004). Intercultural communicative competence as a new objective of foreign language education. In K. van Esch & O. St. John (Eds.), *New insights into foreign language learning and teaching* (pp. 115–130). Frankfurt: Peter Lang.

Stockwell, G. (2007). A review of technology choice for teaching language skills and areas in the CALL literature. *ReCALL, 19*(2), 105–120.

Strauss, P., & U, A. (2007). Group assessments: Dilemmas facing lecturers in multicultural tertiary classrooms. *Higher Education Research and Development Journal, 2*(2), 147–161.

Thorne, S., Black, R. W., & Sykes, J. M. (2009). Second language use, socialization, and learning in Internet interest communities and online gaming. *Modern Language Journal, 93*(S1), 802–821.

14 The E-Job 100 Project
CALL for Increasing Motivation for Learning English

Akiyoshi Suzuki and Teresa Kuwamura

INTRODUCTION

Warschauer and Healey (1998) stated that with the advancement of the Internet and multimedia, current "Integrative CALL" (Computer-Assisted Language Learning) has overcome the principal disadvantage of earlier types of CALL, which was that is was not close enough to real-life communication. Integrative CALL provides learners with an environment in which they can acquire communication skills more spontaneously.

However, in some countries such as Japan, there is a vast untapped potential. The effectiveness of CALL software and e-learning systems is a gold mine that remains unexcavated. Many college students tend to avoid learning English. One of the main reasons is that students believe they will not need English in either their personal lives or in their careers. This is even considered true for some English teachers. As Torikai (2001) points out, "We should begin by considering whether all Japanese really need to learn English or not, and if they do need it, for what reason, and how they should learn it."

Many Japanese college students need to be convinced that it is necessary to learn English before putting their minds to it. The authors are convinced that CALL offers a realistic solution. E-Job 100,[1] which is based on Rogers (1969) "student-centered" educational theory, offers an effective solution. The purpose of E-Job 100 is to create a bridge between students and a suitable CALL system. Our focus is on creating a method to motivate college students in Japan to learn English and to set an example for other countries that might have a similar problem.

BACKGROUND

One of the problems in English education for college students in Japan is a combination of low motivation and low academic ability (see Table 14.1).

Over 50 percent of the students have already lost their motivation to learn before entering college (see Figure 14.1).

Table 14.1   Problems with English Education in Colleges and Universities in Japan (Committee of the Survey, 2003; 787 correspondents; Multiple Answers Allowed)

Item	Percentage of Respondents
(1) Low motivation and academic ability of students	64.5%
(2) Skills of the teacher	29.7%
(3) Excessively high expectations of English education	22.7%
(4) National support for foreign language education	22.1%
(5) Curriculum	21.9%

On the other hand, it is also true that over 80 percent of Japanese precollege students think learning English is important (see Figure 14.2).

Many Japanese students recognize the importance of English in a general way. However, they fail to associate it with themselves.

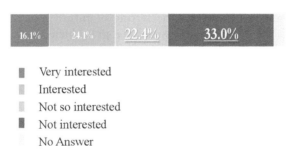

Figure 14.1   "Are You Interested in Learning English?" (Curriculum Research Center, 2005. Correspondents: 30,000 seniors in high school in Japan.)

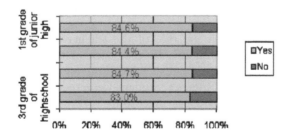

Figure 14.2   "Is Learning English Important for Japanese?" (Curriculum Research Center, 2003. Correspondents: 243,000.)

THE REASON FOR LOW MOTIVATION

According to Suzuki (2007), Japanese students have low motivation due to social conditions. Most Japanese do not need English in their daily lives. However, the Japanese media report that employees in many large Japanese companies need English-language skills. Furthermore, the attitude towards learning English among college students in Japan is diverse, and this is illustrated by their career goals: Not all Japanese college students target jobs at large companies where English is required, according to reports in the mass media. As an example from the school where the authors are teaching, there are some students in the Department of Civil Engineering who want to run beauty salons, and a few other students who want to develop video games, so English-language needs are mixed. In addition, college students in Japan cannot accurately comprehend the real work environment due to a lack of information. Moreover, no research has been done currently in Japan to study a wide range of occupations to determine whether English is needed. Therefore, even when teachers tell their students that they will need English after entering the job market, many of the students tend to take this advice very lightly.

In Japan, some traditional social norms are no longer observed (Kuwamura, 2008). For example, the following phenomena exist: frequent bullying, cynicism, and an increase in the number of students who realize neither the value of study nor the setting of future goals. Furthermore, some students are becoming antisocial due to problems such as feelings of inferiority and rejection by society. Such feelings and behaviors contribute to a lack of motivation to learn.

In response to this situation, the authors have paid attention not only to the students' ability and motivation but also to their sense of independence and their feelings of adequacy. The authors have searched for a relevant theory and come up with an effective and practical solution. Based on the educational theory of Rogers (1969), by focusing on fulfillment of students' personal needs, a CALL program that individualizes learning appears to be the answer.

ROGERS' "STUDENT-CENTERED EDUCATION" AND CALL

Rogers (1969) insisted on the role of the teacher as facilitator and on the students' learning autonomy. Indeed, both of these ideas have been widely accepted in current English education, especially among CALL practitioners. Regarding Rogers' "Student-Centered Education," Dörnyei (2001) confirms its effectiveness. According to Rogers (1995), education should enable students to realize their potential and develop character and self-reliance. The teacher as facilitator gives students materials to determine their level of interest and to develop their effective study skills and self-expression based on their individual needs in class. In addition, the teacher gives students positive reinforcement, including attention, empathy, respect, and praise. Rogers also encouraged a classroom environment in which students feel at ease and participate confidently even if they make mistakes. The teacher uses positive rewards to encourage students to attend class and to express themselves so that they can simultaneously pursue their studies and develop self-esteem, confidence, and motivation. Furthermore, the teacher develops each student's ability to deal with life's challenges and become a whole person.

This type of program has been shown to be effective for Japanese students. Most students in Japan have a passive attitude toward studying English because they fear making mistakes. However, English is a language with strong practicality. In the authors' opinion, the knowledge of English language can be gained only through repetitive practice. Students' learning initiatives and participation are keys to success. It has been shown that English proficiency largely depends on the degree of students' initiative and enthusiasm. The primary responsibility in English education is to encourage students to learn actively instead of expecting to be taught passively. As Johnson and Morrow (1981) state, "A teacher can help, advise and teach, but only the learner can learn" (p. 81).

The explanation of Rogers' student-centered education sounds similar to Curran's educational theory. Both started from "learner-centered education." Indeed, Curran (1972), who did not refer to Rogers by name or to his books, is clearly influenced by him (Brown, 1994, pp. 85–89). However, their educational theories differ in several respects. One of the most important points in Rogers' theory is that a teacher shares the experiences of the students. A teacher should not analyze a student's thought and behavior from his/her own perspective but from that of the student. A teacher comprehends a student's interest, assesses his or her developmental stage, and devises an educational path for each individual. According to Rogers, only in this way can a teacher play a role as facilitator.

A facilitator is one who increases the meaning of education in a student's mind and shapes the future direction for a student. According to the authors' teaching experience, a good facilitator needs to know the particular needs of each individual student. She or he must consider and respond not only to the interests of an individual student but also to the needs of the entire class. Rogers' facilitator both helps students to realize their full potential and facilitates the development of good character and self-reliance.

According to Rogers (1969), "The students who are in real contact with life problems wish to learn, want to grow, seek to find out, hope to master, desire to create" (p. 289). In this way, students become responsible and self-motivated to learn (Brophy, 1998; Gribbs, 1989; Krapp & Renniger, 1992; Sansholtz, Ringstaff, & Dwyer, 1997; Schiefele, 1991). Accordingly, the materials that a teacher gives to students to foster their interest and build their motivation should be real-world examples. Videos showing the use of English in real situations in Japan and authentic documents used in the Japanese workplace have been included by the authors. CALL is the best way for teachers to provide these materials to students and to understand each individual student's needs. Warschauer and Healey (1998) also claim that a teacher should be a facilitator according to Rogers' definition.

Various conditions contribute to reducing the effectiveness of English education in Japan. First, the educational system fails to deal with the belief that students do not need English. Then there is a lack of authentic workplace examples of the use of English. Finally, the students' diversity of values, educational pathologies, and problematic development are not addressed. In response to this situation, CALL, directed by a facilitator according to Rogers' definition,[2] offers an effective solution.

E-JOB 100

Based on the reasoning outlined in the preceding, the E-Job 100 project has been developed by the authors.[3] E-Job 100 is a Web-based learning system in which videos show actual scenes illustrating the use of English by Japanese people in various occupations. Students can choose their favorite jobs and learn English by experiencing an authentic scenario, which helps them to develop their English skills. E-Job 100 allows the teacher to integrate various existing systems and software. It therefore acts as a bridge that allows teachers to use existing educational materials more effectively through use of the Web.

The first goal of the project is to answer the students' question, "Do Japanese people who live in Japan really need English?" Although many Japanese do not need English in their everyday lives, those working in some fields do need it, as in the examples of flight attendants or business employees in international companies. While these examples are well known, there are many professionals whose needs for English are no less real but are less well known, such as beauty salon staff, pharmacists, and musicians.

What is the true degree of English knowledge required by Japanese employees? To answer this question, the authors have researched approximately 150 kinds of jobs to find out whether they require English or not.[4] The authors have asked people in different occupations if they need English, when, how, at what level, how often, and for what purpose: All occupations except that of tax accountant now require the use of English. In fact, most Japanese now need to use some English in their work.

According to the answers to the survey, the authors went to each job site and made a video recording of the real work environment for a day, recording scenes in which English is used. We have edited the video into work and skill scenes of approximately two minutes' duration. In addition, we obtained the original documents that are used in the workers' daily tasks and used them as materials for the students. We have made the video clips and documents available on the Web. Our creed is, "The facts speak for themselves."

Figure 14.3 is a flow chart of E-Job 100. From the top page to the end, the contents include type of job, the top page for each job (Figure 14.4), a page for skills (Figure 14.5), and educational materials (Figure 14.6). The first item on the top page of the job is about what the job involves. One can watch a video of a scene with everyday tasks in which they use English. On the skills page, one can watch the scenes sorted into four skills. On the page for educational materials, we show original materials that the workers actually use in their jobs. There are many types available. In total, pages are being made for approximately 100 types of jobs. That is why this project is called E-Job 100.

To use these pages in class, the authors give students tasks such as to give a presentation or carry out a conversation with a customer and client. The students choose their favorite jobs and complete the task using English. Teachers can use those materials for career education, as an introduction to their English courses, as a goal for student learning, for English for Special Purposes (ESP), and so on.

One of the special features of E-Job 100 is the range of employment sectors. Many occupations in the range are familiar to the students and are even popular but have not been regarded as jobs where English is needed.

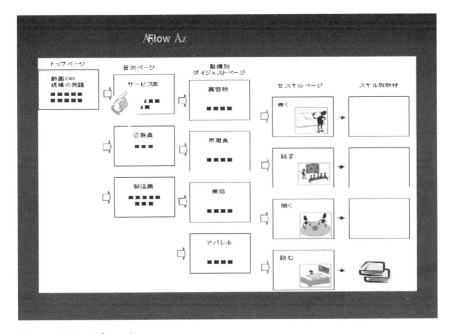

Figure 14.3   A flow chart.

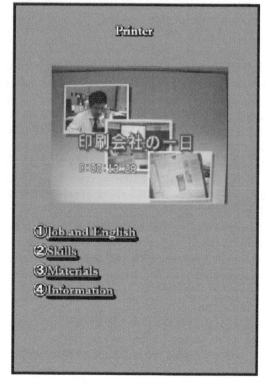

Figure 14.4   Top page for an occupation.

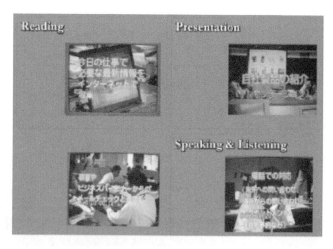

Figure 14.5   Scenes for each skill.

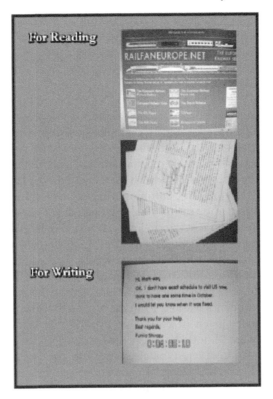

Figure 14.6   Educational materials.

Jobs such as musician, convenience store clerk, and staff for small and medium-size enterprises are all in this category. This aspect arouses the students' curiosity about this set of video educational materials.

In the authors' classes, students are required to play roles by speaking the English needed for their intended future jobs. Students are divided into groups of four or five according to the job categories. Each group needs to do research and make a presentation about their jobs first in English. The rest of the students pretend to be the clients and the customers of the group who is giving the presentation. The listeners ask the speakers various relevant questions after their presentation. If the listeners are academically gifted students, they are required to ask questions in English. The less confident students are allowed to ask questions in Japanese at first and try in English later. After the initial practice, the teacher gives each speaker feedback and asks more questions. The speakers will need to conduct more research on the Internet, rewrite their presentations and memorize them, and then present again. Students may either choose another job every three or four weeks or just concentrate on a single job. As a result of this method, the classroom can be a microcosm of society with its many occupations.

The experience of practicing and making multiple presentations in a microcosm of society gives students the satisfaction of learning useful skills as well as a sense of personal fulfillment and self-confidence.

EFFECT AND CONCLUSION

Every year the authors conduct a questionnaire for students in multiple-choice and free-response format. In the 2005 questionnaire, before the students had used E-Job 100, common answers were "Be snap course," "Be enjoyable," "Be easy," "I don't expect anything," and "I don't like English." In contrast, on the questionnaire in the same year in the last class after the students had used E-Job 100, common answers were "I realized we need English," "I realized the truth," "I need English for myself," "I want to learn English spontaneously," and "I am interested in English." The quality of the class may account for these responses. In 2006, when the students in the class in which E-Job 100 is not used were asked whether they wanted to make a presentation, only 5 students out of a total of 72 wanted to do it. However, when the same question was asked of the class where E-Job 100 is used, 67 students wanted to make a presentation. Typical answers to the questionnaire given in 2007 (78 respondents) before students had used E-Job 100 were "I hope I can get the credits very easily" and "I don't expect anything." However, typical answers to the questionnaire in the same year after E-Job 100 were, "I realized we need English," "I realized the fact," and "I need English for my future." In the multiple-choice questionnaire survey in 2007, 97.2 percent (74 respondents) answered "easily comprehensible," 90.4 percent "Predigested," and 90.2 percent "Interested in this class."

These results have led the authors to the conclusion that CALL has helped to have the truth speak itself. "Not persuasion but showing the facts" by a facilitator from Rogers' (1969) theory is effective for students with low motivation for learning English in Japan. The authors believe that it is effective for Japanese students and that it may be effective in any country that has a similar problem.

NOTES

1. "E" in "E-Job 100" means "electronic," "English," and "Ii" (good) in Japanese.
2. Rogers' facilitator can be effective not only for an individual but also a group that shares a common interest or a problem. In this sense, it can be applied, for example, to Inquiry-Based Learning or Problem-Based Learning.
3. This Internet project has been conducted with the support of the Nippon Telegraph and Telephone Corporation (NTT) in Japan. See http://e-job-100.sakura.ne.jp/

4. On a statistical basis of Career Matrix (http://cmx.vrsys.net/TOP), managed by Japan Institute for Labor Policy and Training, we estimate 95 percent of the Japanese labor force work in approximately 503 different kinds of jobs.

REFERENCES

Brophy, J. (1998). *Motivating students to learn.* Boston: McGraw-Hill.

Brown, H. (1994). *Principles of language learning and teaching* (3rd ed.). Englewood Cliffs, NJ: Prentice Hall Regents.

Committee of the Survey in Japan Association of College English Teachers. (2003). *A multidisciplinary research on the reality of the situation about education of foreign languages and English in Japan—Individual's edition of college teacher of foreign languages and English.* Tokyo: Japan Association of College English Teachers.

Curran, C. (1972). *Counseling learning: A whole person model for education.* New York: Grune and Stratton.

Curriculum Research Center at National Institute for Educational Policy Research. (2003). *Report of the situation of the implementation of the curriculum in elementary and junior high schools in 2001: English in junior high school.* Retrieved from http://www.nier.go.jp/kaihatsu/jissihoukoku/Taro12–9chuei.pdf

Curriculum Research Center at National Institute for Educational Policy Research. (2005). *Report of the situation of the implementation of the curriculum in elementary and junior high schools in 2003: English in junior high school.* Retrieved from http://www.nier.go.jp/kaihatsu/katei_h15/H15/03001051030007004.pdf

Dörnyei, Z. (2001). *Motivational strategies in the language classroom.* Cambridge: Cambridge University Press.

Gribbs, C. (1989). *Alternatives: Games, exercises and conversations for the language class.* Harlow: Longman.

Johnson, K., & Morrow, K. (1981). *Communication in the classroom.* London: Longman.

Krapp, A., & Renniger, K. (1992). Interest, learning, and development. In A. Krapp, S. Hidi, & K. Renniger (Eds.), *The role of interest in learning and development* (pp. 3–26). Hillsdale: Erlbaum.Kuwamura, T. (2008). Comparative study between John Dewey's "child-centered education" and Carl Rogers' "student-centered education." *Bulletin of John Dewey Society of Japan, 49,* 145–154.

Rogers, C. (1969). *Freedom to learn: A view of what education might become.* Columbus, OH: Charles E. Merrill.

Rogers, C. (1995). *On becoming a person: A therapist's view of psychotherapy* (Rev. ed.). Boston: Houghton Mifflin.

Sansholtz, J., Ringstaff C., & Dwyer, D. (1997). *Teaching with technology: Creating student-centered classrooms.* New York: Teachers College Press.

Schiefele, U. (1991). Interest, learning, and motivation. *Educational Psychologist, 26*(3/4), 299–323.

Suzuki, A. (2007). For a new student-centered English education with a high regard for their motivation—moving video picture database: English in diverse job sites in Japan. *Sanken Libraries, 27,* 83–149.

Torikai, K. (2001). "What is English for Japanese?" Commemorative symposium for the publication of Genius English Japanese Dictionary. Retrieved from http://www.taishukan.co.jp/event_genius/event_g.html

Warschauer, M., & Healey, D. (1998). Computers and language learning: An overview. *Language Teaching, 31,* 57–71.

Part IV

Learner Training

15 Pervasive CALL Learner Training for Improving Listening Proficiency

Kenneth Romeo and Philip Hubbard

INTRODUCTION

In the past, one of the barriers to improving listening comprehension was the limited supply of useful materials. The Web has changed that, making an incredibly rich collection of often free audio and video materials available to language teachers and learners. This collection includes dedicated materials designed specifically to support language learning (e.g., Randall's Cyber Listening Lab: http://www.esl-lab.com); authentic materials with dedicated language learning support (e.g., http://www.lingual.net); authentic materials with transcripts, captions, or other aids that were not specifically provided for language learners but that can be useful for them (e.g., http://www.cnn.com/studentnews); and of course the countless unsupported audio and video materials available through commercial media websites and resources like YouTube (http://www.youtube.com).

While the existence of such material is a boon to language teachers and learners, even students who are fairly sophisticated at using digital technology for other purposes may be uncertain of how to exploit these resources effectively for language learning outside of class (Barrette, 2001; Hubbard, 2004; Winke & Goertler, 2008) and may require a significant amount of learner training. The present work reports on the learner training for an advanced ESL listening course taught to international graduate students at Stanford University in spring 2008. The course seems particularly suited for such an inquiry because of the level of the students and the fact that independent listening projects negotiated with the instructor represent a major part of the course homework.

Over the past few years the amount of learner training in listening courses taught by the two of us has been gradually increasing, and beginning with the pilot study (see the following), we decided to foreground the training to the students, making it a more central component. The objective of the research was to explore student responses toward a pervasive learner training approach that sought to make their work with online materials more effective during the course and ideally prepare them for continuing to work on their own after the course ended.

LEARNER TRAINING OVERVIEW

Strategy training for language learners has been broadly implemented since the 1980s. However, the technology environment offers a number of additional opportunities and challenges to learners that require adjustment of established models (e.g., Oxford, 1990). These include (a) acquiring technical skills, both general ones and those specific to individual applications; (b) recognition of the range of options or paths through the material; and (c) foundational knowledge about second language learning along with practice in using that knowledge to make choices among recognized options. To help students acquire some of the requisite knowledge and skills, Hubbard (2004) proposed a set of practice-based Computer-Assisted Language Learning (CALL) learner training principles, as follows:

- Experience CALL yourself. As part of preparation to train their students, it is important for teachers who have not themselves learned languages through computer-based activities to have that experience. This can lead to profound changes in what is trained and how the training is conducted (Kolaitis, Mahoney, Pomann, & Hubbard, 2006).
- Give learners teacher training. If learners are going to make informed choices regarding material and strategies for going through it—that is, take on part of the teacher's role—it is helpful for them to have some of the same base knowledge that professional language teachers have.
- Use a cyclical approach. Both the general concept of learner control and the mastery of specific techniques often take time and repeated exposure rather than the more common "one-shot" training.
- Use collaborative debriefings. Allowing students to discuss their individual homework experiences in groups during the next class promotes reflection and allows them to learn from one another rather than just from the instructor.
- Teach general exploitation strategies. Both dedicated and authentic materials can be used in ways beyond those intended by the designer. For instance, any material with an accurate transcript can be used for dictation practice and to support vocabulary development.

More recently, these principles have been embedded within an evolving conceptual framework recognizing three distinct domains of learner training:

- Technical training: *how* to use the options and controls of both general and specific applications on the computer for language learning purposes. An example is how to control subtitles in various applications. In some cases, subtitles can be toggled on and off with a simple control, but students sometimes need help to find that control.

In other cases, subtitles are embedded in the video permanently, but if learners want to hide them, they can slide the video window down so that the lower part with the text is off the desktop.

- Strategic training: *what* to do to support certain learning objectives, including how to link sequences of strategies (or techniques) into learning procedures. Lingual Net (http://www.lingual.net) for example, provides online video clips with subtitles and recommends watching first with subtitles off for main ideas and then again with subtitles on for details, followed by taking a comprehension quiz, and then watching a third time with the subtitles off again for enjoyment and reinforcement.

- Pedagogical training: determining specific learning objectives and understanding *why* to use certain techniques and procedures to achieve those objectives. This is parallel to the preceding principle "Give learners teacher training." For example, students are not only introduced to "pre-listening" as a strategy, but they are also told about how research in schema activation and top-down processing support this strategy, and why appropriate pre-listening activities can improve both comprehension and retention of new material.

While the first of these areas is unique to the computer environment, the last two can be connected with traditional notions of cognitive and metacognitive strategy training (Oxford, 1990). The main difference is that the notion of pedagogical training here emphasizes the value of understanding the basis for specific techniques and procedures so that informed choices can be made by the individual learner in the same way as a professionally prepared teacher would be making them for a class.

PILOT STUDY

In preparation for the present research, we conducted a pilot study in winter 2008 with a group of 8 students in our course, EFS 693B, Advanced Listening, to test the overall notion of pervasive learner training, along with some of the concepts and data collection procedures. For background, the course is taught each quarter through the English for Foreign Students Program (http://efs.stanford.edu) in the Stanford Language Center. All students are engaged in full-time graduate study: Some of them take this as a course that was required on the basis of an English placement exam taken at the beginning of their graduate study, while others take it voluntarily.

The pilot study was conducted during the final six weeks of the 10-week quarter. During that time, students used new techniques presented by the instructor and enthusiastically adopted many of the pedagogical concepts and strategies introduced. They reported an increased awareness of the listening process and an understanding of effective uses of resources. One surprising result of this study was a realization that students' goals for listening were quite diverse and not always focused on anything more than simple exposure and basic comprehension. Many were already engaged in good listening practices, but some reported rather interesting tendencies, such as an overreliance on text subtitles in their native language. The results of the study emphasized the importance of characterizing learner training so that it could accommodate changes both in students and technology. It also led to some changes in course content, such as increases in direct teaching of strategies, encouragement to engage in exploration, and reflective journaling.

MAIN STUDY: METHOD

The main study took place during the 10-week spring quarter of 2008 (April–June). The subjects were 14 students in two sections of EFS 693B, divided into a morning section (3 students) and an afternoon section (11 students: a 12th student in this section chose not to participate in the research). Students were from Korea, China, Taiwan, Japan, and the Philippines. Most had come to the US the previous September, and all but one (a foreign language instructor in the Language Center) were engaged in full-time graduate study, mainly in engineering degree programs.

There were three parts to the course: in-class listening practice, discussion, and learner training; class homework; and individual projects. The projects were negotiated with the student at the first individual meeting, allowing them to pick objectives and material types in line with their needs and interests. They were required to do a minimum of three 40-minute sessions per week and submit weekly reports specifying the objective, materials, time spent, procedures, and reflective comments (see Appendix 15.1).

The course introduced many techniques for improving listening comprehension, including pausing the media, slowing the playback speed, expanding the player size, doing background research for pre-listening, and listening to materials multiple times with different objectives for each pass. Other techniques were introduced for students to work specifically to improve their proficiency, including listening for meaning, written dictation, and oral summarization, as well as judicious choice of media.

We used a primarily qualitative approach embedded in an action research perspective. Both of the researchers have taught the course that was the setting of this study, and one was the instructor for the classes that contained the subjects. The study itself was undertaken partly in an attempt to improve instruction in the program, so it could very reasonably be categorized as action research, which McNiff (1996) defines as research undertaken by practitioners to improve their practice.

From the beginning, however, our goals extended beyond the particular classrooms where the study took place because our experiences have led us to believe that the implementation of learner training for CALL is something that should be happening much more commonly than is currently the case.

Our goal was to observe how much the techniques helped students improve their listening, or at least helped them positively change the way they interacted with online listening materials. Again, while the learning of the students in the class was always the main consideration in our actions, from the beginning, the study was designed so that the results could be informative for other situations. Specifically, we sought to answer the following questions:

1. What evidence is there that students are using materials reflectively?
2. What have we learned about our students as learners that could affect future training?
3. What evidence is there that students have learned enough to continue on their own?
4. What changes could be made next time?
5. Is the benefit worth the cost in teacher and student time?

Data were collected using a number of different instruments and procedures:

- Pre- and post-surveys. These aimed at characterizing students' current technical proficiency, their prior use of facilitative strategies when using technology for listening, and changes in these at the end of the course.
- Pre- and post-listening test. Students took a 50-item multiple-choice picture identification test as a measure of listening proficiency in weeks 2 and 10 of the 10-week course as a rough measure of progress.
- Individual meeting notes and videos (five per student). Students also met with the instructor for 30 minutes at a time on a biweekly basis (five total), where they would discuss their project activities and any areas where they felt they needed assistance. The first step of most interviews was to elicit a review of the immediately preceding meeting, report, or class session to see how much students remembered. Each subject was also specifically asked if they had decided to do anything different in their listening. During this discussion, suggestions for ways to improve were offered and, when warranted, demonstrated on the instructor's computer. One of the main points of these meetings was often a focus on organization: how to make time to practice listening, how to find resources, and how to use them more effectively. Time was also taken to review the weekly written reports. Finally, students were asked to actually engage with media they had used in order to observe and discuss their techniques and strategies. During this process, they were asked about their comprehension, any

special circumstances were discussed, and, if warranted, suggestions for improvement were made.

- Weekly student reports. Students typically set aside time three to seven days per week to work on individual listening projects. They had a set format for reporting on these sessions (see the Appendix 15.1 for an example), which they would submit weekly by e-mail.
- Notes for each class. These notes (at http://www.stanford.edu/~efs/693b-08) show what materials students were working on collectively in addition to their individual projects and the types and content of in-class training they were receiving.
- End of course interview. The researcher who was not the instructor conducted a 20–30 minute interview during the last week of the course to determine what points had been most memorable to the students.

Data were collected from the weekly reports and from instructor notes and videotapes of the biweekly meetings. Videos were encoded to files and were reviewed with a thorough playback, making written notes in line with categories in the weekly reports. Specific mention was noted of use of any of the techniques that were mentioned in the course. Of special interest were any realizations about specific techniques or about the process of listening in general. Also, since the purpose of the study was to help students improve the effectiveness of their listening practices, attention was given to any mention of changing behavior based on instructor feedback or personal realizations.

LEARNER TRAINING EXAMPLES

As noted earlier, the course was unusual in integrating CALL learner training centrally into the syllabus. A few examples may help make it clearer what that training included and how it was conducted. The full course notes are available at http://www.stanford.edu/~efs/693b-08/notes.html.

Listening Framework

As part of pedagogical training, students were introduced to the following simplified listening framework that distinguished the following types of listening activities, the first more focused on top-down processing, the second on bottom-up processing (Peterson, 2001), and the third on knowledge to underlie the first two.

Learning to Comprehend More Effectively

- Getting the basic meaning
- Retaining important points (notes and memory)

- Interpreting and integrating

Improving Processing

- Comprehending faster speech
- Comprehending a range of accents
- Making processing more automatic: improving accuracy, speed, and capacity

Increasing Language Knowledge

- Sound system (phonology): individual sounds, sound clusters and syllables, linking, reduction, rhythm, and intonation
- Vocabulary (words *and* phrases), including recognizing pronunciation of known items
- Grammar: recognizing the meaning in grammatical endings (like *-ing*), words (like prepositions and modal auxiliary verbs), and structures (like passive or present perfect)
- Discourse: typical organizational structures of lectures, newscasts, discussions, etc.; how speakers introduce and shift topics and comments

The students continued to reference this framework throughout the course in explaining the objectives of specific learning activities they engaged in during their independent listening projects.

Word Frequency for Vocabulary Learning

Many researchers have emphasized the value of word frequency lists in determining which words to devote time to learning (e.g., Nation, 1990). Students in the advanced listening course were introduced to the concept during the fourth week of the course by referencing the well-known General Service List and Academic Word List (Coxhead, 2000). They were subsequently taught and encouraged to run listening transcripts through Tom Cobb's online Vocabulary Profiler (British National Corpus version, which covers frequencies to the 20,000-word level: http://www.lextutor. ca/vp/bnc/), both to determine the lexical difficulty of the material and to identify candidates for learning, generally higher frequency words that they did not know.

Text Support

Locating and using material with text support (captions and/or transcripts) and learning various ways to use that support are important components of the course. The potential value of text support has been well documented in a number of studies (Danan, 2004; Grgurovic & Hegelheimer, 2007), and while concerns persist that this is a shortcut for students whose reading skills are stronger than listening skills, text support makes it much more feasible for our students to use the material independently to build vocabulary, explore grammar, and correct dictations.

Play Speed Control

Some modern media players have the ability to speed up or slow down the play speed of digital audio and video without distorting the sound frequencies in the way that changing the speed of a phonograph record or tape would. By slowing down speech to, say, 80 percent of normal, students are given some additional processing time without compromising the naturalness too severely. Research by Zhao (1997) and McBride (2007) supports the notion that when the learner has control of the speech rate, it can have a positive impact on comprehension. In our course, students are given both technical training on how to use the play speed control and reflective practice to help them determine when and when not to make use of it.

RESULTS AND DISCUSSION

This section reports on group trends and individual differences in the students based on the pre- and post-surveys, student reports, notes, videos from individual meetings, and a final interview. Pseudonyms are used when reporting an individual's data.

Pre-survey

Based on the pre-survey, students in the study had the following characteristics. Students were very comfortable with computers in general, with most selecting the highest level of "I use computers for almost everything I can." Besides lectures and presentations, most of their exposure to English was through authentic media, much of which was accompanied by text resources such as subtitles. Further, for online audio or video, more than half of the students reported manually adjusting the size of the player, indicating that one of the practices we thought was facilitative for learning was already being implemented by these digital natives (Prensky, 2001). Finally, the most common motivation for taking the course was by far a "personal desire to improve listening."

Student Reports and Individual Meetings

Evidence of reflective learning came directly from the weekly reports, which had prompts for stating objectives, procedures, and comments on their individual projects. This was corroborated in the notes taken during individual meetings and review of interview video files. Almost all students reported experimenting with listening, changing media speed, trying dictation, and reading transcripts or captions. Seven reported summarizing with some regularity and two reported regular shadowing (Tamai, 2002; discussed in the following). While some students were quite adventurous with their projects, most of them stuck with a relatively small set of techniques. Most students realized several concepts related to the difficulty of listening media. These realizations can be categorized into:

- Media characteristics: speech rate, audio quality, situation, speaker characteristics
- Memory considerations: clip length, clip familiarity, content familiarity
- Motivation: personal interest, frequency of listening, length of listening.

There is, of course, some overlap in these areas, but for the most part, this is how the instructor and the students identified them. Most students were then able to implement procedures that made use of these concepts to either enhance or challenge their comprehension of the media. The key was, of course, whether or not they were actually motivated to make the effort to challenge their comprehension.

Some students tried variations in each of these areas, as well as different combinations of them. For example, just looking at the main techniques of listening for meaning, written dictation, and oral summarization, almost every student tried these techniques at least once, changing the number of times they used each one per week. Students were also asked to preschedule their study sessions, and while some reported that they did stick to those schedules, several reported that they did not. During week seven, they also experimented with scheduling changes in their study habits, such as the frequency and length of listening sessions. The instructor specifically asked them to compare the effectiveness of six short study sessions of 20 minutes each with three longer sessions of 40 minutes each. The majority reported that they preferred shorter, more frequent sessions, because they felt that they learned more and were able to form better study habits. However, there were three students who felt that 20 minutes was just too short to cover the material in any satisfactory way. In fact, two students actually reported that six longer study sessions of 40 minutes each would have been optimal.

One driving force behind the techniques that students used was their varying individual goals. An interesting contrast can be seen in Chuck and Joe: Chuck reported experimenting with listening to one clip multiple times, reading the transcript, researching background information, shadowing, and dictation. He focused on vocabulary many times in his reports but reported moving from TV shows to news in the media he used because he found it more effective. Joe reported experimenting with most of the same techniques, except for pre-listening research, but added written summarization. In the end he reported preferring to use entertainment to informational media. In this sense, the goals of individual students played an important role in determining what techniques were effective for them. There were many cases of individuals who were ultimately looking for ways to improve their spoken English and would therefore gravitate to media that contained naturalistic native speech, such as TV shows. However, others who were more focused on listening comprehension found that news and other informational media was a much more useful resource.

Some students seemed to have used one particular technique of interest referred to as "shadowing." In most cases, this entails listening to prerecorded media (news or some other entertainment media) and simply following along, repeating the words and sentences that are heard. While there have been studies that show some benefit (Tamai, 2002), it is not clear under what conditions it actually enhances listening comprehension. Of the students who mentioned shadowing as a technique, two in particular explored it in some depth in their weekly listening activities. One of them, Nathan, reported a greater awareness of the processes involved in shadowing over time, and, while he did not stop using it, he used it less frequently. More interestingly, after reducing the amount of shadowing, he tried dictation as a way of increasing his involvement with the material.

Nathan's case can perhaps shed some light on students' gravitation to certain techniques. He had a new mp3 player and was in the habit of downloading podcasts and listening to them during the day. His personal situation also had an influence on his study techniques: He lived with his wife and newborn daughter and reported difficulty finding time to focus on listening outside of the early morning hours. In the end, he found that increasing the frequency of study times, while reducing the length, was the most productive plan for him. This case shows how some characteristics of group diversity develop: Commonalities in personal situations and commonalities in available equipment lead to a natural grouping. Although an instructor could dismiss such trends, saying familial status or purchasing habits should not be allowed to influence academic achievement, it could be argued that finding ways to accommodate such diversity is a much more effective way to reach a larger number of students.

Students in the process of understanding how to improve listening seemed to go through two levels, reflecting the training content. First, they began to realize exactly what made certain media difficult. Many were not exactly aware that characteristics such as the speech rate, content familiarity, and personal interest could be the source of not being able to understand. This realization was reflected in early reports and meetings of almost every subject. At the next level, they were able to implement techniques to make listening easier. These techniques were basically of two types: Some relied on using technology to change their experience with the media (such as slowing down the clip or toggling subtitles on and off), while others involved pedagogical choices that facilitated proficiency improvement (such as repetition and scheduling). For some students over time, these techniques seem to have become internalized and no longer thought of as outside of the listening process. In general, however, while the subjects in this study could be seen as "digital natives," most still do not really know how to use their familiarity with technology to improve their learning without being led through a process of training. For example, we have observed that most recent students in this course expand the media player for videos not because they want to exert greater control, but just because they want the picture to be bigger.

Understanding the process of listening is important in developing and using effective techniques. To a novice, speech media is just flowing sounds, with no footholds for comprehension. The first step is to distinguish familiar patterns and establish word boundaries, separating what can be understood from what cannot. Once these parts are identified, vocabulary issues can be tackled, but, as many students often pointed out, if they do not understand a set of words, it is impossible to look them up without a text reference. Students reported realizing how each individual technique could be used. For example, Marina noted that in multiple listening passes, the first pass is like a warm-up, while the technique of summarization tended to be an overview. Susan reported the more conventional position that reading an overview before listening increased her ability to predict and expect content.

Often, advanced learners such as these already have good listening and good learning practices. As noted earlier, these were assessed in the initial survey, but an interesting reaction to internalization was observed in one subject. In individual meetings, Sam reported reviewing media multiple times and was observed hiding captions, but when asked about techniques he used to improve listening comprehension or proficiency, he did not include these. His idea of a useful technique seemed to be limited to having websites that would test his comprehension, even though he was making use of what was covered in the training.

The topic of subtitles was a very important one for many students. For many foreign students, English media (both pirated and legitimate) is readily available online, and subtitles are so ubiquitous that it is difficult to avoid them. Instructors may encourage conscientious students not to look at them, and even seek out media that does not have subtitles or transcripts available. However, at the same time, it is difficult to ignore how much they help the comprehension process. In their individual projects, students explored this resource by reorganizing their listening, using techniques such as hiding subtitles or reading subtitles first and listening to a passage again. Most concluded that listening without them at least once but then using them to confirm meaning was the most effective strategy. One interesting case was Oliver, who found that the subtitles in the media he was using were not accurate, so he abandoned using them altogether.

Our findings indicate that, rather than ignoring them, it would serve both instructors and students well to identify methods of using (and not using) them to scaffold learning effectively.

Post-Survey and Exit Interview

In a post-survey, students were asked to rank six factors according to the roles that they played in helping them to understand media. The standard deviations of these rank orders showed that speed and number of times listening had the least variation and tended toward the highest end of the range. However, media type (news/movie/lecture), medium (computer/TV/live), and familiarity with content had a much higher variation among students. These results indicate that the only factors students agreed on were speed and number of times listening, indicating that there are large individual differences for other factors.

In order to get a better idea of how the students reacted to the goals of the course, exit interviews were conducted. Perhaps the most notable result of this interview was the extent to which the students gave insightful responses on their own learning processes. Of the 12 students interviewed, 10 gave responses that indicated that one of the most valuable things they learned in the course was a way to approach listening. Several students reported that they suddenly realized that what they had done in the past was simply listening for entertainment and could not really be categorized as an effort to improve their skills, but that, with a small amount of awareness and effort, they could transform those experiences into learning opportunities.

Cost Versus Benefit

As to costs, there is class time lost to training and collaborative debriefings, and student and instructor time in creating and responding to reports. These seem to be outweighed by the benefits. Students were tested at the beginning and end of the course with a 50-item picture identification instrument. The mean score on the pre-test was 59 percent and on the post-test, 70 percent, suggesting that substantial progress had been made (though the source of that progress cannot be confirmed in the absence of a control group). Most telling are the positive student impressions of their own progress and the reported desire from many to continue working independently using the techniques and procedures learned during the course.

CONCLUSION

It is not clear how well this pervasive approach would work with a skill other than listening, with less advanced students, or with students lacking a certain level of technical proficiency. In addition, the small number of participants, the specialized setting, and the fact that much of the data utilized was self-reported all suggest caution in generalizing these results. Nevertheless, for this group at least, the value of learner training appears to be supported. Based on the results reported here and the instructor's experience the following year, the course is being taught experimentally in the 2009–2010 academic year in a blended learning format, meeting just one day a week, with the other day replaced by additional online listening activities, both group and individual.

There are clearly many areas for further research indicated in this study. In particular, techniques such as shadowing, dictation, and oral summarization give varying degrees of useful practice, but it is not clear how these techniques work on a psycholinguistic level and under what conditions they would be most effective. While it may be obvious that the use of subtitles and transcriptions short-circuit the comprehension process, it is not clear how their interaction with audio and video media can be used to promote successful proficiency improvements. Finally, it is important to note that technology and students' familiarity with the tools used in learning are moving targets. For example, just between our pilot study and the main study, there was a large shift away from software media players to embedded Flash-generated players, which often eliminate learners' ability to change the size of the player to gain more control. Any approach to promoting effective teaching and learning must be based firmly on sound pedagogical principles to guide instructors and students in their decisions in an as yet unknown range of choices.

In addition to the specific results from our study, we hope to have shown that learner training is potentially a very important topic for the future. Online media, text as well as audio and video, are becoming more and more prevalent, with many universities now putting lectures on the Internet for a variety of reasons, including convenience. As students become more comfortable with the online environment, the time spent learning on their own increases, and it is important to guide them to effective study habits. Online materials can be just information, but especially for language learners, they can also be an especially effective way to improve proficiency.

REFERENCES

Barrette, C. (2001). Students' preparedness and training for CALL. *CALICO Journal*, *19*(1), 5–36.

Coxhead, A. (2000). A new academic word list. *TESOL Quarterly*, *34*(2), 213–238.

Danan, M. (2004). Captioning and subtitling: Undervalued language learning strategies. *Meta: Translator's Journal*, *49*(1), 67–77.

Grgurovic, M., & Hegelheimer, V. (2007). Help options and multimedia listening: Students' use of subtitles and the transcript. *Language Learning & Technology*, *11*(1), 45–66.

Hubbard, P. (2004). Learner training for effective use of CALL. In S. Fotos & C. Browne (Eds.), *New perspectives on CALL for second language classrooms* (pp. 45–67). Mahwah, NJ: Lawrence Erlbaum.

Kolaitis, M., Mahoney, M. A., Pomann, H., & Hubbard, P. (2006). Training ourselves to train our students for CALL. In P. Hubbard & M. Levy (Eds.), *Teacher education in CALL* (pp. 317–334). Amsterdam: John Benjamins.

McBride, K. (2007). *The effect of rate of speech and CALL design features on EFL listening comprehension and strategy use.* Unpublished doctoral dissertation, University of Arizona. Retrieved from http://www.slu.edu/~kmcbrid8/documentos/McBride.Diss.pdf

McNiff, J. (1996). *You and your action research project.* London: Hyde Publications.

Nation, I. S. P. (1990). *Teaching and learning vocabulary.* New York: Newbury House.

Oxford, R. L. (1990). *Language learning strategies: What every teacher should know.* New York: Newbury House.

Peterson, P. (2001). Skills and strategies for proficient listening. In M. Celce-Murcia (Ed.), *Teaching English as a second or foreign language* (3rd ed., pp. 87–100). Boston: Heinle.

Prensky, M. (2001). Digital natives, digital immigrants. *On the Horizon, 9*(5), 1–6.

Tamai, K. (2002). On the effects of shadowing on listening comprehension—Keynote lecture at the 3rd Annual Conference of JAIS. *Interpretation Studies, 2,* 178–192.

Winke, P., & Goertler, S. (2008). Did we forget someone? Students' computer access and literacy for CALL. *CALICO Journal, 25*(3), 482–509.

Zhao, Y. (1997). The effects of listeners' control of speech rate on second language comprehension. *Applied Linguistics, 18*(1), 49–68.

APPENDIX 15.1 EXAMPLE STUDENT REPORT

EFS 693B Independent Project Report #3
Name: xxxx
Date: 5/4/2008
General objectives: To improve listening for meaning

Session	Objective	Materials	Date/Time	Procedure	Comments
1	Listening for meaning	Video Arcade http://www.englishbaby.com/lessons/4516/real_life/video_arcade	5/01/08 20:00–20:30	Listen first, and take the quiz. Listen again to find the points I missed previously. Finally find the new words.	In this class, there are several new words about video games, but I am not familiar with them.
2	Dictation	Hunting http://www.elllo.org/english/0851/T881–Jake-Hunting.htm	5/02/08 19:30–20:10	Take the dictation for several parts of the conversation.	Since elllo is comparatively easier in terms of speed of speech, it is a good material for me to take the dictation.
3	Listening for meaning	Trouble in Paradise http://www.englishbaby.com/lessons/4517/eavesdropping/trouble_in_paradise	5/03/08 21:00–21:25	Listen first and take quiz. Read the transcript to find the new phrases and finally listen for several times to figure out the new phrases.	Since I have already been familiar with this soap opera (relationship between the actors and actress), it become much easier for me understand their conversation.
4	Build vocabulary	It's Raining Men http://www.english-baby.com/lessons/4432/eavesdropping/it_s_raining_men	5/04/08 9:00–9:20	Read the transcript first, find the new words, and listen to the conversation.	Finding the new words first will help me to concentrate on the part containing them, and make it easier to understand the meaning.
5	Listening for meaning	Broken Bulb http://www.englishbaby.com/lessons/4350/eavesdropping/broken_bulb	5/04/08 9:20–9:50	Listen to the conversation, take the quiz. Find new words. And finally listen for several times to try to understand everything.	Since this class does have too many new words, it is comparatively easier, but I should care about the meaning outside their conversation.

Ideas for next week: keep on improving the ability to listen for meaning.

16 Guiding the E-Learner in Foreign Language and Communication Courses

Maija Tammelin, Berit Peltonen, and Pasi Puranen

INTRODUCTION

The use of various e-learning modes has increased considerably in foreign language and communication courses in higher education in recent years. In this chapter we use the term "e-learning" as an umbrella term for various ways of using computers and the Internet for learning (cf. Littlejohn & Pegler, 2007); consequently, the terms *e-learner*, *e-teacher*, and *e-tutor* are used. The two e-learning modes that this chapter is mainly based on are those of blended learning and online learning. We use the term *e-teacher* in connection with blended learning and the term *e-tutor* when reference is made to online courses. By *blended learning* we mean courses that use a mix of approaches ranging from classroom teaching to a variety of uses of technology, whereas by *online courses* we refer to courses that take place exclusively online, whether the students attending the course live at a distance or are campus-based. Even our online courses, however, include one mandatory kickoff session in class at the start of the course.

While the e-learning options are becoming a regular part of the language curricula, it seems that the emphasis on the teacher and the teacher's role is being shifted onto the role of the learner. Consequently, the crucial role of guidance in e-learning is being increasingly recognized (see, e.g., ODLAC, 2008a, 2008b, 2008c). As a result of these developments, language teachers are facing the challenge of guiding their e-learners as effectively as possible in order to help them get the most out of their learning experience. Although it seems that in many parts of the world the "net generation" (Oblinger & Oblinger, 2005) is competent in using the media and new technologies, especially in connection with their outside school activities, such competencies do not automatically make the "digital natives" (Prensky, 2005–2006) efficient e-learners. E-learners, therefore, need to be provided with sufficient and effective guidance and training.

In 2007 the Department of Languages and Communication at Helsinki School of Economics launched a collaborative project on the guidance of e-learners (Peltonen, Puranen, & Tammelin, 2007, September) for the purpose of enhancing language learners' e-learning skills. The main aims of our chapter are (a) to present the components of effective guidance that we identified as a result of our collaborative project, (b) to give practical tips to e-learners and e-tutors, (c) to present an example of how guidance is provided in one of the department's blended learning courses, and (d) to give recommendations to teacher trainers and institutions providing language education.

COMPONENTS OF EFFECTIVE GUIDANCE

We carried out the department's guidance project from 2007 to 2009. It was a collaborative project in which we used as our main data the following: learner feedback, our archived course logs and materials, our own observations and experiences in our own blended learning courses in Spanish and Swedish, and English-language online courses in Academic Writing, Managerial Writing, and Communication for Corporate Social Responsibility. On the basis of our data we first defined what we meant by *effective guidance* and what we regarded as its aims. We found good guidance to consist of the following three main points: giving time, attention, and respect to the learners. The main aims of guidance are to improve and maintain the learners' motivation, to empower the learners, and to reduce the number of possible course dropouts. We see that guidance provided to e-learners includes four main components that center on the following issues: (a) orientation for e-learning, (b) e-learning skills and the roles of the e-learner, (c) the roles of the e-teacher/e-tutor, and (d) guidance for interaction, peer reviewing, and utilizing feedback.

Maintaining the learners' motivation until the end of an e-learning course plays a central role in guidance. This needs to be taken into account in all course-related activities, starting from planning the course and its learning tasks to providing the students with final feedback. Compared with traditional classroom teaching, motivating e-learners presents different types of challenges. A central factor in motivating learners and creating a positive atmosphere is the tutor's consistent presence online. The tutor can be present in many different ways and sometimes even a small "sign of life" can make the learner feel that he/she has not been left alone. For creating a sense of presence the tutor can use, for instance, short messages sent to all participants, a discussion forum, chat, a blog, or even different kinds of color codes in learners' assignments. The fact that the tutor is present by observing, commenting, encouraging, and, if needed, also by reminding and criticizing, has a direct impact on how the learners' motivation and interest in learning can be maintained throughout the e-learning course. As for maintaining motivation, it is also important to plan the assignments so that longer assignments, in particular, can be completed through smaller subtasks or sections on which the tutor can give feedback and guidance to learners and thus boost the learners' learning process during the entire course.

One useful practical tool for following up on the learners' learning processes is a blog-type online learning diary. For instance, the tutor can guide the writing of the diary, when needed, with the help of analytical questions to the learners. In this way the tutor can encourage the learners to reflect on their own learning processes and receive immediate student feedback on the online assignments. The digital learning diary can be individual or, for instance, shared with a pair or a small group, in which case the diary enters a peer dimension and can therefore offer new and different perspectives into learning.

With the help of guiding comments, feedback, reflection, and questions to the learners—along with overall strong online presence—the tutor not only strengthens the learners' learning process and increases the learners' motivation but also makes his/her own pedagogical thinking visible and makes the objectives of the course assignments more transparent for the learners. This meta-cognitive guidance is important from the perspective of how the learners experience the meaningfulness of the assignments. This again affects the learners' motivation and thereby the functioning and success of the whole course.

Orientation for E-Learning

Learners need to have a clear idea of what to expect from an e-learning course. Does the course take place fully online, or is the course format a blended one consisting of a mix of approaches, activities, and use of e-tools? It is important to ensure that all course participants have the basic information and communication technology (ICT) skills needed for studying in an e-learning course. Some learners may need guidance in improving even their basic ICT skills. The face-to-face course kickoff session is highly important for providing instructions for studying in an e-learning course, be it a blended learning or an online course. The kickoff session is also important for creating a sense of belonging to the group and a positive atmosphere.

The tutor can contribute to the learners' orientation to the course by being in touch with the learners even before course commencement, in connection with the enrollments or by opening up the course site in advance. The tutor can send various written messages, use the discussion forum, or send video clips or sound greetings to the course participants. The main challenges for the tutor at the beginning of the course include presenting and stressing the following: (a) the course aims and sub-aims, (b) the idea of autonomous learning and the importance of the course timetable and deadlines, and (c) the importance of a positive learning environment.

E-Learning Skills and the Roles of an E-Learner

E-learners need guidance to make them aware of the skills they need and how their roles as e-learners may differ from their traditional classroom roles. An e-learner is able to:

- communicate effectively in an online environment
- be aware of his/her own e-learning skills: to set goals for oneself, to evaluate one's learning outcomes
- control his/her own self-motivation
- work autonomously within a given timetable
- work alone and in a group
- avoid superficial learning and aimless "surfing" on the Internet.

After identifying the e-learning skills required from e-learners, we came up with the following examples of guidance that can be given directly to e-learners as practical tips:

- Mark down the deadlines of the assignments in your calendar/cell phone. Make yourself a realistic timetable after you have read the assignments and received the teacher's instructions. Observe the deadlines and remove the unnecessary activities from your calendar before the deadlines.
- Be aware of your personal time-management skills; don't make your timetable too tight.
- Concentration is important when you work on the assignments; keep your thoughts away from issues not requiring your immediate attention. Avoid useless surfing on the net.
- The basis for the ability to concentrate is that you know why and for what purpose you are studying. Not being sufficiently aware of the objectives is often the reason for the problems with managing your time. Make the objectives of your learning clear to yourself.

The Roles of an E-Teacher/E-Tutor

In order to be able to provide effective guidance, the e-tutor needs to be aware of his/her own role in the learner's learning and study process. Ideally, an e-tutor should be able to serve as a model of an exemplary e-learner. The tutor should be able to take on many different roles, including the roles of an advisor and a supporter of the learners' study goals, a motivator and coach, a "personal trainer," a producer of content when needed, and very importantly, a creator of a positive and supportive atmosphere (Tammelin, Peltonen, & Puranen, 2009, June).

The online tutor's central skills also include the ability to "listen" and find meaning in what the learners have to say on the net. The online tutor can promote, in many different ways, the learners' learning process so they can reach their learning goals. If the learner meets with obstacles or problems regarding the assignment or his/her own learning, the tutor can help by giving clear instructions or guiding the learner through questions that can help the learner find the answers him/herself. The tutor also often needs to address learners' negative feelings on the net. They can be related to the assignments, fellow learners, or the tutor. The tutor's "first-aid" kit can include listening to and sympathizing with the learners' problems. Sometimes even sleeping overnight can help restore the learner's ability to behave sensibly and even out the biggest outbursts of emotion.

After identifying the e-learning skills required from e-teachers/e-tutors, we came up with the following examples of guidance that can be given as practical tips:

- Estimate the workload on the learners required by the assignments and indicate the average time needed for completing the assignments.
- Try to make the instructions for the assignments as clear as possible so that the materials and the tools for completing the assignments are easily accessible on the net.
- Make sure you can be reached for questions and can respond within a reasonable time. When the deadline approaches, be prepared to guide your students even at short notice.
- Remind your learners with sufficient lead time and frequently of the assignment deadlines by using different digital media.
- Give your learners a model timetable in which you indicate what the learner should have completed by which dates so that the assignments will be ready on time.
- Reserve enough time for commenting on the learners' assignments and giving meaningful feedback.
- Always keep in mind that you, as the tutor, are a model of a good online learner for your learners.

Interaction, Peer Reviewing, and Feedback

As interaction and e-communication can still be difficult for some learners, they may need guidance for coping with different forms and channels of interaction such as discussion forums, chat, group tasks, social media, and so on. E-learners also need guidance to carry out their peer review assignments as these reviews play an important role in most online and blended learning courses. Furthermore, learners need guidance for utilizing tutor and peer feedback.

CASE: SWEDISH FOR BUSINESS

In this section we present a blended learning course called Swedish for Business as an example of how guidance is provided in a course. The starting level of the language proficiency of the students attending the course is B1 in accordance with the European Framework (Common European Framework of Reference for Languages [CEFR], 2007). The course lasts for seven weeks. The contact hours in class are used for oral presentations, and all written work is conducted in an online environment. The total amount of course work for the students is calculated as 80 hours.

The requirement for performing the oral exercises successfully in class is that the students have mastered the needed business vocabulary. The course handout includes texts and related exercises on different business topics such as accounting, commerce, marketing, and banking. Although the learners study the texts by themselves, the teacher guides them to independent learning with his/her online comments on the texts.

The learner can also turn to the teacher with his/her questions about the texts. The learners place the written assignments in their digital folders and the teacher checks and comments on them. After each topic has been addressed, the learners complete one individual assignment and a topic-related vocabulary test. The course site also offers additional material related to the topics in the form of video clips and other written material. In this way the teacher tries to make sure that the learner knows enough topic-related vocabulary when the topic is addressed by the oral presentations.

The course participants are divided into small groups that set up their own companies for which they create their own websites. The participants then give oral presentations about their companies in class. The material to be presented must be online a couple of days before the oral presentation so that the teacher can correct the most blatant errors in the presentation material. After the oral presentation in class, the learners discuss the content of the presentation; in other words, the learners use the vocabulary that they have learned.

The teacher's feedback and guidance is sent to the learners individually as a sound file after the classroom presentation. The learners have their own folders for individual assignments and feedback. This system also functions as a kind of learning diary. The learner can improve his/her oral presentation by practicing his/her pronunciation and intonation on the department's Karaoke Language Center website, which is a website meant for self-study. It contains video clips in which the teacher reads texts related to different business topics and the learner can practice reading the texts by imitating the teacher's model voice. The learner can practice reading the texts in advance for as long as possible because the "video teacher" does not get tired of speaking. The course ends in job interviews during which the learners apply for a job in their peers' companies. The more active the company has been, the more applications they will have received. After the interviews, the companies publish the names of those who were appointed for the open jobs. Being appointed equals direct positive feedback from the peers.

After successfully completing this course, the learners can choose another elective blended learning Swedish course in which they study in specific topic-related groups in collaboration with another group of students from another Finnish university. The groups communicate with each other via video-conferencing and the use of a Learning Management System (LMS) platform. Various net meeting tools are used for conducting this collaboration and a video annotation tool called Victor is used for giving feedback. With the help of Victor, the students comment on both their own group's meetings and the other groups' negotiations that have been carried out via video-conferencing. The groups produce final reports on their topics (e.g., related to finance, marketing, business law, stock market) in collaboration with their team members.

The Helsinki group's members also participate in a full-day conference meant for the students attending Swedish courses in universities in the Helsinki region and they make excursions to companies that operate mainly in Swedish in Finland. The students report on these visits in the course blog. Not only does the teacher comment on the blog, but the students often refer to other students' writings in their own texts. Commenting is always more active the more interesting the student's writing is. The students also follow the news about the Swedish economy from online newspapers and journals in addition to the news video clips available on the net. The students write about at least one topic per week, and they also need to comment on at least one other student's text. Again, the more interesting the student's writing, the more comments it receives from peers. The teacher gives weekly feedback on the writings. The teacher's summary contains instructions for improving language structures, comments on the content, and possible links to extra materials. As in the previous course, the students place their individual feedback in their own folders, and this feedback thus functions as their own learning diary. At the end of the course, the student evaluates his/her course performance with the help of a digital matrix and places the evaluation in his/her personal folder. The teacher uses the same evaluation matrix and compares the two evaluations. In general, based on the feedback the student has received during the course, the students have a rather realistic idea of their proficiency in written and oral Swedish. They tend to underestimate their skills rather than overestimate them.

Because of the short duration of the course (seven weeks) and the amount of intensive course work the course involves, the participants need a great deal of teacher guidance and feedback. The teacher's work starts the moment he/she receives the enrollment lists one week before the start of the course and continues long after the course. The teacher gives guidance *before* the course regarding course information and practical instructions. Guidance *during* the course is related to technical support and the students' learning process. Guidance and feedback *after* the course focus on evaluating the learning outcomes and raising the students' awareness of their needs for lifelong learning. The Swedish for Business course has shown that students appreciate guidance that includes individual (especially) oral online feedback as well as regular, up-to-date, and critical feedback.

IMPLICATIONS FOR LANGUAGE EDUCATION
PROVIDERS AND TEACHER TRAINING

The aspects of guidance that we identified as the result of our collaborative project need to be recognized not only by the e-teachers and e-tutors themselves but also by the teacher trainers who prepare new language teachers for their professions that nowadays also require teaching skills in e-learning environments. Many current language and communication teachers involved with blended learning and online teaching feel that their workloads have increased. Therefore, they may not welcome any more pressure that would increase their availability in the capacity of an "omnipresent," "ubiquitous" guide. Finding a balance between the increased need for effective and efficient guidance and the teacher's/tutor's possibility to provide it is therefore challenging. Technology can help meet this challenge if institutions providing language education recognize that teachers need to be provided with institutional support (e.g., technical support and training—see Tammelin, 2004), which often is insufficient. Teachers may not even have knowledge of or access to the use of new versatile e-tools for giving guidance and feedback for their e-learners.

CONCLUSION

In this chapter we have addressed the important role of guidance for e-learners in language and communication learning and presented the results of our collaborative guidance project. The data for the project were collected from our blended learning courses in Spanish and Swedish and English-language online courses in Academic Writing, Managerial Writing, and Communication for Corporate Social Responsibility. The data consisted of learner feedback, our course logs, and our own observations and experiences. In this chapter we presented the components and main aims of effective guidance along with practical tips for e-learners and e-teachers/e-tutors. Finally, we described one blended learning language course in detail as an example of how guidance is given throughout that particular course.

The results and recommendations arising from our project are based on practical evidence rather than theory. Therefore, more elaborate research is required, especially into the role of guidance in e-learning and, in particular, interaction between the learner and the teacher/tutor.

REFERENCES

Common European Framework of Reference for Languages. (2001). Retrieved from http://www.coe.int/t/dg4/linguistic/CADRE_EN.asp

238 Maija Tammelin, Berit Peltonen, and Pasi Puranen

Littlejohn, A., & Pegler, C. (2007). *Preparing for blended learning*. London: Routledge.
Oblinger, D., & Oblinger, J. (2005). *Educating the net generation*. Retrieved from http://www.educause.edu/educatingthenetgen
ODLAC. (2008a). *Institutions' guide*. Retrieved from http://www.elearningguides.net
ODLAC. (2008b). *Learners' guide*. Retrieved from http://www.elearningguides.net
ODLAC. (2008c). *Teachers' guide*. Retrieved from http://www.elearningguides.net
Peltonen, B., Puranen, P., & Tammelin, M. (2007, September). *Guiding through aligning: Models and practices for online teachers and learners*. Poster session presented at EUROCALL 2007 Conference, University of Ulster, Coleraine, Northern Ireland.
Prensky, M. (2005–2006). Listen to the natives. *Educational Leadership, 63*(4), 8–13. Retrieved from http://www.ascd.org/authors/ed_lead/el200512_prensky.html
Tammelin, M. (2004). *Introducing a collaborative network-based learning environment into foreign language and business communication teaching: Action research in Finnish higher education. Media Education Publications 11. Department of Applied Sciences of Education. University of Helsinki.* Helsinki: Yliopistopaino. Retrieved from http://www.helsinki.fi/~tella/mep11.html
Tammelin, M., Peltonen, B., & Puranen, P. (2009, June). *The role of the ubiquitous tutor in fostering independent learning*. Paper presented at the Independent Learning Association Conference, Hong Kong.

Part V
Teacher Education

17 The Use of ICTs in Foreign Language Teaching

The Challenges of a Teachers' Education Program

Carla Barsotti and Claudia Martins

INTRODUCTION

Contemporary society is in a process of great change; people presently have access to a myriad of technologies, from small daily use objects to sophisticated computers and electronic gadgets. Information and communication technologies (ICTs) play an important role in this context. As pointed out by Kenski (1993) and Moraes (1997), they provide fast and easy access to information, allowing people to follow the changes of a world in permanent evolution. The influence of these resources on education cannot be ignored. Bringing these resources to the school environment is a way of enriching classroom activities, bringing them closer to the students' reality and making them more meaningful for the students. It is imperative for teachers to incorporate the use of technologies in their classroom practice in order to create a learning environment adequate for the students' needs.

In Brazil, a country where the majority of the population does not have access to any kind of ICTs, there are some teachers who are constantly looking for professional growth and are willing to overcome the difficulties that may arise on the way. There are many aspects involved in teaching foreign languages, but the focus of this investigation was the profile of foreign language teachers and some of the issues concerning the integration of ICTs in their everyday teaching. This chapter presents the results of two concomitant surveys conducted with foreign language teachers who attended CELEM—*Curso de Especialização em Ensino de Línguas Estrangeiras Modernas*—the Specialization in Foreign Language Teaching Course at Federal University of Technology, Paraná (UTFPR), which is the first technological university in Brazil. The main objectives of this chapter were to investigate the teachers' profiles and also their ICT knowledge, experiences, and skills development. The goal was to offer one specific example of research whose results may provide course developers with insights for improving teachers' education programs.

We will provide first an overview of education and foreign language teaching in Brazil, followed by a description of the graduate course in which the research took place. Then we will present the first survey, about the foreign language teachers' profile, and the second about the relationship between foreign language teachers and the use of ICTs.

THE BRAZILIAN FOREIGN LANGUAGE TEACHING CONTEXT

The 1996 Educational Guidelines and Directives Law

Until 1996 Brazilian states could decide when and how a foreign language would become part of the primary school syllabus. In 1996 the Brazilian government, with the support of the Ministry of Education, approved the Educational Guidelines and Directives Law (LDB—*Leis de Diretrizes e Bases da Educação Nacional*), which divided education into preschool education for 0–6-year-olds, not compulsory; basic education, which comprises primary education (first through ninth grades), compulsory for children from 7 to 14 years old; and secondary education (first through third grades) (Lei no. 9:394, 1996). After secondary education the students may apply for higher education and continue their studies.

The 1996 LDB determined that at least one foreign language must be taught from fifth grade upwards, with the choice of language to be left to the school and the local community according to the capacity of the institution. A second foreign language should be offered in secondary school wherever possible, and again the choice is up to the school and the community. It is advisable that the choice of second language offered should take into account the diversity of local demands, the cultural background[1] of the people in the area, and work market needs, once the learners may look for positions in the area.

Also according to the LDB, special classes can be created in order to develop specific subjects like foreign languages and some others. These special groups are characterized as extracurricular activity groups, where students with a similar level of knowledge, but sometimes at different ages and from different school grades, are taught together.

Nevertheless, due to the small number of hours and unprepared teachers who sometimes have only superficial knowledge of the subject matter and poor pedagogical skills, the foreign language classes—instead of preparing the students to achieve an overall proficiency—turned into reading classes where the main objective is to decode written passages to answer tests. This situation made the students, whose families could afford it, look for private language institutes and courses that offer better prepared teachers and usually bring the desired results.

The National Curriculum Parameters
(PCNs) and the 2005 Spanish Law

In order to guide the teaching of different subjects the National Council for Education then created the National Curriculum Parameters (PCN) (Ministério da Educação [MEC], 1999), which suggests some procedures for specific subject areas.

For the Languages, Codes, and its Technologies area, where foreign languages are inserted, the document emphasizes the practical character that foreign language teaching should have, once languages are now recognized as fundamental for human communication. Of course, languages are the means to get information, and to get in contact with different ways of thinking, feeling, and conceiving reality. The parameters suggest, among other things, that the learner should be prepared for choosing the appropriate register, and for recognizing and using verbal and nonverbal strategies for communication. Besides that, the student should know the foreign languages and use them as access tools for getting information about the world and other cultures (MEC, 1999).

Having foreign languages inserted in one area implies that they are no longer isolated topics. Rather, they are integrated with the other curricular disciplines demanding interdisciplinary activities in language classes, that is, activities that allow the learners to communicate in an adequate way when dealing with a myriad of topics in different situations.

In 2005 a new law came into force making it mandatory for schools to offer Spanish-language classes. The intention of the Ministry of Education is to make Spanish available to all students in secondary school. It may also be included, optionally, in the full curriculums of primary school (fifth through eighth grades). According to this law, the Spanish language must be offered by the regular school system during normal school hours, but student registration is optional. The idea was to implant it gradually in the full curriculums of senior secondary school within five years from the publication of the law. The law also emphasizes the need for implanting Foreign Language Centers whose programs must necessarily include Spanish (Lei no. 11.161, 2005).

Although the law intended to make Spanish an option or to add a second modern language to the curriculum, some schools have divided the English classes' hours in half in order to include Spanish classes.

Public and Private Schools and Foreign Language Teachers

In Brazil there are public schools (state, municipal, or federal) that are free of charge, and private schools that charge the students a substantial fee. Unfortunately, this is not the only difference, since there is also a belief that the quality of teaching is usually better in the private sector. To teach in the public school system, teachers are required to have a university degree in the subject they intend to teach. Besides that, there is a public examination with written tests and curriculum vitae analysis. For foreign language teachers there is also a specific language test and some questions on foreign language teaching methods.

Foreign language teaching, both in private and public schools, is believed to be ineffective for real communication because the classes are usually oriented to teaching reading. Both public and private schools can have their Foreign Language Centers where the teaching of a foreign language can be a more complete experience, preparing the learners for real communication.

Private language institutes are another important option for learning foreign languages in Brazil. According to Walker (2005, p. 40), "Brazil is remarkable for its enormous and highly developed private language institute sector [. . .] outside the normal educational structure." These institutes offer a variety of programs such as semi-intensive, intensive, immersion, and special courses that can be taught to small groups or on a one-to-one basis.

The most popular foreign language taught in Brazil is English, followed by Spanish and some others like French, German, and Italian. Among undergraduate modern language students English is by far the most popular major. Nevertheless, due to some poor university programs, there is in Brazil a lack of qualified professionals for teaching all foreign languages: It is not uncommon for schools and language institutes to have difficulties in finding such professionals. So as a strategy for improving the teaching of foreign languages in Brazil it is essential for foreign language teachers to continue their studies and training.

CELEM

UTFPR is a regular institution that offers technical, undergraduate, and graduate courses besides extension courses for the community. In teacher education one of the courses offered is CELEM.

CELEM is a *lato sensu*[2] course created in 2004 as a result of the perception that in Curitiba, Paraná, there were no specialized courses for foreign language teachers once they graduated, other than *stricto sensu*[3] programs, which are usually longer and require a deeper knowledge in the field. The course is intended to help develop participants' critical views about foreign language teaching and also to inspire and motivate scientific academic research. The goals of such a course are to offer participants an opportunity to develop their understanding of the processes involved in foreign language teaching and also to acquaint them with new methods and technologies available for improving such processes. CELEM also promotes the exchange of knowledge and experiences in the area, fostering the development of research and studies. This theoretical and practical knowledge aims at the improvement of teaching through the pedagogical development of foreign language teachers.

To take part in such a course the candidates must hold a university degree, not necessarily in the foreign language teaching area, and preferably work or have experience in foreign language teaching. It is expected that candidates have already mastered the foreign language they teach or are willing to teach. The selection criteria include a thorough analysis of candidates' curriculum vitae, undergraduate course report, and compatibility with the course research areas.

The course program was designed to enable foreign language teachers to improve and broaden their knowledge, complementing their academic formation. It was originally planned for 360 hours of classes, which are both theoretical and practical. Among the subjects taught are Neuropsychology, Linguistics, Intercultural Issues, Literature, Foreign Language Teaching Methodology, Technology in Foreign Language Teaching, and Assessment. To receive the specialist certification the students must complete the course and also write a monographic work on a course-related theme.

THE SURVEYS

Considering the aforementioned information the following questions about the foreign language teachers enrolled in CELEM were framed:

- Who are they: What is their academic background, age, and how long have they been teaching?
- Do these teachers have enough knowledge to incorporate technologies in their teaching?

In order to answer the questions two surveys were conducted with CELEM's participants at UTFPR at two different points. Survey 1 aimed at identifying the academic and professional background of the participant teachers as well as some of their personal data. This survey has been conducted every year, since the first offering of CELEM in 2004, in the first discipline of the course, Foreign Language Teaching: Methodology and Techniques. Survey 2 aimed at identifying how much the course participants knew about ICTs and what basic abilities they had. It has been taking place since 2006 during the discipline Technology in Foreign Language Teaching.

Survey 1: The Foreign Language Teachers

The students were selected to CELEM through some specific criteria, as previously discussed. However, it was noticed that they seemed to have very different backgrounds, both academic and professional. According to André (2002), teachers are beings who keep on building values and beliefs, and they act according to some personal characteristics that distinguish them from each other. With that in mind, we sought to identify some of the features of the foreign language teachers who had enrolled at CELEM searching for professional and academic development.

In order to determine the profile of the aforementioned teachers, from 2004 to 2006 a documental investigation was conducted through the analysis of their curriculum vitae and application forms as a way of collecting data for this survey. The information collected was mostly about gender, age, academic background, professional background, and foreign languages taught. To obtain a broader and deeper picture, in 2007 a questionnaire was elaborated.

The questionnaire incorporated the topics previously obtained through the documental investigation mentioned earlier and also included some items partially based on the Teacher Self-Observation Form, adapted by Brown (2001). It aimed at looking in detail at the academic and professional backgrounds of CELEM's participants, as well as identifying their beliefs concerning the teaching and learning of foreign languages. It was completed by the 2007 and 2008 CELEM participants. The questionnaire was organized in two different sections. The first was about the participants' academic preparation concerning knowledge of the foreign language and pedagogical principles, international certificates obtained, specific training received, work experience, and self professional image. The questions and items in this part were open-ended, which enabled participants to write freely about the topics. In the second section of the questionnaire the participants were asked to check the alternatives they considered truthful from a list of 15 statements. The statements were about teachers' and students' classroom behavior, foreign language learning and teaching beliefs, methodological principles, teaching techniques, the LDB, and the PCN. The questionnaire was used as a first-day classroom activity. After completing the second part of the questionnaire the students were expected to carry on a brief group discussion to explain their positions and opinions on the topics.

It was noticed that when answering the questionnaire, despite having been told that the activity was an icebreaker, some participants did not feel at ease and were worried about providing correct and appropriate answers. The influence of the students' reaction on the final results was not investigated, since it was unexpected. This issue deserves further investigation.

Results

In the five years (2004–2008) there were 126 students enrolled, being 17 percent male and 83 percent female. This reinforces a Brazilian cultural belief that teaching, especially the teaching of foreign languages, is mostly a feminine career, with low salaries frequently not enough to support a family (Santos, 2008). The participants' ages ranged from 23 to 61. Nevertheless, most of them were in three different age groups: 35 percent were between 21 and 30; 33 percent were between 31 and 40; and 26 percent were between 41 and 50; with 6 percent older than 51.

Despite the fact that all CELEM participants work or intend to work in the area of foreign languages, 74 percent had majored in Languages and 26 percent majored in areas such as Psychology, Journalism, Engineering, and others. In Brazil, private language institute teachers are not always required to hold a language degree: Sometimes a degree is not needed for someone to be hired to work as a teacher. About half of the participants (52 percent) had been working in the area for about five years by the time the questionnaire was answered; 22 percent had been working for between 6 and 10 years; 9 percent between 11 and 15 years; 8 percent between 16 and 20 years; and the others (9 percent) had been working for between 21 and 35 years.

It was determined that English was by far the most commonly taught foreign language, totaling 76 percent of all participants. As for the other participants, 12 percent taught Spanish, 9 percent French, 7 percent Portuguese, 4 percent German, 4 percent Italian, and 1 percent Japanese. It should be noticed that the addition of these percentages will result in a figure higher than 100 percent due to the fact that some participants were teaching more than one foreign language.

In the years 2007 and 2008, a total of 56 participants answered the questionnaire. In the open-ended section it was found that 55 percent of the participants had experienced the language in a foreign country, while 45 percent had not. Concerning the reasons for pursuing foreign language teaching as a profession the participants mentioned: like teaching (32 percent); enjoy interacting with people (30 percent); like the foreign language (21 percent); identify with the foreign culture (20 percent); want to share their experience of foreign language learning (11 percent); and lack of routine (9 percent).

Table 17.1 illustrates what statements, from the second section of the questionnaire, the participants considered truthful.

It is important to explain here that the statements in Table 17.1 were chosen to provoke discussion and debate among participants. During their discussion it was noticed that some of the participants, even some of those who checked item 9, were not familiar with the law (LDB) or the parameters (PCNs). Item 10 stood out with 100 percent of the participants agreeing that the teacher may have great influence on students' motivation and this can influence both the teaching and learning of a foreign language.

Table 17.1   Survey 1 Questionnaire Results: Students Who Think the Statements Are Truthful

STATEMENTS	TRUTHFUL
1. The foreign language teacher must have a near-native knowledge of the language.	70%
2. S/he is responsible for the students learning and for their attitude towards learning.	50%
3. S/he must always correct all errors and mistakes the students make.	12%
4. Learning is a result of teaching.	30%
5. Teaching can be assessed taking into consideration what the students learn.	62%
6. The teacher must choose one best methodology to use in class.	46%
7. Teachers do consider the methodological characteristics when planning their classes.	66%
8. When the institution authorities impose a methodology to be used there is standardization.	50%
9. The foreign language teachers are prepared for using in class what the National Curriculum Parameters (PCNs) suggest.	18%
10. There are ways to guarantee that the students' foreign language knowledge will be about the same in the whole country.	11%
11. The choice of a good book guarantees successful classes.	7%
12. A class plan is important for a successful class.	63%
13. There is no need of planning for the experienced teacher, neither when the school nor when the textbook provide a class plan.	4%
14. A class plan must be strictly followed.	5%
15. The teacher may have great influence on his students' motivation and this can influence both the teaching and learning of a foreign language.	100%

Survey 2: The Teachers from the Sample and the ICTs—Results and Analysis

With the introduction of the discipline Technology in Foreign Language Teaching in CELEM in 2004, it was noticed that not all teachers taking the discipline were able to do certain basic tasks with some ICTs: The group was made up of teachers with different levels of ICT knowledge. The same happened in 2005. There was a need to try to identify how much the course participants knew about ICTs, and what basic abilities they had.

A questionnaire was then prepared based on Davies' ICT "can do" lists (2006). According to Davies, foreign language teachers who want to integrate ICTs into their teaching should be familiar with the Windows operating system and a series of other software applications. He lists 19 applications, and for each there is a range of essential tasks that teachers should be able to carry out to feel comfortable working with that software. Davies selected the tasks and applications according to their usefulness for teaching foreign languages. In order to adapt and use the lists, Davies was contacted by e-mail; he agreed, asking only that his name and the copyright message in English and Portuguese were displayed at the bottom of the document, as well as the indication that the lists originated at the ICT for Language Teachers website (http://www.ict4lt.org). From the 19 applications originally listed, 7 were selected: Windows, Word, browsers, e-mail software, PowerPoint, Excel, and antivirus and security software. These 7 applications were chosen because they were the most basic.

The lists were then translated into Portuguese and adapted. In Part 1 of the survey participants were asked to indicate their level of knowledge under each heading on a scale of 1 to 3, 1 being basic, 2 intermediate, and 3 advanced. In Part 2, participants were asked to place a tick in the box in the right-hand column if they could do something, leaving it blank if they did not know how to do it. In Part 3, participants indicated their understanding of statements concerning aspects that are essential under each selected application, checking only the ones that they knew about. Table 17.2 is an adapted sample of the three parts of the questionnaire.

Data were collected from CELEM groups in 2006, 2007, and 2008. The total population was 72 teachers. The questionnaire was given to the participants in the classroom and they were asked to answer it at home and bring it back in the following classes. To avoid possible distortions in the answers given, the participants were not asked to identify themselves. The response rate was 87 percent: That is, 63 students answered the questionnaire.

Table 17.2   Example of the Three Parts of the Questionnaire: PowerPoint

---

PART 1
I would describe my ability to use PowerPoint as (1–3)

PART 2
Now indicate what you can do: Tick (√) for "yes," leave blank for "no." I can:
Start PowerPoint.
Exit PowerPoint.

PART 3
Essential things that I understand:
I understand that certain color combinations in slides must be avoided in order to make slides legible: e.g., avoid red/green.
I understand that fonts must be of a certain size in order to be legible—at least 24-point.

Table 17.3   Level of Knowledge on a Scale of 1 to 3 (1 = Basic / 2 = Intermediate / 3 = Advanced)

	1	2	3	Didn' t answer	Wrote 0	Total
Windows	5%	33%	57%	5%	0%	100%
Word	3%	37%	50%	10%	0%	100%
Browsers	17%	40%	32%	11%	0%	100%
E-mail software	11%	49%	30%	10%	0%	100%
PowerPoint	33%	33%	25%	6%	2%	100%
Excel	49%	27%	13%	10%	2%	100%
Antivirus and security software	51%	19%	10%	13%	8%	100%

Part 1

In Part 1 of the survey participants were asked to indicate their level of knowledge of the application. Although instructions were clear, 2 percent of the students decided to write 0 for PowerPoint and Excel and 8 percent did the same for antivirus and security software. However, 0 was not offered as a possible answer. It was inferred that participants wanted to make it clear that they had no knowledge at all of the applications. Some of the results obtained showed that 30 percent of the students considered their level of knowledge of e-mail software as advanced. Although the Internet has been increasingly used by all sectors of society, only 32 percent of the participants indicated their level of knowledge of browsers as advanced. Results concerning PowerPoint, Excel, and antivirus and security software are the ones that stand out: Respectively, 25 percent, 13 percent, and 10 percent of the participants consider their level of knowledge of these applications to be advanced. Table 17.3 shows the results obtained in Part 1.

Part 2

In Part 2 of the survey participants were asked to tick the tasks they knew how to do. Table 17.4 shows the number of tasks for each application.

Table 17.4   Number of Tasks for each Application

Windows	18 tasks
Word	39 tasks
Browsers	26 tasks
E-mail software	25 tasks
PowerPoint	23 tasks
Excel	35 tasks
Antivirus and security software	11 tasks

Due to the large number of tasks that comprised this part of the questionnaire, the following analysis will focus on the tasks whose results stood out for the high rate of affirmative as well as negative answers. It was not the purpose of the present investigation to carry out an analysis of the results of all the tasks proposed by Davies (2006) in his ICT "can do" lists, but to give an overview of the teachers' ICTs abilities and skills.

Concerning their knowledge of Windows, the participants answers indicated that they could not do the following tasks: *Find a file that I have mislaid* and *Format a floppy disk* (19 percent); *Use Windows Explorer to examine the contents of a disk and of different folders* and *Use the Windows task bar to toggle between applications* (14 percent); *Restore a window* and *Move or copy a file from one disk to another* (10 percent). The tasks with 100 percent of affirmative answers were: *Maximize a window*, *Minimize a Window*, and *Open a Windows application*—that is, start a computer program under Windows. However, 2 percent of the participants answered they could not *Close a Windows application*—that is, terminate a computer program under Windows. It was not expected that participants would be familiar with formatting a floppy disk since this resource has been replaced by CDs, flash drives, and so forth. However, it appears contradictory that they could open a Windows application but could not close it.

When asked about Word, some of the tasks participants did not know how to do were *Insert an audio file into a document* (62 percent), *Make hidden formatting characters visible or invisible* (51 percent), and *Convert existing text to a table* (43 percent), among others. There were no tasks in this section with 100 percent affirmative answers. The tasks with the highest rate of affirmative answers (98 percent) were *Exit Word, Save a document that I have typed, Print a document*, and *Open a document that I have previously saved*.

Results from Part 1 and Part 2 about Windows and Word were compared; difficulties in doing the tasks were not many. The percentage of participants who could not do certain activities is not significant, nevertheless, it still surprises that some basic tasks could not be done. Although participants indicated that they were able to do almost all the tasks, they did not feel confident enough to state that their level of knowledge of these two applications was advanced. In analyzing the results from Part 2 it was expected that the percentage of participants with an advanced level of knowledge would be higher, but this was not the case. There are not enough data to explain this verification.

More difficulties were found in the use of browsers than in the previous applications. The results confirmed what was found in Part 1 of the survey. Some of the tasks that participants did not know how to do were *Remove "web clutter" from my computer* (92 percent), *Unzip a downloaded ZIP file* (46 percent), and *Copy a graphic or picture into another application* (37 percent), among several others. The only task that 100 percent of the participants answered they knew how to do was *Exit a browser*. Once again a discrepancy was verified since 98 percent did not know how to *Start a browser*.

When using e-mail software most of the difficulties found were related to discussion lists: 68 percent of the participants could not *Resume receiving mail from a discussion list*, 60 percent could not *Temporarily suspend mail sent to me via a discussion list*, and 49 percent could not *Join a discussion list* or *Leave a discussion list*. Discussion lists are a very useful application for foreign language teachers because they allow communication and collaboration among professionals in the area, besides providing forums for international exchange of ideas, questions, and experiences. The only task that 100 percent of the participants answered they knew how to do was *Delete an unwanted incoming message*. For the tasks *Check for an incoming message* and *Read an incoming message*, 2 percent of the participants answered they did not know how to do them.

Some of the tasks participants did not know how to do with PowerPoint were *Insert a video file into a slide* (60 percent), *Insert a sound file into a slide* (56 percent), or *Remove transition and animation effects from a presentation* (43 percent), among several others. There were no tasks with 100 percent affirmative answers. The tasks with the highest rate of affirmative answers were *Start PowerPoint* and *Exit PowerPoint* (87 percent).

The use of Excel by language teachers offers several advantages and provides some ease in doing certain tasks. However, Excel was one of the applications whose results from Part 2 of the survey confirmed the low rate of participants (13 percent) with an advanced level of knowledge in Part 1. Some of the tasks participants did not know how to do were *Calculate an average of a column or row of figures* (70 percent), *Convert a set of figures into a graph or chart* (67 percent), and *Sort a set of cells into order, based on a selected column* (63 percent), among many others. There were no tasks with 100 percent affirmative answers. For the tasks *Start Excel* and *Exit Excel*, respectively 87 percent and 89 percent of the participants answered they could do them.

The item antivirus and security software was the application with the lowest level of knowledge in Part 1 (51 percent basic, 19 percent intermediate). The results in Part 2 confirmed what was shown in Part 1. Most of the tasks had an affirmative response rate below 50 percent. Some of the tasks the participants did not know how to do were *Configure my anti-adware/ spyware software* (83 percent), *Install e-mail filtering software on my computer* (79 percent), and *Configure my firewall software* (78 percent), among many others. The conclusion is that in relation to the security of their computers participants needed more orientation and appropriate training.

Part 3

Part 3 of the survey verified the section "Essential things that I understand," where some statements are made about the various applications.

Participants were to check only the statements they knew. There were statements for four of the seven applications.

For browsers, there were eight statements and participants could understand most of them. For instance, 94 percent could understand that computer viruses can be transmitted via hostile websites and that up-to-date antivirus software is essential while they are browsing the web, and 86 percent could understand that their computer can be "hacked" while browsing the web and that a firewall is essential. It was concluded that participants are aware of the importance of protecting their computers. However, they do not know how to do so, as seen in the results obtained in Part 1 and Part 2 of the antivirus and security software. The biggest difficulty here was that 88 percent of the participants could not understand how frame-based websites work. The terminology here is probably the problem.

Concerning e-mail software, there were five statements and participants could understand most of them. In four of these statements the rate of understanding was more than 87 percent. However 51 percent answered that they could not understand basic "Netiquette."

There were two statements for PowerPoint (see Table 17.2). The first statement was understood by 83 percent of the participants and the second was understood by 79 percent. Despite the difficulties shown in Part 2, most participants could understand these two essential statements.

For the item antivirus and security software there were eight statements. Most of the participants (90 percent) understood that it is essential to update their antivirus files regularly. The difficulties were in relation to understanding the terminology used in the area. For example, for the statement "I understand the term 'hoax virus,' and I know how to avoid being tricked by people who send me information about hoax viruses," 65 percent of the participants answered that they did not understand it; for the statement "I understand the term 'spyware,' and I know how to remove it from my computer," 68 percent answered they did not understand it; for the statement "I understand the term 'adware,' and I know how to remove it from my computer," 78 percent answered they did not understand it; and finally for the statement "I understand the term 'spam,' and I know how to avoid being 'spammed,'" 49 percent answered they did not understand it. The results obtained in this part confirmed those obtained in Part 1 and Part 2 about antivirus and security software.

FINAL REMARKS

The use of technological resources can help foreign language teachers to make their classes more dynamic, efficient, and attractive. Nevertheless, the use of such resources per se does not guarantee change, as many of the teachers are not ready to explore them properly. As Moraes (1997) points out, it is crucial for teachers to be updated not only on their subject matter,

254 Carla Barsotti and Claudia Martins

but also on the new teaching technologies and methodologies. However, the results of the second survey showed that CELEM's foreign language teachers' knowledge about ICTs is not enough to facilitate and improve their teaching practice, for, as confirmed by survey 2, some of them are not comfortable or familiar with some basic ICT applications and their possibilities.

The second survey also showed that the level of knowledge about ICTs varies greatly among the participants: While some teachers from the sample had difficulties doing tasks considered "essential" by Davies (2006), others had basically no problems. This confirmed what had been noticed about the teachers' ICT abilities observed in the 2004 and 2005 CELEM classes. The heterogeneity of the groups in relation to the use of ICTs proved to be not a matter of chance but a regular feature when foreign language teachers from different academic and professional backgrounds are put together in one class.

Since the two surveys started being conducted and the results analyzed, some measures have been taken to improve not only CELEM, but also the qualifications of other teachers. For instance, the discipline Technology in Foreign Language Teaching has already been implemented with some changes. Now, 10 hours of this discipline are dedicated to exploring the usage possibilities of basic applications, such as Word, in foreign language teaching. The focus of the discipline shifted from a theoretical to a more practical one. Despite the fact that CELEM does not have its own computer laboratory, this discipline is now taught in a computer laboratory that allows students to carry out hands-on activities. CELEM teachers of practically all the disciplines have also been asking participants to use PowerPoint creatively and originally when giving their oral presentations, as a way of making them familiar with this basic ICT and taking advantage of its best features. It is a way to show them that once they get acquainted with PowerPoint they can also have advantages when using it in their language classes and avoid "death by PowerPoint."

In 2007 and 2008, courses on the use of ICTs were given to the UTFPR teachers of the department responsible for CELEM and also to teachers of different institutions. This was at the suggestion of some CELEM participants who worked at these schools and felt the necessity of multiplying the knowledge acquired at CELEM at their workplaces.

The results of the two surveys described in the present chapter proved to be useful for promoting the initial changes mentioned before. Some outcomes may only be known in the future. Some have already been felt, such as when courses were given to colleagues to enhance their practice by using ICTs, and when CELEM's students realized there was the need to share with other teachers from their workplace the knowledge on ICTs they had gained when doing CELEM.

The assessment and adjustments of teachers' training courses are necessary measures for keeping up with the world changes and evolution of technology. Besides that, new generations of students, born in the techno-logical era, are very comfortable with most electronic gadgets, which have a short life span and are replaced by more modern ones all the time. So teachers who want to be part of this evolutionary process must be open and willing to participate in this ongoing process.

It was noticed, however, that this investigation had some limitations. The sample size was small and local—126 participants from the same course—which prevents the generalization of the results obtained. Also, the fact that the results from the two surveys were analyzed separately and the data were not correlated limited the possibilities for obtaining deeper and broader results. So, a future direction of this project is to use the top-ics from survey 1 as variables to be correlated with the data obtained from survey 2. This might very likely provide relevant information concerning foreign language teachers and their relationship with ICTs. It will then be possible to know whether age, gender, specific training received, or work experience has any connection with ICTs abilities, and so forth. From this point on, the present study should be conducted in other institutions and courses, as a strategy to guarantee a broader sample and to check whether the results obtained so far will be confirmed.

NOTES

1. This is due to the fact that Brazil, after being discovered by the Portuguese in the 1500s, received groups of immigrants from Europe and Asia.
2. According to the GFME, "Two types of graduate programs are recognized by the Brazilian Ministry of Education. *Lato sensu* or 'specialization' courses award recognized certificates and require at least 360 hours of course work or approximately two years. These courses are characterized as 'continuing education.' *Lato sensu* courses require an undergraduate degree to enter and do not require a thesis to graduate" (pp. 306–307).
3. According to the GFME, "*Stricto sensu* courses award a Master's or Doctor-ate degree. Approximately two years of study and a thesis are required for a master's degree, and approximately four years, including a dissertation, are required for a Doctorate" (p. 307).

REFERENCES

André, M. (2002). Formação de professores no Brasil (1990–1998) [Teacher train-ing in Brazil]. *Série Estado do Conhecimento n. 6* [State of Knowledge Series no. 6]. Retrieved from http://www.publicacoes.inep.gov.br/arquivos/formacao_de_professores_148.pdf

Brown, H. D. (2001). *Teaching by principles: An interactive approach to language pedagogy.* New York: Longman.

Davies, G. (2006). *ICT "can do" lists for teachers of foreign languages.* Retrieved from http://www.ict4lt.org/en/ICT_Can_Do_Lists.doc

GFME. (2006). Global guide to management education 2006—Brazil. Retrieved from http://www.gfme.org/global_guide/pdf/305-312%20Brazil.pdf

256   *Carla Barsotti and Claudia Martins*

Kenski, V. M. (1993). O ensino e os recursos didáticos em uma sociedade cheia de tecnologias [The teaching and learning resources in a society full of technology]. In M. R. N. S. Oliveira, (Ed.), *Didática: ruptura, compromisso e pesquisa* [Didactics: rupture, commitment and research] (pp. 127–147). Campinas: Papirus.

Lei no. 9.394, de 20 de dezembro de 1996. (1996). Dispõe sobre as diretrizes e bases da educação nacional D.O.U. de 23 de dezembro de 1996 [Provides for the guidelines and bases for national education]. Retrieved from http://portal.mec.gov.br/arquivos/pdf/ldb.pdf

Lei no. 11.161 de 05 de agosto de 2005. (2005). Dispõe sobre o ensino da língua espanhola [Provides for the teaching of the Spanish language]. Retrieved from http://www.planalto.gov.br/ccivil_03/_Ato2004–2006/2005/Lei/L11161htm

Ministério da Educação. (1999). *Parâmetros Curriculares Nacionais* [The national curriculum parameters]. Brasília, DF: MEC/Semtec. Retrieved from http://portal.mec.gov.br/seb/arquivospdf

Moraes, M. C. (1997). *O paradigma educacional emergente* [The emerging educational paradigm]. Campinas: Papirus.

Santos, E. A. (2008). Profissão Docente: uma questão de gênero? [Teaching profession: A gender issue?]. *Fazendo Gênero 8—Corpo, Violência e Poder* [Doing Gender 8—Body, Violence and Power]. UFSC. Retrieved from http://www.fazendogenero8.ufsc.br/sts/ST8/Elizabeth_Angela_dos_Santos_08.pdf

Walker, S. (2005).*The landmark review of ELT in Brazil*. Retrieved from http://www.britishcouncil.org.br/elt/downloads/Newsletterweb_files/Newsletterweb_files/LandmarkReview2005_revised_.pdf

18 "We Argentines Are Not as Other People"

Collaborative Learning Online in an Underserved Country

Marie-Noëlle Lamy

INTRODUCTION

A persistent challenge has faced tutor trainers and tutors at my adult learner institution since the inception of communicative online teaching in the mid-1990s. Language tutors who were very experienced at teaching languages in face-to-face tutorials were at that point invited to forge new skills in order to teach using real-time communication software for group work. Technical training provided by the institution soon proved insufficient, as even experienced teachers could not transfer their competencies straightforwardly to an online environment. More tools were developed to take account of the requirements of their discipline, such as Web-based toolkits and guides to good practice, which fulfilled the basic needs of many (more than 100 language tutors trained with these tools in the first decade and a half of our online operation) but left others unsatisfied and seeking further development (Lewis, 2006). Meanwhile, in research of a more generic kind, Peraya and Viens (2005) encapsulated the nature of the desired new competencies with the coinage "technopedagogical," and argued against simplistic reliance on training guides, as "these often interminable lists say more about the culture's objects than about the culture itself as a vital element of intervention" (p. 7). Technopedagogical development, they proposed, was cultural and depended on how individual variables, such as values, fears, motives, and "representations" (or perceptions) and structural variables, such as functions and roles, came together to form the culture of educators and educational managers. In 2007, I was able to put some flesh on these abstractions, as I took the opportunity to turn a commission from a Latin-American university wishing to upskill its language teachers, into a practical and theoretical investigation into the nature of change in teacher education.

SOCIOPOLITICAL BACKGROUND

In a historical account of educational policy in Latin America, Schugurensky and Davidson-Harden (2003) explain the situation in today's Argentina by going back to the "Córdoba reform," fought for by students of the Universidad de Córdoba in 1918, which saw the instigation of tuition-free education. Thereafter a dual public–private system has flourished and according to INDEC, the National Institute for Statistics and Census (http://www.indec.gov.ar/), 78.8 percent of Argentinean students were enrolled in public universities in 2004 against 22.2 percent in the private sector.

Distance learning and ICT have different roles to play in each part of this divided landscape. In the public sector, which is committed to charging no fees, the development of distance education services represents a huge financial commitment that institutions have trouble meeting. Nevertheless the government of Argentina became active in pushing ICT in 1995, when it set up the management system University Interconnection Network to offer national and international connectivity, as well as training courses. This took a long time to disseminate, as it was viewed with suspicion by end users whose trust in government was always fragile, and was particularly badly shaken by the 2001 economic disaster. Now, however, according to Finquelevic (2003):

> [t]he Ministry of Culture and Education, through the Secretariat of University Policies (SPU) has encouraged the implementation of a national infrastructure, on which was built the larger academia network in the country: 33 National Universities are connected to this network, which provides them national and international connectivity. (2003, section III E, para. 8)

However, in two national conferences held in 2005 and 2006 speakers stressed obstacles: slow recognition and insufficient reward for teachers participating in technology-mediated activity and difficulty in justifying the time taken (Acuña, Lucero, Marilef, & Plaza, 2006; Bianco, 2005).

Meanwhile, private digital networks have also started operating in Argentina's higher education sector, making the overall picture harder to capture. Clearly, private sector developments are more efficient because they are backed "by big companies and their foundations, both local (Noble Foundation; Argentine Banks Association) and multinational (Microsoft Argentina; Coca Cola; Santillana; Fundación Telefónica, etc)" (Pini & Gorostiaga, 2008, p. 439) but such organizations favor market-led practices that demand that their teaching staff accept a productivity-driven working environment and deliver evaluation-driven curricula.

Overall, then, the early 2000s were a period of great change in the expectations placed on higher education teachers in Argentina for the development of e-learning, but the political context is very difficult for teachers in each sector.

INSTITUTIONAL BACKGROUND—THE UNIVERSITY OF CÓRDOBA FACULTY OF LANGUAGES

This study was conducted in conjunction with the Universidad Nacional de Córdoba (UNC), 700 km north of Buenos Aires, which enjoys a very good national reputation as far as the teaching of languages is concerned. Students follow undergraduate programs, without fees. Master's and PhD programs are also available but postgraduate students are self-financed. Among these are a master's program in English with a focus on Literature or on Applied Linguistics, a master's in Translation Studies, a PhD in Language Sciences, and a specialization in Translation Studies. Some of these courses are of interest to teachers as part of their ongoing credit-bearing professional development, and accumulation of credits can be used towards improvement in job conditions. Among the positive factors are the levels of equipment (exceptionally good for Argentina: one computer room with 20 PCs, and 25 classrooms with various technological resources, although no way, at the time of the study, of involving the interactive oral skills). However, among the concerns are what academics perceive as administrative lack of vision and insufficient recognition of teachers' efforts. A department for distance education in languages has been created, in response to which 2007 saw the launch of a CPD course on the use of educational platforms (Moodle and E-ducativa) for teaching languages, followed in 2008 by a course for online tutors (roles, tasks, and challenges). In 2009 teachers were offered workshops on how to use Internet resources and technology in their classes: on virtual environments and on the design of activities for virtual environments. Plans for further workshops on the construction and design of conceptual maps and on the production and editing of audiovisual resources had also been made, but had to be abandoned due to staffing problems.

The online course discussed in this chapter took place in 2007, in this context of fast change, using the platform E-ducativa, which provided asynchronous and synchronous text-based tools, supplemented by the use of Skype for synchronous oral communication in small groups. The participants were 16 in-service teachers (13 teachers of English and 3 teachers of French). They had little experience of using IT for teaching although some were fluent and keen text chat users in their private lives. All were female native speakers of Spanish, aged between 30 and 60, recruited for the course across the country's public and private universities, and some cumulated their university post and posts in public or private high schools. Henceforth, I refer to them as *trainees*.

An Evolving Brief

The UNC initially asked me to design and teach a 20-hour qualifying course to "raise awareness of ICT" among language teachers. As trainees would get no release from their full-time jobs and as UNC could only offer to fund me for a short visit from Europe, it was agreed that the course would be offered in blended mode, starting with a five-week online phase facilitated by me at a distance, followed by a visit to UNC during which I would run a two-day face-to-face workshop, concluding with a second distance online phase (taking place over two weeks). This pragmatic decision was also in keeping with the core topic of the course, which was "teaching online." Hence my design would be based on experiential learning, backed by reflection and collaborative small-group work.

As preparation progressed, it gradually became clear through successive Skype briefings with staff managers at UNC that behind the request for awareness-raising lay another concern for me to address in the design of the course. South American language teachers, according to the brief, tended to have limited involvement with "communicative" methods, being themselves the product of a transmissive education system. Research agreed with this perception: Celani and Collins (2005) studied critical thinking within interactions in an online course for Brazilian trainee teachers and found that communication overwhelmingly took the form of trainee questions addressed to their tutor, with no peer discussion or resolution of issues raised. The authors concluded that "[these trainees'] histories, both personal and educational, do not offer much room for reflection [. . .] Their previous background is one of received knowledge as something complete, unquestionable, to be transmitted as it was received" (p. 43). Keller, Lindh, Hrastinski, Casanovas, and Fernandez (2009) also found that 110 technology teachers at the Universidad Nacional de Tecnologia (with headquarters in Buenos Aires but operating countrywide) "primarily accept and use the features of learning that influences their traditional roles the least, as the transition to a new role might be too challenging" (p. 67). Thus the integration of communicative practice into the repertoire of my trainees now became an important objective, which could be accommodated, alongside the more technological one, within the experiential collaborative model that I had in mind.

Course Design in Response to the Brief

Experiential learning (Kolb & Kolb, 2005) relies on engagement in a cycle of experiencing, reflecting, conceptualizing, testing, and so on, iteratively. This cycle was chosen as the basis for the course pedagogy for two reasons, one practical and one principled. Firstly, it is relatively undemanding in terms of time spent reading materials, as it relies instead on the learner reflecting on events that are happening to her during the course contact hours. This answered the practical issue of the trainees' limited time, and their unavailability for absorption of large volumes of content. Secondly, I decided to ground the cycle in the trainees' collective experience, as this pedagogical design was best adapted to the specific course context: The trainees were members of a shared culture as teachers in the Argentine higher education system, whilst the tutor was not. It was therefore important that the trainees' own perceptions, rather than the teacher's "knowledge," be encouraged to emerge and become the material with which the participants would work.

To maximize the trainees' exposure to communication online as part of their experiential learning, the course contained peer-to-peer (tutorless) and group-to-tutor interactive tasks at every stage, and several of the assignments including the final one reflected this. Among the marking criteria sent to the students was the stipulation that "[a]nswers should take into account the collective work of the group (the individual's answers, taken over the duration of the course, should contain at least two references to the work of the group)."

To ensure that reflection on communicative experiences took place, individual e-readings (including website browsing and analysis) were prescribed at regular intervals and reported on in assignments. Along with the course forum, the most important instrument in the training was the trainee's e-portfolio. Each trainee collected her reports and assignments in an e-portfolio, in this case a Word file, where the tutor also recorded her feedback and marks. The e-portfolio's contents were thus added to as the course progressed, shuttling back and forth between the tutor and the trainee. As some of the assignments were reports of peer-to-peer group conversations via E-ducativa's chat facility or via Skype, to be used as objects of study and analysis, the assignment's author was not the only person with an interest in seeing the tutor's comments: All the peers involved in the original conversation could be assumed to wish to see the feedback as well. For this reason, trainees were encouraged—but not compelled—to upload their portfolios to a shared area for "mutualization" of feedback. At the end of the course, with the trainees' prior agreement, the tutor mutualized the trainees' perceptions by posting a report that included integral reproduction of their final essays. This assessment strategy was designed to ensure that the course pedagogy (socio-collaborative, with individual and shared reflection) was supported by the way that trainees were assessed, in conformity with Knight's (1995) and Thorpe's (2000) findings on assessment design.

All activities were conducted in the trainees' professional languages (English for the teachers of EFL, French for the others) and course materials were collected or created in each language. Two of the trainees were able to take advantage of both collections.

RESEARCH QUESTIONS

The research objective was to determine whether the experiential learning design of the course, framed as it was within a collaborative process, provided support for the transformation of the professional practices of established teachers. The research questions were aimed at identifying the obstacles to such transformation. Three types of obstacles were hypothesized:

- Technical/developmental obstacles: What role might the under-provision or unreliability of ICT in Argentina play in hindering transformation?
- Political obstacles: How did institutional constraints affect the potential for transformation?
- Ideological obstacles: What was the impact of the trainees' own educational cultures on their approach to transformation?

RESEARCH METHODOLOGY

The chosen research methodology prioritized the use of the learners' own words and discourse as reflected in their productions. The corpus was collected from the trainees' e-portfolios where, as explained earlier, they told the story of their collective and individual experiences on the course and incorporated transcripts from their group conversations. The final assignment was also a synoptic piece, in which personal evaluation was part of the task. Its instructions read as follows:

> This is a synoptic assignment, i.e., it goes back over the whole of your course experience, to help you reflect on it. You must revisit your Portfolio and the Readings and resources that you studied. Write an essay (1,500 words minimum) answering the question: "If I was designing a short online course for familiarizing face-to-face language teachers with distance teaching, what would I do differently from the course that I have just studied, what would I imitate from it, and why?" You are invited to constructively critique the course. You must back up your positive or critical arguments with examples taken from your own experience or from your readings.

This part of the assessment strategy had a double rationale. As well as the aim of matching the assessment closely to the learning mode experienced by the trainers, the requirement for students to write this report for marks lowered the risk of drop out, consequently ensuring a fuller set of research data as well as better completion rates (in the event, no drop out was observed). An inherent danger in this strategy was that some trainees might build in a favorable bias to please their tutor. To address this, course design took into account research on the use of reflection in assessment by adult learners, documented by Anson (1994), Macdonald (2003), and Thorpe (2000), who had not found that bias was among the weaknesses of such an approach, although insufficient scaffolding by markers was. For example, Thorpe reports that when asking, "Which part(s) of questions 1 to 3 did you find difficult to answer and which did you find easier? Why do you think that was?"(p. 82), a wide range of unpredictable responses were offered, which tutors did not at first know how to mark, until they had had a chance to discuss with course designers ways to handle reflective assignments and the element of subjectivity inherent in them. In the current course, scaffolding was achieved through providing example trainee answers and model marker feedback responses.

Two Types of Semantic Analyses

Two complementary forms of semantic treatment were applied to the data: an automatic analysis of the whole corpus using Tropes (a piece of semantic analysis software developed by French researchers, now commercialized by Acetic/Semantic-Knowledge; see http://www.semantic-knowledge.com/) and a manual scrutiny of a sub-corpus using the Appraisal method of discourse analysis. These choices are now explained in greater detail.

The choice of the Tropes discourse analysis software was determined by the need to use an existing high-performance language semantic analysis program built to handle French or English data with equal ease, an important feature as trainee data comprised texts in each of these languages. At the time of this project, Tropes operated in these two languages (to which, by the time of writing, Spanish and Portuguese have been added). Its search engine automatically identifies the key themes structuring texts. Under Tropes, each significant word is part of a semantic chain. For instance, a query on the word *election* will retrieve sentences from documents containing the closely related words *campaigning*, *ballot*, and *vote*. Unlike a concordancing program, Tropes does not need an item to be physically manifested in the data. Instead it relies on underlying semantic principles, so in the case of the preceding words, it assigns them to a superordinate category "Politics," even though the lexical item *politics* may not explicitly appear in the corpus. To help Tropes to highlight the themes in a corpus of texts, the software can draw on 20,000 semantic subcategories and assign them to superordinate categories, such as Politics. (The initial letter of each category name is capitalized in the rest of this chapter, to distinguish a category from its corresponding lexical item.) Tropes can return both frequency and "relational" results (i.e., showing which semantic categories relate most strongly to which others).

However, two limiting factors soon became apparent: (a) in Tropes, words are classified according to their most frequent meaning, not their contextualized uses, for example, the word *target* would be automatically identified as belonging to the category Military, but not to the category Language; (b) Tropes' dependency on frequency does not suit it to the analysis of themes that may be realized through few linguistic resources with little redundancy across the texts, yet may be supported by rhetorical strength, such as an emotional metaphor or an appeal to the reader for empathy. Conversely, categories too closely fitting the main purpose of the texts are overrepresented and yield results that are too ubiquitous to provide a basis for useful insights. In the present case this applies to the category Education, which came out in top of the categories rankings in the analysis and will be left out of the discussion that follows. All these conditions made it necessary to carry out additional analyses of the data, further to the automatic Tropes report. Firstly, the concern was with adjusting Tropes' quantitative findings in order to take contextualized meanings into account. To this purpose an additional reading was carried out using some of the software's tools to reinterpret some of the results. I am calling this a "semi-automated" reading, since it relied on taking in information returned by the software, rereading the full texts to assess possible distortions due to the software's bias against contextual meanings, then running further edited automatic searches accordingly. Secondly, a fully manual analysis was needed, in which the focus would be on close reading of the source data in order to detect themes that were not handled well by the software yet were cultural representations rhetorically presented by the trainees as important to them or to their audience. The analytical framework chosen for this purpose was Appraisal analysis, a form of discourse analysis seeking to identify evaluative meanings, which grew out of Systemic Functional Linguistics. Appraisal analysis has "arisen through extensive research into the nature of evaluative meaning" (Coffin & O'Halloran, 2006, p. 83) and it has been used successfully with different types of small-scale corpora (Bednarek, 2009). The way it was operationalized in this study will be explained shortly.

AUTOMATIC ANALYSIS AND DISCUSSION

The corpus, made up of the complete set of final assignments, comprised 24,000 words. In examining the 10 most strongly represented categories as reported by Tropes, it is seen (Table 18.1) that the frequency rankings can be grouped into five bands: Band I contains the only category with more than 1,000 words assigned to it; Band II holds the only category with more than 500 words assigned to it; Band III has within it three categories with around 300 words assigned to each; Band IV has between 100 and 150 words assigned to each of its two categories; and, finally, Band V contains categories with a small number of words assigned to them, between 15 and 30.

Leaving aside the category Education, in the top band, as advised earlier, I will comment on the four next bands in decreasing order of frequency.

Communication is the only category in the second band. The words that have been flagged by Tropes as explicitly mentioned in the source data are *communication* (as a lexical item), *debate*, *chat* and *discussion*,

Table 18.1   The 10 Most Frequent Semantic Categories in the Corpus

Band	10 most frequent categories	Words assigned to the category
I	1. Education	1,139
II	2. Communication	541
III	3. Social Group	304
	4. Language	303
	5. Time	300
IV	6. Cognition	157
	7. Feeling	104
V	8. Environment	30
	9. Europe	25
	10. Technology	15

conversation, and *greeting*. Related themes include Planning, Interaction, and Social Group. Extracted contexts (one of the facilities offered by this software) show contextual associations within the semantic category Communication to be dynamic and human-centered, rather than technical, for example: *understanding by real true communication, sustaining communication, when communication gets disrupted, students have to interact again, communication is sought at all costs, to profit from the flow of communication on the spur of the moment, interacting with real live native speaker in real-life communication situations, new modes of teaching including the simplest Internet communication media like the e-mail and audio/video-conferencing.*

Celani and Collins (2005) revealed that their participants' interpretation of the meaning of "communication" was not collaborative but instead was reduced to information elicitation. In this connection it is worth noting that nothing in the automatic or in the semiautomatic reading of the UNC corpus indicates a relationship between Communication and Information.

In the third band the theme with top frequency is Social Group. Words explicitly mentioned in the texts include *community, forum, cooperative, cooperation, collaborative, collaboration, support,* and *team*. In this corpus, the category Social Group also has strong relations with the categories Communication, Organization, and Feeling.

An undervalued item in Band III is Language, a semantic category that can therefore be assumed to be almost as representative of the trainees' preoccupations as is Social Group. In fact, given that these trainees were all language teachers, it was perhaps a little unexpected that Language did not appear higher up in the rankings. Almost equally important to them was the theme of Time, although in this case a semiautomated reading of the corpus revealed that the trainees discussed two different topics (a) real-*time* online teaching, and (b) demands made by the training on their *time*—thus muddying the content of the category and diminishing its usefulness for the study.

In Band IV, the category Cognition (represented by the lexical items *mind, thinking, knowing*, and *knowledge*) ranked top of the band by a very small margin over Feeling, again an interesting finding, implying that although these teachers did associate these lexical items with learning, they did not give them priority over the communicative dimension of learning, and they conceptualized learning as partaking in Cognition and Feeling equally. The appearance of Feeling in the top 10 categories warrants a little more scrutiny. Highlighted terms in that category were *fear, anxiety, empathy, confidence, self-esteem*, and *success*. Major related semantic categories were Education and Communication and Law (the latter as a result of a lengthy discussion about a language role-play, on criminals and lawyers, invented by the trainees during the face-to-face workshops), while the category Behavior was a much less well-represented semantic relation.

In the lowest-frequency band in the table, the significance of the categories Environment, Europe, and Technology was reassessed after the semiautomated reading of the results. Environment was on the list because of several occurrences of the phrase "virtual environments," and also because of three mentions of "supportive environments." Europe featured because much mention was made of English and of Córdoba (identified by the—European—software as a European city). Finally, the unexpected statistical nonsignificance of the category Technology could be explained by the fact that the software only assigned the words *technology, computer*, and *computing* to that category, ignoring many occurrences of *chat*, which it assigned to the category Communication instead.

According to the automated and semiautomated readings of the data, it can be seen that these trainees represent their world as one where success in teaching and learning is predicated on communication, social activity, and attention to affect. The reduced role played by semantic categories such as Cognition or, to name some that were at the bottom of the frequency list, Academic Degree, Test, or Failure, supports the interpretation that these trainees did not evince the expected interest in the transmissive, evaluation-driven system that had been associated with South American education and educators in the literature and in the course briefing.

Manual Analysis and Discussion

As mentioned earlier, Tropes cannot capture categories associated with very low-frequency lexical items. Yet some of these may be framed within rhetorical contexts lending them significant weight. One such cultural representation came strongly out of the manual reading of the data (and inspired my title): It concerned the idea of "being from Argentina." A mini-corpus of extracts featuring the keywords *Argentina, Argentine(an), South America(n)*, and *(this/our) country* was therefore put together and subjected to Appraisal analysis. Appraisal analysis relies on identification of the linguistic exponents of the functional concepts Engagement, Attitude, and Graduation, with Attitude being subdivided into three subsets: (positive or negative) Affect, (positive or negative) Judgment, and (positive or negative) Social Valuation. As will be seen in the examples that follow, grammar and lexis can both play a role in making these notions available to readers and listeners.

Engagement is in evidence when the text's reader is presupposed to share the writer's worldview. As Coffin and O'Halloran (2006, p. 84) point out:

> one important dimension of APPRAISAL is that it maps a set of resources which, rather than being simply viewed as a means for a speaker or writer to make 'personal' comments on the world, is viewed as a set of interpersonal tools for developing solidarity between a speaker/writer and their audience.

In the current data, for example, an assignment written for the European tutor contains this reflection by a participant concerning her views on the ideal conditions for designing distance courses:

> maybe if the training program is designed with a European or Canadian dimension, with proper time devoted to the study, then maybe that is possible.

She explicitly provides a value judgment—"proper"—to describe European (and Canadian) procedures, and implicitly constructs her European reader as a sharer of that judgment.

Affect is an expression of the writer's or speaker's emotions and feelings. For example, *love* conveys these explicitly in:

> I also attended a three-month course on Interpretation at the Faculty of Languages 10 years ago. This is a field which I love.

Judgment is characterized by language expressing the writer's or speaker's view on the rights and wrongs of human behavior, for example, the slur on the diligence of Argentinean students in:

> Argentinean students [. . .] are not very much used to read carefully to follow instructions.

This example also illustrates the Appraisal method's ability to capture contextual semantic effects at sentence level. Lexical items that may be value neutral in their denotation can become connoted negatively or positively because of the occurrence of another item further along the written or spoken chain. Here the adverb *carefully* serves to orient the statement "Argentinean students [. . .] are not very much used to" into a negative judgment on the students, rather than, for example, an empathetic one, as would have been the case if she had written, "Argentinean students [. . .] are not very much used to blindly obeying rules." In the data and figures that follow, I refer to this semantic reorientation mechanism as *disambiguation*.

Like Judgment, Social Valuation reflects values invested into the discourse by the writer/speaker, specifically ones that have a bearing on social phenomena. Consider, for example, the following quotation, in which the interpretation of the adjective *complex* (a neutral word, in that "a complex situation" may be a good, *rich* one, or a *bad*, inextricable one) is reinterpreted as a negative by the use of the verb "to face," which connotes difficulty or potential conflict:

> [i]n Argentina, in general, most teachers face a complex situation.

Finally, Graduation expresses values of intensity (low or high) and can be evidenced in adverbs and a variety of hyperbolic and hedging stylistic devices. This example uses a double adverbial phrase to increase the intensity of the claim:

> Argentinean students [. . .] are not very much used to read carefully to follow instructions.

Figures 18.1 (a) to 18.5 (b) illustrate the type and distribution of the evaluative meanings explicitly and implicitly embedded in the mini-corpus, "Argentina." In the figures, abbreviations refer to the following Appraisal analysis constructs, realized by linguistic items found in the mini-corpus: E (for *Engagement*, shown in italics), J (for *Judgment*, in gray), SV (for *Social Valuation*, underlined), and G (for *Graduation*, plain).

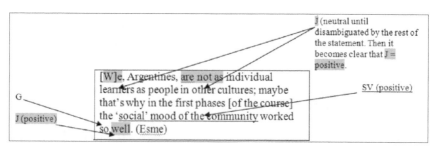

Figure 18.1 (a)   On being a learner.

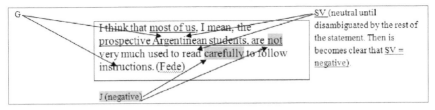

Figure 18.1 (b)   On being a learner.

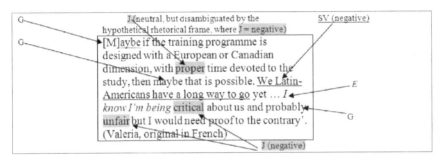

Figure 18.2   On designing distance courses.

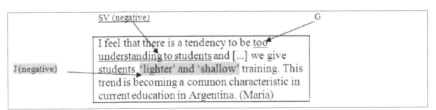

Figure 18.3   On pedagogy.

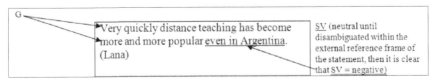

Figure 18.4   On educational cultures.

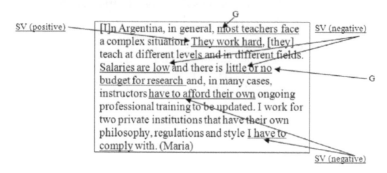

Figure 18.5 (a)   On professional conditions.

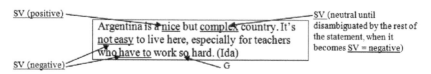

Figure 18.5 (b)   On professional conditions.

From this analysis it can be seen that by far the two most frequent Appraisal values across the mini-corpus are Graduation (providing hedging to the many unquantified claims made), and Attitude, via its subsets Judgment and Social Valuation, both overwhelmingly negative. These negativities are expressed in relation to the referents "us" (meaning the trainees, in the context of Figure 18.1 [a]); "the prospective Argentinean students" (Figure 18.1 [b]); "we Latin-Americans" (*we* meaning *educators* in the context of Figure 18.2); those involved in "education in Argentina" (Figure 18.3); institutions determining teachers' professional circumstances (Figure 18.5 [a]); and Argentina as a country (Figure 18.4 and Figure 18.5 [b]). The two examples of positive Social Valuation refer to "the Argentines" (Figure 18.1 [a]) and "Argentina" (Figure 18.5 [b]).

In other words, the talk about Argentina is characterized by a split between the professional context (negative) and the socio-geographical context (positive) that serve as the two main frames of reference for the keywords *Argentina, Argentine(an), South America(n),* and *(this/our) country.*

Summary of the Discussion

I have described a two-pronged approach to data analysis that, in relying on a mix of automatic and manual methods to allow for the capture of both low- and high-frequency linguistic exponents of underlying semantic structures, has cast some light on the three research questions that guided this investigation.

In response to the first question, it can be seen that technical/developmental factors are absent from the representations offered by the trainees. Technology-related themes that might have been expected to feature, such as unstable connections, inadequate bandwidth, or scarcity of computers on campus were not evidenced, nor were discussions on the quality of the technology in general. Technophobia featured as a topic at first, as one participant displayed anxiety about using the tools. However, this was soon resolved as others rallied round with practical help, and the only traces of this episode that were left in the data were group self-congratulations about the power of mutual support. In conclusion, according to the study, technical issues are not a significant factor in the professional transformation of online teachers. These findings accord with Keller et al. (2009), for whose cohort from the Universidad Nacional de Tecnologia (UNT) "most of the barriers are related to organizational management more than purely technological issues" (p. 78). Although Keller et al.'s informants were technology teachers and their confidence with technology is less surprising, they too ranked lack of opportunity to update technical knowledge as the main obstacle to their use of ICT tools with students.

This links in with the second question, which relates to the role of political and institutional agencies. Like their UNT colleagues above, the UNC cohort's thoughts about the role of politics and educational institutions were well represented in the corpus, and this role is overwhelmingly framed as an inhibitor of transformation. For both Keller et al.'s (2009) informants and the UNC teachers in our study, lack of opportunity to update is ascribed to lack of time due to working conditions, particularly to cumulating posts, a situation made unavoidable by low salaries, according to the informants.

Such findings (orientation to technology but failure to appropriate the tools) may be interpreted as a reflection of the state of transition that the Argentinean education sector was beginning to experience at the time of data collection for the study, with infrastructural progress preceding political-institutional change, leaving university teachers with the contradiction of up-to-date and functioning tools that they were not adequately encouraged or supported to use.

The final question was premised on the hypothesis that the trainees' own educational cultures might constitute an ideological obstacle to transformation. This question received a clear answer through the automatic analysis, where little evidence was found to support claims by staff managers and by some researchers that the teachers were uninterested in pedagogies that did not conform to the transmissive learning cultures to which they themselves had been exposed. Instead, evidence arose from the data allowing the interpretation that these teachers are reflectively aware of the contradictions that structure their professional circumstances—the informant in Figure 18.5 specifically links dual post-holding with "different" pedagogical cultures, which it is her uncomfortable duty to conform with—and that they overwhelmingly construct their professional world through notions such as community, social group, and feeling, showing them to be reflective socio-constructivists regardless of reputation.

CONCLUSION

Besides these insights, some practical observations may also be made. Firstly, the practical achievements of the trainees throughout the course, their enthusiastic engagement in answering its increasing technological demands, and their collegiate response to one "techno-anxious" peer, have shown that low personal technological skills at the start of training are not a significant obstacle to professional development as up-to-date online practitioners. It will be remembered that the course was designed as an experiential learning environment, which meant that one's own technological difficulties or those of a peer were grist to the reflective mill. The teachers understood the value of learning from such hiccups, which might affect their own future online students. They were therefore inclined to persevere and overcome them. These principles of course design might profitably be reused in future continuing professional development for teachers.

Secondly, semantic analysis of teacher productions has helped show that they perceive obstacles to their development as linked to the socio-institutional conditions in which they work. This perception, whilst a perennial of labor relations, with its connotation of blaming the boss, takes on significance against a contemporary background of governmental and institutional attention to technological provision in education. That teachers perceive themselves as being unsupported regardless of markedly enhanced technological provision in their still reputedly underserved country is an indicator that they, at least, do not confuse educational technology with education, and that they should be listened to, if the common mistake signaled by Warschauer (2008) of overreliance on computer experts in ICT development projects is to be avoided.

Finally, the insights arising from this study underline Peraya and Viens' (2005) view of technopedagogical change as shaped by the interplay of cultural variables, prominent among which are "representations," or perceptions. They also confirm the conclusion that a coresearcher and I reached in our search for a definition of "online learning cultures" (Goodfellow & Lamy, 2009), where we drew attention to the fact that the "participants" in online learning cultures include the institutions themselves. Two traditional ways way of viewing the institutions are as inhibitors of development—as do the informants in this chapter—and conversely as facilitating actors. However, a somewhat different dimension is introduced if we consider the interaction between learners/teachers on the one hand, and agents of institutions on the other. "The identities that learners develop through engagement with [. . .] the national, institutional, corporate, professional, disciplinary and peer-group practices that frame the whole undertaking of learning online " (Goodfellow & Lamy, 2009, p. 171) are permanently being constructed and reconstructed. In the case study in this chapter, they are constructed as resistance and creativity. A possible follow-up project might be to use this investigation's methodology to look at the perceptions of those on "the institutional side" of the online educational culture that has been under scrutiny here. Deriving from this, but beyond the scope of this chapter, are further questions for research into organizational learning.

REFERENCES

Acuña, A., Lucero, M., Marilef, M., & Plaza, J. (2006). La Historia de la EAD en la UNCo: Un largo camino recorrido y otro tanto por recorrer. In *Proceedings from ¿Edudiseños o Tecnodesignios? IV Seminario Internacional—II Encuentro Nacional de Educación a Distancia*. Universidad Nacional de Córdoba: Editorial Asociación de Profesores de la Facultad de Ciencias Exactas e Ingeniería de la Universidad Nacional de Rosario. Retrieved from http://rueda.edu.ar/06_publicaciones/pub-digitales/edu-o-tecno.rar

Anson, C. M. (1994). Portfolios for teachers: Writing our way to reflective practice. In L. Black, D. A. Daiker, J. Sommers, & G. Stygall (Eds.), *New directions in portfolio assessment: Reflective practice, critical theory and large-scale scoring* (pp. 185–200). Portsmouth, NH: Heinemann-Boynton/Cook.

Bednarek, M. (2009). Corpora and discourse: A three-pronged approach to analyzing linguistic data. In M. Haugh (Ed.), *Proceedings from 2008 HCSNet workshop on designing the Australian national corpus* (pp.19–24). Somerville, MA: Cascadilla Project.

Bianco, A. C. (2005). Resistancias de los docentes en los procesos de incorporación de las nuevas tecnologías a la educación. Reflexiones a partir de una experiencia. In *CD of Proceedings from Congreso Internacional Educación Superior y Nuevas Tecnologías*. Universidad Nacional del Litoral: Centro MultiMedial de Educación a Distancia.

Celani, M. A., & Collins, H. (2005). Critical thinking in reflective sessions and in online interactions. *Applied Linguistics in Latin America, 18*, 41–57.

Coffin, C., & O'Halloran, K. (2006). The role of appraisal and corpora in detecting covert evaluation. *Functions of Language, 13*(1), 77–110.

Finquelevic, S. (2003). *ICT and economic development in Latin America and the Caribbean*. Paper presented at the World Summit of Cities and Local Authorities on the Information Society, Lyon, France, 4–5 December. Retrieved from http://www.cities.lyon.fr/en/devecoAL.html

Goodfellow, R., & Lamy, M.-N. (2009). New directions for research in online learning cultures. In R. Goodfellow & M.-N. Lamy (Eds.), *Learning cultures in online education* (pp. 170–183). London: Continuum Books.

Keller, C., Lindh, J., Hrastinski, S., Casanovas, I., & Fernandez, G. (2009). The impact of national culture on e-learning implementation: A comparative study of an Argentinean and a Swedish university. *Educational Media International, 46*, 67–80.

Knight, P. (1995). *Assessment for learning in higher education*. London: Kogan Page.

Kolb, A. Y., & Kolb, D. A. (2005). Learning styles and learning spaces: Enhancing experiential learning in higher education. *Academy of Management Learning and Education, 4*(2), 193–212.

Lewis, T. (2006). When teaching is learning: A personal account of learning to teach online. *CALICO Journal, 23*(3), 581–599.

Macdonald, J. (2003). Assessing online collaborative learning process and product. *Computers and Education, 40,* 377–391.

Peraya, D., & Viens, J. (2005). Culture des acteurs et modèles d'intervention dans l'innovation technopédagogique. *International Journal of Technologies in Higher Education, 2*(1), 7–19.

Pini, M. E., & Gorostiaga, J. M. (2008). Teacher education and development policies: Critical discourse analysis from a comparative perspective. *International Review of Education, 54,* 27–443.

Schugurensky, D., & Davidson-Harden, A. (2003). From Córdoba to Washington: WTO/GATS and Latin American Education. *Globalization, Societies and Education, 1*(3), 321–357.

Thorpe, M. (2000). Encouraging students to reflect as part of the assignment process: Student responses and tutor feedback. *Active Learning in Higher Education, 1*(1), 79–92.

Warschauer, M. (2008). Whither the digital divide? In D. L. Kleinman, K. A. Cloud-Hansen, C. Matta, & J. Handelsman (Eds.), *Controversies in science and technology: From climate to chromosomes* (pp. 140–151). New Rochelle, NY: Liebert.

19 Electronic Portfolios in a BA CALL Course

Supporting Reflective and Autonomous Learning

Salomi Papadima-Sophocleous

INTRODUCTION

There has been great interest worldwide in autonomous learning and in the use of electronic portfolios (henceforth, e-portfolios) in different learning areas such as finance, strategic management and marketing, politics and government, fine arts, and education. Learning how to learn and learning how to learn autonomously and have the ability to reflect on previous learning and demonstrate such learning in the form of tangible work are these days very important skills in general, and in teacher education in particular, and should be part of the main goals in teacher education. However, this is an area that has undoubtedly lagged behind other skills such as reading and writing and that needs to be systematically included as an integral part of learning. Substantial research needs to take place in order to find out the success of such practice. This chapter describes the integration of e-portfolios as a tool for reflective and autonomous learning in a teacher education course, and more specifically in a Computer-Assisted Language Learning (CALL) course in a private university in Cyprus, part of a BA in an English Language and Literature undergraduate degree. It establishes, through students' reflections, how effective such integration has been.

AUTONOMOUS LEARNING

Autonomous learning is considered to be a lifelong learning skill. Holec (1981, p. 3) defines autonomous learning as the "ability to take charge of one's own learning." Little (1991, p. 4) describes learner autonomy as the learners' acceptance of their own learning and "a capacity for detachment, critical reflection, decision making, and independent action." Learner autonomy is also defined as the ability to take personal or "self-regulated" responsibility for learning (Benson & Voller, 1997). It is the presence of initiative in learning, of sharing in monitoring progress, and of evaluating the extent to which learning is achieved (Schunk, 2005). Typically, learners who exercise autonomous learning understand the purpose of learning, accept responsibility for their learning, share in the setting of learning goals, take the initiative in planning and executing learning tasks, and regularly review their learning to evaluate its effectiveness (Little, 2003).

LEARNER TRAINING

Trim (1988, p. 3) states:

> No school, or even university, can provide its pupils with all the knowledge and the skills they will need in their active adult lives. It is more important for a young person to have an understanding of himself or herself, an awareness of the environment and its workings, and to have learned how to think and how to learn.

This is quite applicable in teacher training as well. Teacher trainees need to be trained to learn how to think, how to learn, how to reflect and evaluate their learning, how to evidence it (demonstrate such learning in the form of tangible examples of work), and how to continue to learn autonomously. All these need to be an integral part of their training. Teacher trainees need to be aware and apply reflective and autonomous learning if they are to be able to foster that in their learners. Little (1995) argues:

> It is unreasonable to expect teachers to foster the growth of autonomy in their learners if they themselves do not know what it is to be an autonomous learner; in determining the initiatives they take in their classrooms, teachers must be able to apply to their teaching those same reflective and self-managing processes that they apply to their learning.

PORTFOLIOS

Portfolios in General

Portfolios are used in a variety of fields: finance, strategic management and marketing, politics and government, fine arts, and education. Each specific area determines the type of portfolio used. For example, in finance the portfolio is a collection of institutional or individual investments. In strategic management and marketing, it is a collection of company products, projects, services, or brands offered for sale. In politics and government, it is the post and responsibilities of a cabinet minister or other head of a department. In the arts (painting, architecture, or fashion modeling), it is prior work (photographs, magazine clippings, or other physical evidence of the trade). From these areas, it is very clear that the purposes, and as a consequence, the content of portfolios, are completely different in each case.

Portfolios in Education

Portfolios in education have been around for a long time, long before the digital age. There is a vast variety of definitions of the portfolio in education, a field that has developed and that demonstrates the increase and the multiplicity of the portfolio's use (Barrett, 2000a, 2000b, 2002, June; Bird, 1990; Gibson & Barrett, 2003; Lorenzo & Ittelson, 2005; Paulson & Paulson, 1994; Paulson, Paulson, & Meyer, 1991). A portfolio is a container of documents that provide evidence of someone's knowledge, skills, and/or dispositions (Barton & Collins, 1993, p. 203). It also constitutes a collection (or archive) of reflective writing and associated evidence, which documents learning and that a learner may draw upon to present his or her learning and achievements (Richardson & Ward, 2005). Portfolios appear to represent a move toward learner-centered, self-directed, peer-to-peer, and autonomous learning. As Georgi and Crowe (1998) explained, "Portfolios can motivate students to learn because they have the power to make connections between theory and practice and to select items for the portfolio that express their purpose and design" (p. 75).

Digital or E-Portfolios

Student e-portfolios were born out of print-based portfolios (from the mid-1980s) in mainly art, English, and communication studies. They gained status in higher education during the mid-1990s (Lorenzo & Ittelson, 2005), are now stored in digital form, and are known as digital, computer, or electronic portfolios.

Digital portfolios are selective and purposeful collections of student work, records of learning, growth over time (Barrett, 2000a, 2000b), and they change on the part of the student. They are multimedia representations of learning achievements. They may include text, photographs, illustrations, diagrams, spreadsheets, Publisher and PowerPoint presentations, digital images, videos, music and sounds, voice recordings, and links to useful and interesting websites. They are student-centered, promote active learning and student responsibility, and constitute a showcase of work and reflection. Portfolios provide information to students, parents, teachers, and members of the community about what students have learned or are able to do. Portfolios can be student, teaching, and institutional documents (Lorenzo & Ittelson, 2005).

In teacher preservice education, digital portfolios give students the opportunity to create digitized presentations of their work and skills, and evidence of their competencies. Portfolios bring together curriculum, instruction, and assessment. Some e-portfolios are created with the use of specific programs or systems, off-the-shelf software or customized systems that involve designing a networked system or buying a proprietary software package or online service. According to Grant (2005), they may be "proprietary or open source, [. . .] web based or [. . .] stand alone on a users PC" (p. 75).

Research in the Use of Portfolios

There is a wide body of theoretical research that advocates the use of portfolios in education (Cotterill, McDonald, Drummond, & Hammond, 2004; Dewey, 1983; Paulson & Paulson, 1994; Paulson et al., 1991; Sweet, 1993), in teacher education (Barrett, 2000a, 2000b; Bird 1990; Wolf & Dietz, 1998), and in EFL teaching and learning (Council of Europe, 2001a; Rea, 2001; Wang & Cheng, 2003). The study reported here investigated a case in Cyprus, where preservice language teachers studying CALL engaged in e-portfolio development as an integral part of their learning and their development of reflective and autonomous learning.

FOREIGN LANGUAGE TEACHING AND THE TEACHER TRAINING CONTEXT IN CYPRUS

Foreign Language Education in Cyprus

Cyprus, an island in the eastern part of the Mediterranean Sea, was a British colony from the end of the 19th century until 1960 when it became a republic. As a result, many Cypriots speak English. According to Country Report Cyprus (2004, p. 19), foreign language teaching constitutes one of the five pillars of the educational system of the Republic of Cyprus. Based on the Council of Europe (2001b) perspective, Cyprus language education includes mother tongue/first language, minority languages, and foreign languages.

School Language Program and Autonomous Learning

In the public sector, "Modern Greek is studied throughout primary and secondary education" (Language Education Policy Profile, Cyprus, 2003–2005, 2005, p. 14). At the same time, Cyprus shows its considerable commitment to foreign languages:

> Study of the English language is compulsory from the fourth year of the primary school to the first year of the Lyceum. English and French are compulsory for all three grades of the Gymnasium and in the first class of the upper secondary. At the second year of the Lyceum students choose two foreign languages out of seven (i.e. English (the most

favorite option), French, German, Italian, Spanish, Russian and Turkish) to be studied during the second and third year of the Lyceum. (Language Education Policy Profile, Cyprus, 2003–2005, 2005, p. 14)

In addition, there are many private schools where students are taught mainly in English or another foreign language; "English is the sole language of instruction in 17 out of 34 private secondary schools in Cyprus" (Language Education Policy Profile, Cyprus, 2003–2005, 2005, p. 17). Moreover, "supplementary private tuition outside school hours is widespread. Most parents (estimated at over 80 percent) whose children attend public schools resort to seeking private classes (frontistiria) for them in the afternoon" (Language Education Policy Profile, Cyprus, 2003–2005, 2005, p. 15).

Language Programs at Tertiary Level

There are three government and three private universities in the Republic of Cyprus. The government universities offer their courses in Greek and the private universities in English. They offer mainly two types of language-related courses: Bachelor of Arts in a language and literature, and language courses as compulsory or elective courses in degrees of different nature. For example, the Department of English Studies at the government University of Cyprus (UCY) offers an undergraduate degree program BA in English Language and Literature. English may also be taken as a minor by students from other departments at UCY. At postgraduate level, an MA in Teaching English as a Foreign Language and research PhDs in Linguistics, Literature, and Translation are offered. The Department of French Studies offers a main language program (French Studies, Modern Languages and European Studies Program, Master in French Studies, and Doctorate in French Studies) and secondary programs (French Studies, German Studies, Gender Studies, and European Studies). There is also a Turkish and Middle Eastern Studies Department. Furthermore, the UCY Language Center provides foreign language instruction for all students of the university, offering courses in English, French, Italian, Spanish, German, Russian, and Turkish to meet compulsory language requirements and elective options. The Language Center also provides language instruction and professional teacher training support through its fees-based Adult Education Program. Language for specific purposes courses are tailored to the needs of business and government service communities. The language-teaching program also provides advanced language maintenance courses and training in instructional technology to practicing language teachers. The government Cyprus University of Technology offers English for Academic Purposes (EAP) and English for Specific Academic Purposes (ESAP) for all students as part of the compulsory language requirements of all courses offered in the 10 different departments, and elective options in a variety of languages. It also offers courses in Greek as a second language to foreign students. In addition, it offers a variety of language courses to administrative and teaching staff, professionals, and other interested people in the community. All courses are tailor-made to learners' needs. The languages department of the private University of Nicosia offers a Bachelor of Arts in English Language and Literature. The Language Center of the same university offers a range of languages to meet the compulsory or elective requirements of different courses. These languages include French, German, Italian, Russian, and Greek as a second language. The private European University also offers a Bachelor of Arts in English Language and Literature and English courses to meet the language requirements of different degrees. The private Frederic University offers Greek language electives. The government Open University of Cyprus offers a Bachelor in Hellenic Civilization.

Language Teaching and Learning, Autonomous Learning and Technology

Many developments in language policies, curriculum design, teaching, learning, and assessment, both in Europe and Cyprus, have been facilitated by reference to instruments and documents of the Council of Europe (2001a), such as the *Common European Framework of Reference for Languages* (CEFR), and the *European Language Portfolio* (Language Education Policy Profile, Cyprus, 2003–2005, 2005, p. 7). For example, there was a partial introduction of the European Language Portfolio and an introduction of Language Rooms in a number of schools.

The full implementation of technologies has gained top priority (Country Report, Cyprus, 2004, p. 17). The aim was to encourage students to become autonomous language learners, ensure more efficient learning potential to the full at their own pace, promote and enhance the idea of lifelong language learning, and promote European intercultural awareness and communication identity. Amongst other innovations, the upgrading of the program for better use of the school library, improving, supporting, and upgrading the language rooms, and introducing new syllabuses, enhance autonomous learning (Country Report, Cyprus, 2004, p. 18). All these indicate clearly that autonomous learning is gradually becoming an integral part of language education in Cyprus.

Language Teacher Training

There is also evidence that autonomous learning has started to be addressed in teacher training. The University of Cyprus offers preservice and in-service courses for languages, thus providing assistance and guidance to newly appointed language teachers in preparation for their induction into the state school system. Theses courses have, as their objective, the training of educators in using and applying contemporary strategies, techniques, and approaches in their teaching. The latest teaching and learning theories are introduced and discussed. Amongst others, included in the basic content of the preservice course are the use of the Language Room and the European Language Portfolio. Amongst the methods discussed is autonomous learning (Country Report, Cyprus, 2004, pp. 22–23). At the University of Nicosia, the use of portfolios and the application of autonomous learning constitute integral parts of two courses: Teaching English as a Foreign Language (TEFL) and CALL.

THE STUDY

CALL E-Portfolios: Developing Reflective and Autonomous Learning

The BA in English Language and Literature offered at the University of Nicosia is taught in English and one of its aims is to prepare future teachers in the areas of TEFL and CALL. An integral part of the CALL course is to train students to become autonomous learners through the use of technology in general and through the use of e-portfolios in particular. The whole teaching and learning activity evolves around the use of student digital portfolios. These are used to evidence student development and encourage reflective and autonomous learning. This study aimed at investigating the development of reflective and autonomous learning of the CALL students through the use of e-portfolios.

Participants

Participants were 7 fourth-year BA in English Language and Literature undergraduate degree students. They had already studied literature- and linguistics-oriented courses for seven semesters, including Applied Linguistics, Teaching English as a Foreign Language, and Basic Computer Knowledge. CALL is an eighth semester course. Two of the students were male and five were female. These CALL students participated in this study as a regular class activity. They ranged in age from 18 to 21, with a mean age of 19 years. All of them were Greek Cypriots and all spoke Greek as their first language. They had studied English at primary and secondary levels and also as part of their BA and were learners of English as a foreign language. They were all of C2 level of the CEFR of language competence.

Principles of Portfolio Development

In order to fully respond to the challenges of the current pedagogical thinking, Nunes (2004, p. 328) based the development of portfolios in an EFL classroom on the following two principles: (a) portfolios have to be continually in the making and document work in progress, in other words, they have to be developed in action; and (b) portfolios should document the reflective thought of the learners. Based on those two principles, the CALL class embarked on a program of portfolio development. The objectives of this study were to find out how the record of student reflection in the digital portfolio could contribute to a more informed approach towards reflective and autonomous learning, leading to lifelong learning.

Rationale for the Use of E-Portfolios with this Group of Students

In language teacher education and in the specific area of CALL, the idea is to prepare future teachers who would: (a) be aware of the theoretical and practical trends, (b) have practice in applying theories, and (c) have the ability to reflect on their learning and develop an ability for autonomous and lifelong learning. These were the backbone of the development of the CALL course at the University of Nicosia.

Each task was based on specific criteria that students were expected to meet. Students could submit drafts and resubmit work for improvement through the semester. Assessment was formative. The final product was submitted on a CD, on an individual basis.

Physical Evidence of Reflective and Autonomous Learning

The following was the type of exploratory work students undertook that helped them develop their teaching, critical, and reflective skills, and their skills in autonomous and continuous learning:

- Observation notes of the use of CALL in TEFL classes
- Needs analysis of a specific TEFL teaching situation and the use of CALL
- Annotated review of language websites, with exercises for different language areas (writing, speaking, listening, reading, pronunciation, grammar, vocabulary, expressions and idioms, culture, etc.)
- Evaluative review of two language software programs and two language websites
- The use of two ICT tools in TEFL: theory, examples, and students' own developed examples
- TEFL teaching material development using two different tools (word processor, PowerPoint, webpage creator, MSN, etc.)
- Collaborative, comparative review of two electronic testing tools (collaboration using at least two electronic collaboration programs and keeping a record of the collaboration)
- Development of a digital portfolio, showcasing their learning
- The bibliography and general and specific resources used while researching a topic, which could be used for future references
- Personal profile

- Reflection—the process of student reflective learning included the following:
  - Pre-course entry review of CALL learning
  - Reflective journal during the course
  - Post-course self-evaluation.

METHOD

Introduction of Portfolios

The portfolio provided a framework for the whole course. At the start, the lecturer introduced the notion of e-portfolios to the students, stating the educational aims. She explained that the aims of portfolios were to document each student's progress (as measured by their subjective feelings and the amount of effort they put into the course) and their achievement (as measured by the marks given during the semester). These were based on student work that constituted: (a) learning and evaluation (this included reflective journal, peer evaluation, and end-of-course self-evaluation), (b) development of an evaluation rubric, (c) annotated evaluative review of Internet TEFL teaching activities, (d) evaluative review of a Web 1.0 or Web 2.0 technology and how it is used in TEFL, (e) comparative collaborative online review of L2 testing software, and (f) the development of student e-portfolio, as well as any other information each student believed was relevant. In this way the course began and ended with a portfolio focus. Therefore, besides including completed individual and group work, the portfolios could also contain any other type of material students believed to be important for their learning process (pictures, texts, articles, and other material that had a special meaning for the students) and, above all, reflections on whatever they believed to be important for them as learners and individuals.

From the first week of the semester, students were asked to engage in reflection. They were introduced to the notion and were given examples of each kind of reflective task they were going to be involved in during the duration of the course (review of previous learning, reflective journal, and end-of-program self-evaluation). They were asked to reflect on their previous learning and use of English and technology in writing. They were also given a written example of such a reflective review of learning by their lecturer. During the course, classroom time was also dedicated to the explicit training of learning strategies, having students describe, model, and give examples of the strategies they used to carry out particular tasks, as well as by presenting, describing, and providing practice of new strategies so that they became aware of alternatives.

Eventually, these techniques bore fruit, transforming the portfolios into a curriculum for reflecting before (review of previous learning), during (reflective journal), and after learning (end-of-program self-evaluation), that is, a central curricula framework for the development of the students' meta-cognitive awareness. So, after a somewhat "shy" beginning in portfolio development, in the end, the students produced a comprehensive portfolio with solid evidence of their learning and a substantial record of the process of their reflective learning and their development of autonomy.

RESULTS AND DISCUSSION

Although the majority of the portfolios produced by the students illustrated the idiosyncrasies of their authors and were "unique and single creations," some commonality was also noticed as far as the focus of their work was concerned, though its language and substance are different. A content analysis of the portfolios (based on one of the principles used by Nunes, 2004, p. 328, for the development of portfolios in an EFL classroom) and carried out by the author, displayed the emergence of several recurring issues that the learners referred to mostly in their reflection, as well as the two principles of portfolio development referred to previously.

One of the principles of portfolio development mentioned earlier in this chapter is reflection; for the current study, only entries that brought the dimensions and levels of the students' reflective thought to light were selected. In attempting to identify what the students most reflected on, the entries were grouped according to the issues that repeatedly appeared, and this highlighted four areas: syllabus, instruction, learning, and assessment. The following are examples and quotations of student reflection about these four areas.

Syllabus

Under *syllabus*, we grouped the reflections on the content included in the syllabus, in terms of their relevance for the students, for example:

> Student Quote 1 (IS)
> Assessment, evaluation, problem solving, contemplation, collaboration, experimentation, and technology are just a few words, which summarises this course . . . Learning does not have to be boring or difficult, and with the help of technology, learning becomes easy and pleasurable. In addition, I learned how to think as a future teacher but as a student as well. (end-of-program self-evaluation)
> In summarising this course, the only thing I must say is that I learned things of great significance to me as a future teacher of English. I learned all the methods of teaching; their advantages and disadvantages, the importance of technology in teaching, all the various ICT tools and their meaning in learning, how to evaluate them, how to use them and many

more. In conclusion, I feel very proud of the work I have done and of the choice I made in selecting this course. Now I am thinking of doing my masters in CALL. (Reflective Journal, Wednesday, 5/10/2006)

Student Quote 2 (NM)
When I first heard about CALL, I did not have a clue about what it was or what it was dealing with. I was a little frustrated when I realised that it was about computers and that's because I never had a good relationship with them. My opinion though, started to change with the passing of time as we were introduced in the fields of CALL in more depth. What made this class more interesting was the fact that the course blended theory with application. (end-of-program self-evaluation)

Student Quote 3 (SL)
Through this course I learnt so many things. I found out how to create websites. I learnt how to evaluate different software programs and websites. I made a research with children and found out how to use Microsoft Excel . . . to get the research results . . . on charts. I knew how to make PowerPoint Presentations and how to work with Microsoft Word but I found out new things about these two tools. I cooperated with a classmate [. . .] to do the comparative review. I reflected my previous experience on computers and I put on [. . .] paper my estimation and my comments about this class. In this class, I felt so free to talk and I wouldn't mind even if what I said was something stupid. (end-of-program self-evaluation)

From these representative samples of student reflections on the CALL syllabus, it is apparent that at the end of the course students were clearly aware of its content and of what they learned. They expressed their appreciation of the importance of technology in language teaching; they realized that learning can be pleasurable. Moreover, they became aware of their transformation from teacher trainees to future teachers.

Instruction

In the area of *instruction*, we included the students' reflections on teaching aids and materials, teaching methods, instructional activities, strategies, and tasks. Three examples of the several entries considered in this category appear in the following:

Student Quote 1 (IS)
Today we performed some listening activities. The lecturer proved exactly her point [teaching listening through a listening activity]. (Wednesday, 03/22/2006)

Student Quote 2 (NM)

Today we were given a handout, that included methods and techniques which could help us in teaching. To be more specific, the handout introduced us in how technology has entered and is part of our daily lives. Also we [. . .] learned how to use computers in language learning and know how computers and ICT can enhance teaching and learning of areas such as grammar, speaking and writing, reading and listening comprehension, vocabulary, cultural and intercultural communication. In this lesson . . . we had seen how to use technology [in TEFL] and we visited some [TEFL] activities on the Internet which were very interesting and helpful. (Reflective Journal, Day 11, 3/08/2006)

During this lesson we talked about WebQuests. It is really amazing when you discover that there are such topics as web quests which are not only interesting and helpful but also effective and allow students to be self-sufficient and depend only on themselves. (Reflective Journal, Day 21, 3/27/2006)

In the area of instruction, the representative entries of student reflections record student realization that the following are important: (a) to use the appropriate methodology, (b) to make learning relevant to student everyday life, (c) to make it meaningful, and (d) to include various types of instruction methods, materials, and techniques to make teaching and learning more successful.

Learning

Entries grouped under the heading *learning* included reflections on the contents dealt with in class, on the students' weaknesses, strengths, needs, and learning strategies. The reflections that follow illustrate some of the issues referred to by the students:

Student Quote 1 (IS)

When I chose this course, I knew I was in for a new experience. I chose [it] because I was in the search of new knowledge. I wanted to learn something new and exciting because from all my classes I know what to expect but also I know the boring way of teaching . . . and the boring lecture. In this course the tests were abolished, everything I learned was via problem solving and evaluation, while simultaneously I was being taught and I did not even realise it up until now! It was fun and exciting despite the pressure of time and the stress. In a few words, this course was exhilarating. I have learned the history of teaching methods, boring and exciting, I also learned the advantages and disadvantages of every method and how to use these advantages for my own benefit. In a few words, I was taught how to be a teacher.

Student Quote 2 (NM)

I always had fun when I created something by myself. Imagine how proud for myself I felt when I managed to create my own E-portfolio. That was something I considered impossible to do but it is also something I achieved through CALL . . . In conclusion, CALL, is not only a course that teaches you how you can use the technology to teach English as a foreign language. It is also a course through which I improved my knowledge in computers, I learned how to capture the important points and summarise them, how to collaborate electronically with others and write an excellent paper, but I also learned that impossible is nothing. As my grandmother used to say, "When there is a will there is a way." (end-of-program self-evaluation)

Student Quote 3 (MS)

Taking a look at different TEFL websites I had the benefit of finding out some very interesting language exercises, and learning how to create some of my own . . . I believe that websites like those are the future of language teaching. I found them very useful, and fun. I enjoyed doing those exercises myself.

In the preceding sample entries regarding student reflection about learning, it is evident that students realized through their own CALL learning experience how much one can learn, and how important it is to learn through active involvement, through activities that turn learning into fun and make learning a successful endeavor. Students also realized that they can be proud of the results of their learning and can feel a sense of achievement. Moreover, they have learned how to gradually become autonomous learners.

Assessment

Under *assessment*, we grouped reflections on the students' competence and skills, their performance in classroom tasks and in conventional tests, as well as reflections on the portfolio itself. Examples of some of these entries appear in the following:

Student Quote 1 (IS)

This was our last class and the presentation day . . . We talked about how each of us evaluated this course but also how we evaluate ourselves. It was interesting enough that we all learned what we were supposed but individually we all learned how to think as teachers and how to be good ones also. Sadly, it is the end yet I feel very proud of myself, of the work I have done and of all the new things I have learned! (Reflective Journal, Wednesday, 5/10/2006)

This course has indeed changed the way I think about myself as a future teacher but also as a current student. I have to admit, that at the beginning I was so panicked and afraid that I would not make it to the end. Here I am today feeling proud of myself of what I have achieved. (end-of-program self-evaluation)

Student Quote 2 (SL)

This course was so interesting and honestly I am very proud of the work I have done. I will be very proud presenting my website to the others and say: "Look! This is my work. Look at what I have achieved through CALL lesson." However, I put a lot of effort to finish all this work . . . At first, I didn't believe in myself and thought I couldn't manage to finish, BUT I'm here alive and very proud, because I made it!!! To be honest, the idea of using CALL in TEFL would be something very good and will attract many customers, in case I will open an Institute of English. I will reconsider the idea of having other courses of CALL or seminars or even be specialised in CALL in order to use it in my future job. It will be another qualification in my Curriculum Vitae. (end-of-program self-evaluation)

Student Quote 3 (MS)

My conclusion about this course, and about me as a student in this course, is that you need a lot of organisation, and once you give the right time for each assignment and do them when you are assigned to do, everything will be alright and much easier to handle. If you leave them at the last moment, you just panic and cannot do the work that has to be done, properly. I as a student should have worked harder and devote more time on this course and the exercises, because as it seems they are very interesting and we all learned from them. This was a course that we could actually use in the future as teachers . . . with this course we learned how to use the computer and the internet as a tool for TEFL, and that is the future of education: Computers and CALL. (end-of-program self-evaluation)

Student Quote 4 (ES)

Each one of us had to present our webpage with as many documents he or she could include in his or her e-portfolio. It was a good experience because by seeing others' work I could pick up some points which could be helpful for mine. (Reflective Journal, Week 13, 5/8/2006)

Student reflections on assessment revealed the following: (a) their awareness and appreciation of the competences and skills they acquired during and through the course, (b) their pride in their performances and achievements, and (c) their reflections on the different aspects of their work as a whole, and on their portfolios as a whole, and on the future potential of using CALL in their teaching as future teachers of English.

Table 19.1 shows the number of entries each area had in the portfolios of the 7 students who participated in this study. Although there were 7 students in the class, only 6 participated in the portfolio study in a systematic way.

Table 19.1   Areas of Students' Reflections—Number of Entries

Students	Syllabus	Instruction	Learning	Assessment
LC	7	6	2	2
GE	not completed the course due to health reasons			
SL	6	16	5	3
NM	19	19	12	9
MS	7	7	8	1
IS	23	20	6	12
Total No. of Entries:	62	68	33	27

Areas of Students' Reflections

As Table 19.1 clearly demonstrates, most reflective thoughts produced by the students in their portfolios focused on the domains of instruction (68 entries) and syllabus (62 entries). For assessment there were only 27 entries, and for learning only 33 entries. All entries related to syllabus mainly describe students' interest in the course content, even those of 2 students who found the load somewhat heavy. While there were some references to some parts of the course as being boring (3 students mentioned that the number of language websites reviewed made this activity somewhat monotonous and suggested reducing the number), students' reflection on syllabus and instruction mainly described their positive feelings about the course content, the variety of teaching strategies, materials used, and the activities they were involved in. They also commented on the flexibility in changing aspects of the instruction that did not work as effectively as expected. Although there were some references to students' learning, these mainly concentrated on their weaknesses rather than their strengths, and on strategies they could use to overcome them. Students stated their preference for portfolios as a tool for assessment rather than tests and exams. Students systematically reflected on the way they worked; their work; the knowledge, skills, and experiences they gained from the course; in which areas they could have done better and in what way; and the future prospects of such achievements.

The Value of Reflection

The students' reflections revealed different levels of understanding of issues and learning processes. They also revealed a development of their understanding of self-reflection towards a more systematic and conscious control of their meta-cognitive processes (see *syllabus* student quote 2, *learning* student quotes 1 and 2, and *assessment* student quotes 1 to 4). Their reflections on the syllabus and on instruction provided very useful information to the lecturer on how students feel about the content, materials, and strategies, and what their preferences were. The process also enabled students to develop a critical awareness of the value of their studies. Students' reflections on learning not only provided useful information about their preferred learning styles, needs, and difficulties, but also helped them develop into reflective and autonomous learners. Finally, their reflection on assessment helped them develop their meta-cognitive skills, and encouraged them to become more autonomous learners. Reflecting on their work and the way they worked helped them evaluate themselves and come up with ideas for improvement.

CONCLUSION

This study concentrated on the specific case of incorporating e-portfolios as an integral part of a CALL course, aiming to support reflective and autonomous learning and prepare future teachers of English to become more reflective and autonomous lifelong learners. As current research in the use of e-portfolios (Barrett, 2000a, 2000b; Bird, 1990; Cotterill et al., 2004; Dewey, 1983; Council of Europe, 2001b; Paulson & Paulson, 1994; Paulson et al., 1991; Rea, 2001; Sweet, 1993; Wang & Cheng, 2003; Wolf & Dietz, 1998) and autonomous learning (Benson & Voller, 1997; Holec, 1981, Little, 1991, 1995, 2003; Schunk, 2005) and our study suggests, as an instrument promoting reflection and autonomous learning, the portfolio can develop into a valuable tool in enabling students to become more in control of their learning, more aware of their learning processes, more critical of themselves, and more able to make the link with their previous, current, and future lifelong learning.

REFERENCES

Barrett, H. (2000a). Create your own electronic portfolio: Using off-the-shelf software to showcase your own or student work. *Learning & Leading with Technology, 27,* 14–21.

Barrett, H. (2000b). *Electronic teaching portfolios: Multimedia skills + portfolio development = powerful professional development.* Association for the Advancement of Computing in Education. Retrieved from http://electronicportfolios.com/portfolios/site2000.html

Barrett, H. (2002, June). *Introduction to the forum.* Paper presented at International Society for Technology in Education (ISTE)'s Forum on Assessment and Technology, San Antonio, TX.

Barton, J., & Collins, A. (1993). Portfolios in teacher education. *Journal of Teacher Education, 44,* 200–210.

Benson, P., & Voller, P. (Eds.). (1997). *Autonomy and independence in language learning.* London: Longman.

Bird, T. (1990). The schoolteacher's portfolio: An essay on possibilities. In J. Millman & L. Darling-Hammond (Eds.), *The new handbook of teacher evaluation: Assessing elementary and secondary school teachers* (pp. 241–256). Newbury Park, CA: Sage.

Cotterill, S. J., McDonald, A. M., Drummond, P., & Hammond, G. R. (2004). *Design, implementation and evaluation of a 'generic' e-portfolio: The Newcastle experience. ePortfolio 2004 (Generic ePortfolio).* Newcastle upon Tyne: University of Newcastle.

Council of Europe. (2001a). *Common European framework of reference for languages: Learning, teaching, assessment.* Cambridge: Cambridge University Press.

Council of Europe. (2001b). European language portfolio. Retrieved from http://www.coe.int/t/dg4/portfolio/default.asp?l=e&m=/main_pages/welcome.html

Country Report, Cyprus. (2004). *Language education policy profile.* Cyprus: Ministry of Education and Culture.

Dewey, J. (1983). *Experience and education.* New York: Collier Books.

Georgi, D., & Crowe, J. (1998). Digital portfolios: A confluence of portfolio assessment and technology. *Teacher Education Quarterly, 25*(1), 73–84. Retrieved from http://www.csub.edu/~dgeorgi/projects/digital.htm

Gibson, D., & Barrett, H. (2003). Directions in electronic portfolio development. *Contemporary Issues in Technology and Teacher Education, 2*(4), 559–576. Retrieved from http://www.citejournal.org/vol2/iss4/general/article3.cfm

Grant, S. (2005). The electronic portfolio domain: A suggested set of interrelated technical definitions. Retrieved from http://www.inst.co.uk/clients/jisc/techedef.html

Holec, H. (1981). *Autonomy and foreign language learning.* Oxford: Pergamon.

Language Education Policy Profile, Cyprus, 2003–2005. (2005). Language education policy profile. Strasbourg: Ministry of Education and Culture, Cyprus.

Little, D. (1991). *Learner autonomy: Definitions, issues and problems.* Dublin: Authentik.

Little, D. (1995). Learning as dialogue: The dependence of learner autonomy on teacher autonomy. *System, 23,* 175–181.

Little, D. (2003). Learner autonomy and second/foreign language learning. *Subject Centre for Languages, Linguistics and Area Studies Good Practice Guide.* Retrieved from http://www.llas.ac.uk/resources/gpg/1409

Lorenzo, G., & Ittelson, J. (2005). An overview of e-portfolios. *Educause Learning Initiative.* Retrieved from http://net.educause.edu/ir/library/pdf/ELI3001.pdf

Nunes, A. (2004). Portfolios in the EFL classroom: Disclosing an informed practice. *ELT Journal, 58,* 327–335.

Paulson, F. P., & Paulson, P. (1994). Assessing portfolios using the constructivist paradigm. In R. Fogarty (Ed.) (1996), *Student portfolios: A collection of articles* (pp. 27–45). Palatine, Illinois: IRI Skylight Training and Publishing.

Paulson, F. P., Paulson, P. R., & Meyer, C. A. (1991). What makes a portfolio a portfolio? *Educational Leadership, 48,* 60–63.

Rea, S. (2001). Portfolios and process writing: A practical approach. *Internet TESL Journal, 3*(June). Retrieved from http://iteslj.org/Techniques/Rea-Portfolios.html

Richardson, H., & Ward, R. (2005). *Developing and implementing a methodology for reviewing e-portfolio products: A report to the JISC. (Version 1.0).* Wigan, UK: The Centre for Recording Achievement. Retrieved from http://www.jisc.ac.uk/uploaded_documents/05 percent20epfr percent20REPORT percent20version percent201.0 percent20final.doc

Schunk, D. H. (2005). Self-regulated learning: The educational legacy of Paul R. Pintrich. *Educational Psychologist, 40,* 85–94.

Sweet, D. (1993). Student portfolios: Classroom uses. *Education research consumer guide*. Office of Research, Office of Educational Research and Improvement (OERI) of the U.S. Department of Education. Retrieved from http://www.ed.gov/pubs/OR/ConsumerGuides/classuse.html

Trim, J. L. (1988). Preface. In H. Holec (Ed.), *Autonomy and self-directed learning: Present fields of application* (p. 3). Strasbourg: Council of Europe.

Wang, H., & Cheng, L. (2003). Portfolio assessment for ESL writing. *Contact: Newsletter of the Association of the Teachers of English as a Second Language (TESL) of Ontario, 29*(3), 50–54.

Wolf, K., & Dietz, M. (1998). Teaching portfolios: Purposes and possibilities. *Teacher Education Quarterly, 25*, 9–22. Retrieved from http://www.teqjournal.org/backvols/1998/25_1/1998v25n103.PDF

20 Voices from EFL Teachers
A Qualitative Investigation of Teachers' Use of CALL

Seijiro Sumi

INTRODUCTION

The term "normalization" (Bax, 2003) has been gaining attention from CALL researchers and has aroused considerable discussion among them. According to Bax, normalization is the stage in which the use of technology is truly integrated into teaching practices and the physical existence of technology goes unnoticed.[1] For example, a wristwatch, a pen, and shoes are all technologies, yet we hardly even recognize them as technologies because they have become normalized in our everyday practice.[2] Bax called normalization the final stage of CALL and this concept has provided a new theoretical perspective on the use of technology in foreign language teaching.

Warschauer (1998) also mentioned that:

> The truly powerful technologies are so integrated as to be invisible. We have no "BALL" (book-assisted language learning), no "PALL" (pen-assisted language learning), and no "LALL" (library-assisted language learning). When we have no "CALL," computers will have taken their place as a natural and powerful part of the language learning process. (para. 11)

However, the stage of integration and normalization has yet to be achieved in most educational settings (Chambers & Bax, 2006). A number of studies have been carried out to identify factors that contribute to hindering the use of technology. For example, Kessler (2007) conducted a Web-based survey of 108 graduates of MA TESOL programs, and concluded that poor quality and limited quantity of CALL-related teacher preparation programs had a significant effect on teachers' (non)use of technology. In the Japanese context, Edasawa, Takeuchi, and Saeki (1994) conducted a large-scale survey of 454 schools in which LL facilities had been used, and pointed out the factors that prevented teachers from using technology in foreign language teaching, such as difficulties in using the facilities and lack of supports.

Zapata (2004), however, criticized the previous studies and claimed that it was important to investigate teachers' actual use of technology in the "context" where technology was used. She stated that "most of the existing studies have been based on instructors' self-reported perceptions and application of instructional technology, but have not investigated actual classroom use or the institutional and pedagogical factors that influence that use" (p. 340). According to Zapata (2004), teachers' perceptions of and readiness for the use of technology in the classroom were not considerations detached from the real world in which they live, but were collectively constructed results that were deeply rooted in local practices. Similarly, Egbert, Huff, Mcneil, Preuss, and Sellen (2009) insisted, referring to Jung (2005) and Kern (2006), that teachers played a vital role in integrating technology well into instruction and determining the success of the CALL classrooms. They also emphasized the importance of investigating CALL practices from teachers' perspectives in a given context, including teachers' voices, observations, and concerns, saying "most important, studies neglected to look at the context, specifically those areas on which teacher voice and experience could shed light for explanation of the phenomena under investigation" (p. 765). Lafford (2009), summarizing previous CALL studies, stressed that it was significant for CALL studies to identify the factors that impede teachers' use of technology and hinder integration and normalization of the use of technology from teachers' perspectives in given local contexts.

THE PRESENT STUDY

The purposes of this study are (a) to investigate the factors that impede "integration" (Warschauer, 1998) and "normalization" (Bax, 2003) of the use of technology in foreign language teaching from teachers' point of view, and, based on the findings, (b) to propose a perspective that integrates technology into teaching practices.

Participants and Environment

Interviews were carried out with 24 participants in this study. All of them were English instructors (12 males and 12 females) experienced in using LL or CALL facilities (i.e., technologies) in the Japanese EFL context. Except for one who was teaching at a junior high school,[3] all of them were teaching at tertiary institutions. The participants were selected because of their wide teaching experience and experience in using LL or CALL facilities and computers. The average length of teaching career was 14.79 years (max. = 30, min. = 1, SD = 8.64 [years]) and of experience of using computers was 17.79 years (max. = 30, min. = 5, SD = 7.11 [years]). Among them, a total of 23 instructors used computers every day and quite often. Nineteen of them had experience in using LL facilities, and 16 of them had experience in using CALL facilities.

To get more detailed information, classroom observation was conducted at five universities. The universities were chosen based on the results of the interviews, and took into consideration the technological settings in classrooms and students' levels of English.[4] Also, in this study, an in-depth explanation of two classes was provided among the five classroom observations, as examples of typical LL and CALL classrooms settings in the Japanese EFL context (Cases 1 and 2).[5]

The classroom setting of Case 1 was based on a standard LL system, which is one of the longest-lived and best-selling LL systems. The instructor in charge of Case 1 had six years' teaching experience at the university and 10 years experience in using computers. The purposes of the Case 1 course were to improve students' listening ability and to enhance their grammatical competence in English. One lesson lasted for 90 minutes. There were 18 students in Case 1. Students' English ability was relatively low, with Test of English for International Communication (TOEIC) scores ranging from 200 to 400.

The classroom setting of Case 2 was based on an advanced CALL system. The instructor in charge of Case 2 had 25 years' teaching experience and 26 years' experience in using computers. There were 40 students in Case 2. The purpose of the course was again to improve students' listening ability. One lesson lasted for 90 minutes. Students' English ability was intermediate, with TOEIC scores ranging from 400 to 600.

METHOD

Data Collection

A semi-structured interview was adopted for this study because it allowed interviewees to elaborate on particular issues and introduce new ones (Thornton & Sharples, 2005). Each interview lasted 30–60 minutes per participant, and interviews were recorded and later transcribed by the author with the participants' permission. Major questions asked during the interview were regarding (a) their present use of technology, (b) the factors that might affect the use of technology in the classroom, and (c) their perception of (or reaction to) using technology in foreign language teaching. Interview data were collected from January 2007 to February 2008, and all interviews were conducted in Japanese and translated into English by the author. Table 20.1 shows the list of the participants.

Based on the findings obtained through the interviews, classroom observation was conducted at five universities to investigate difficulties in the use of technology within the classroom context, with the permission of the instructors in charge.

Table 20.1   The List of the Participants

No.	ID	Gender	Years in teaching English	Years in using computers	Experience in using LL facilities	Experience in using CALL facilities
1	01_F01	F	4	18	yes	yes
2	01_M01	M	30	15	yes	no
3	01_F02	F	14	24	yes	yes
4	01_F03	F	22	9	yes	no
5	01_F04	F	6	26	no	yes
6	01_M02	M	13	10	yes	no
7	01_M03	M	25	26	yes	yes
8	01_M04	M	25	20	yes	yes
9	01_M05	M	30	30	yes	yes
10	01_M06	M	27	30	yes	yes
11	01_F05	F	6	9	yes	yes
12	01_F06	F	15	20	yes	yes
13	02_M01	M	19	23	yes	yes
14	02_M02	M	6	10	yes	no
15	02_M03	M	20	25	yes	no
16	02_F01	F	6	20	yes	no
17	02_F02	F	12	15	yes	no
18	02_F03	F	20	25	yes	yes
19	02_F04	F	1	5	no	yes
20	02_F05	F	4	9	no	yes
21	02_M04	M	16	15	no	yes
22	02_M05	M	16	17	yes	yes
23	02_M06	M	5	11	yes	yes
24	02_F06	F	13	15	yes	yes

In the classroom observations, instructors' actions during lessons were recorded from multiple perspectives by applying a triangulation procedure to the data collection process. Triangulation is one of the research methodologies that make it possible to examine the complex structure of practices from multiple sources (Dörnyei, 2007; Takeuchi, 2003). Two video cameras were set up to record instructors' behavior during lessons. The first video camera was set up to capture instructors' operation of the LL or CALL system; the second was set up in the rear of the classroom to shoot the whole classroom. Field notes were taken in Japanese by the author during lessons and later translated into English by him. Follow-up interview sessions were held after lessons to investigate what and how the instructors were thinking while they were using technology during the lesson.

Data Analysis

A part of the grounded theory approach procedure (Corbin & Strauss, 2008) was used in the analysis of the data collected through the interviews. According to Corbin and Strauss, this approach is "a specific methodology developed by Glaser and Strauss (1967) for the purpose of building theory from data" (p. 1), and the analysis in the approach is "a process of examining and interpreting data in order to elicit meaning, gain understanding, and develop empirical knowledge" (p. 1).

In general, the process of the grounded theory approach can be divided into four steps: (a) open coding, (b) axial coding, (c) comparative analysis, and (d) conceptual saturation (Corbin & Strauss, 2008; Harada, 2003). According to Corbin and Strauss (2008, pp. 159, 195), each step is defined as follows:

(a) Open coding: Breaking data apart and delineating concepts to stand for blocks of raw data
(b) Axial coding: Crosscutting or relating concepts to each other
(c) Comparative analysis: Comparing incident against incident for similarities and differences
(d) Conceptual saturation: Acquiring sufficient data to develop each category/theme fully in terms of its properties and dimensions and to account for variation.

In this study, the steps from (a) to (c) were applied. To maintain objectivity in the coding process, inter-rater reliability of all the coding results between the author and a postgraduate student who is majoring in foreign language education was calculated: It was at 82.5 percent. Intra-rater reliability was also calculated, showing 93.0 percent of agreement. The author decided that the results were at an acceptable level of agreement, as 70 percent agreement seems to be the benchmark (Potter, 1996). Disagreements between the raters were discussed and solved between the two raters. MAXQDA 2007 (Kuckartz, 2007) was utilized as a tool for analyzing the data. The software has been developed especially for qualitative analysis (Corbin & Strauss, 2008; Lewins & Silver, 2007).

To analyze the instructors' use of technology in a context in which technology was actually used, video observation data were digitalized and segmented according to the critical aspects of a lesson. Each segment of a lesson was labeled by four features: (a) time, (b) description of action, (c) equipment in use, and (d) scene. These features were generated in accordance with Goodwin and Goodwin (1996), who observed a work-place in an airport, and divided workers' actions into three categories—timelines, description of situation, and tools that workers used—in order to capture workers' actions as a whole. Based on their idea, the four features were formulated by the author and used to categorize teachers' actions in this study. These four features allowed us to capture instructors' successive actions with timeline data and pictorial images and to observe the "entire world" in which teachers were actually involved. These four features also made it possible to investigate how difficulties in the use of technology emerged along with instructors' actions within the classroom context.

RESULTS

Interview

As a result, three factors that seemed to be impeding the use of technology in foreign language teaching were found:

1. Technology factor (with 4 sub-factors)
2. Environment factor
3. Institution factor (with 2 sub-factors).

Technology Factor

The factor includes (a) gaps in intention between system developers and instructors, (b) system instability, (c) operation complexity, and (d) con-strained technology settings.

A first problem that most instructors complained about were the gaps between what system developers thought that instructors wanted to do and what they in reality wanted to do in lessons.

> It may be OK to have a fully functional CALL system. A company says that you can do this and that. But I am not sure if I can use all of those features in lessons. I just want to use a simple networked classroom instead. (01_M03_52–53; translation mine)

> There is a gap between system developers and instructors with regard to the merits of the use of technology in classes. It takes me a lot of time to adjust myself to the system's features. (01_F04_40–41; translation mine)

A number of instructors also reported that operation complexity is another problem. Figure 20.1 presents a line of control devices that are placed in

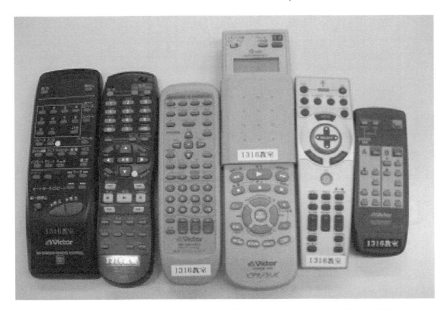

Figure 20.1 From the left, control devices for audio, DVD, amplifier, VHS, projector, and an unknown device, all placed in a single CALL classroom.

a CALL classroom. To use a VTR, a DVD, or a CD player in the CALL classroom, instructors need to manipulate a corresponding control device. The problem of operation complexity especially occurs when an instructor alternately uses several players in succession. System developers tend to install all the devices that are expected to be used during lessons within the limits of the available budget. As a result, each player in the system has a different control device, and this makes operation complex. Norman (1988) criticizes such a phenomenon as "creeping featurism," which means adding features that increase the system's complexity more and more, so that eventually the system becomes unusable and unstable.[6]

Figure 20.2 presents a typical example of CALL system interface design. The video and sound input resources that are set in different circuits make operating a system difficult for instructors. For example, in order to play a DVD, an instructor needs to select video and sound input resources separately and almost simultaneously. This system setting is clearly different from our "mental model to play the DVD," which gives us predictive and explanatory power for understanding how to play the DVD (Norman, 1983). In addition, there are usually three sets of output combinations, such as students' monitors and headsets, instructor's monitor and headset, and room monitor and loudspeakers. As a consequence, countless numbers of buttons are placed on a console box, and instructors need to control them swiftly during lessons. Instructors commented as follows:

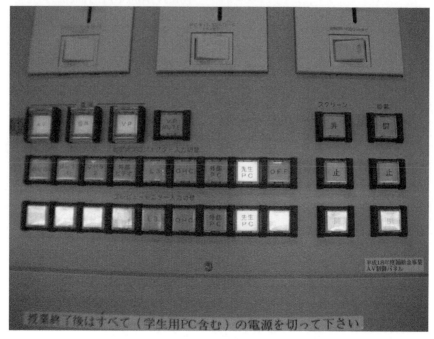

Figure 20.2   Teachers need to select input resources by pushing buttons swiftly during lessons.

You know, there are many buttons. I have never figured out which is which. It is a mess. (02_F01_67–67; translation mine)

DVD, VTR, CD, and Tape; every player has a different control device. (01_F04_50; translation mine)

Environment Factor

This factor contains no subcategory. Most of the instructors' comments centered on the CALL/LL classroom size. In the Japanese context, CALL classrooms are usually designed to accommodate a large number of students. Classroom size, therefore, is often bigger than typical classroom sizes. In addition, classrooms are crammed to the maximum with desks, chairs, and computers. As a result, they impede smooth interaction between an instructor and students. Figure 20.3 is a picture taken in an LL classroom. There was almost no space left between aisles. What is worse, the students put their bags in the aisle, so that the instructor could hardly walk around the classroom; smooth interaction with students during the lessons was thus hindered.

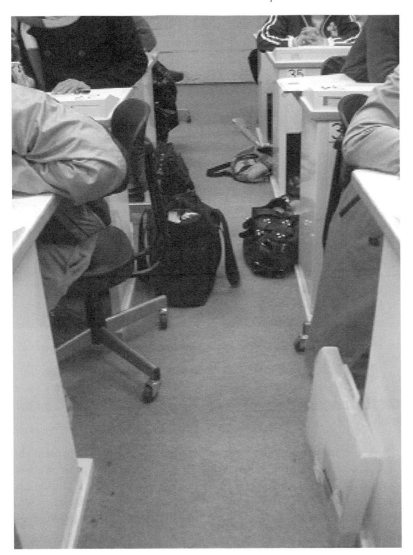

Figure 20.3   A picture taken in an LL classroom.

There is little space available around students, so that they have no choice but to put their bags in the aisle beside them, which prevents the instructor from having smooth interaction with students during lessons.

Figure 20.4 shows an overall picture of a CALL classroom. The classroom was designed to accommodate about 60 students and each student had an individual computer, so that almost no space was available for interaction between the instructor and the students.

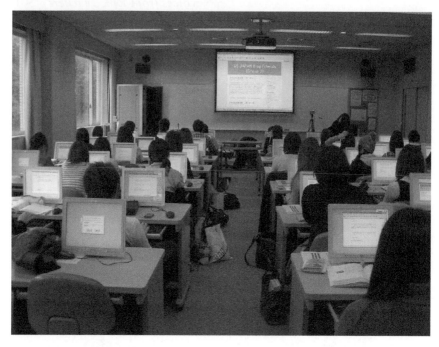

Figure 20.4   A CALL classroom, showing how difficult it is for the instructor to see students' faces and have smooth interaction with them.

The instructor who was using the classroom said in the interview as follows:

> If you want to conduct student-centered learning, I do not think a CALL classroom is suitable for that. CALL classrooms are better suited for drill practices and individual learning. I think human inter-action is important for language teaching, but it is really difficult for me to have it with students in a CALL classroom. (01_M06_25–26; translation mine)

In another interview, an instructor commented as follows:

> I can barely see the students' faces because of the classroom size. (02_F01_44; translation mine)

Institution Factor

Lastly, the institution factor, which includes the lack of (a) teacher support and (b) teacher training, should be explained. This factor was also identi-fied in Chambers and Bax (2006). Most instructors interviewed said they would like to have some sort of support or teacher training in the use of technology in foreign language teaching.

> We definitely need a support system for the use of technology during lessons. That is, full-time staff who can provide technical advice. (01_M03_69–70; translation mine)

> If we had a person who could take care of technical problems in CALL classrooms, we could save a lot of time and concentrate on teaching. (02_F06_96; translation mine)

An instructor who wanted to have teacher training in the use of CALL said the following:

> I am willing to use my pocket money, if I could have teacher training in the use of technology. But the university doesn't offer such training for staff. (01_F05_73; translation mine)

Summary of Interviews

In the interviews, it became clear that instructors use facilities in a limited way, adjusting their teaching styles or lesson plans to the environmental and technological settings in the classroom. In addition, many instructors believe that using computers for foreign language education is useful, but LL or CALL facilities are not necessarily utilized as intended and are often regarded as impeding face-to-face interaction between an instructor and his/her students. Instructors also tend to be excessively fearful in using technologies for teaching because system features and interface design of CALL facilities are extremely complicated. The following instructor's comment seems to summarize succinctly a dilemma that may be shared by many instructors in the Japanese EFL context:

> If I could use technology appropriately during lessons, it could help my students understand better and I could make my lessons more appealing. But, in reality, I am just worried about using it in a way that goes beyond my current skills. I do not want to waste my time just on handling devices during lessons, so I use them as far as I can handle them. (02_F01_31–33; translation mine)

Classroom Observation

Case 1

Figure 20.5 shows the system setting of Case 1. The system was designed and upgraded based on a standard LL system, which is one of the longest-lived and best-selling LL systems. The system can handle six types of input

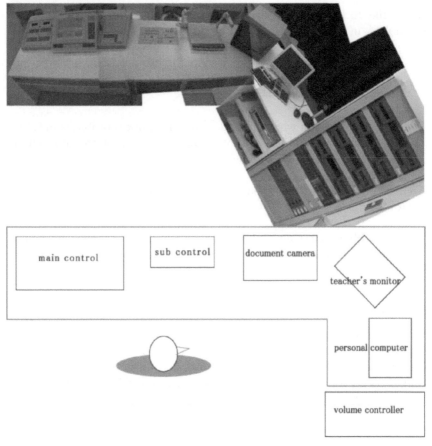

Figure 20.5   The Case 1 system setting. To handle many input and output combinations, the system has the subcontrol unit. However, operation of the main control is not synchronized with the subcontrol unit, so that a teacher has to manipulate both units simultaneously to play video or audio devices.

resources such as (a) cassette, (b) VHS, (c) DVD (CD), (d) LD, (e) document camera, and (f) PC. The system can also handle six types of output resources such as (g) students' monitors, (h) students' headsets, (i) students' cassettes, (j) a room projector, (k) room speakers, and (l) an instructor's monitor. Accordingly, in this room, more than 30 input and output combinations are available, which makes operation extremely difficult (Figure 20.6).

This problem is evident when the instructor makes the shift from one device to another, for example, from a DVD to a PC. Table 20.2 describes the instructor's action and operation of the system while he was giving students a dictation task. He showed the students some scenes from a movie on a DVD, and the students tried to fill in the blanks on a handout provided. He gave the students some time so they could check their answers, and then

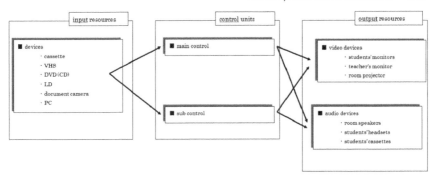

Figure 20.6   This shows the system configuration of Case 1.

he changed the input resource from a DVD player to a document camera to check students' answers. Although this is a very common teaching procedure that we often see and do in LL or CALL classrooms in the EFL context, the instructor had to go through five steps as quickly as possible with this system.

To play the DVD again, the instructor needed to go back through the same procedure. This back-and-forth action from the DVD to the document camera was observed 14 times during the lesson in this case. Even though the instructor got used to this operation, he made a mistake on 2 occasions of the 14 in this lesson. In addition, consistent rules for labeling the buttons did not exist on the Case 1 system interface, so that different labels were printed on a pair of buttons such as "VHS1" on the main control and "S-VHS" on the subcontrol, or "VID1" on the main control and "書画" (labeled in Chinese Characters, "Document Camera") on the subcontrol, although both buttons in each pair refer to the same device. Inconsistent interface design and labeling made operation much more difficult.

Table 20.2   A Procedure for the Use of an LL System during a Lesson

Time	Description of action
0:13:07	Pause the DVD with the remote control.
0:13:11	Put the handout on the document camera.
0:13:16	Press the button on the main control's touch panel, and change the video resource from "VHS1" (DVD Output) to "VID1" (Document Camera Output).
0:13:17	Press the "OK" button on the main control's touch panel, and confirm the video output resource.
0:13:20	Press the button on the sub control unit, and change the video resource from "S-VHS" (DVD Output) to "書画" (named in Chinese Characters, "Document Camera").
0:13:23	Give the students instructions looking at the teacher's monitor.

Case 2

Figure 20.7 shows the system setting of Case 2. The system was designed based on an advanced CALL system. The distinguishing feature of this system is that the system can send digitalized data such as CD sound files and DVD video files to the students' PCs, and the students' PCs can record data on their hard disk drives. Once recording is finished, the students are able to study on an individual basis.

Because of the way that various components were installed, however, the system configuration had become extremely complicated. What made the system difficult to use was that the output device unit (including CD, DVD, and VHS players), the input control unit, and the output control unit were all separately arranged around the instructor's console. Hence, the instructor had to manipulate three units to play just a single DVD in the classroom. In addition, each unit had a different interface design and inconsistent labels, so that the instructor needed to figure out the system setting every time. Table 20.3 describes the instructor's actions and operation of the system while he was playing a DVD and trying to send the DVD's data to students' PCs and the projector.

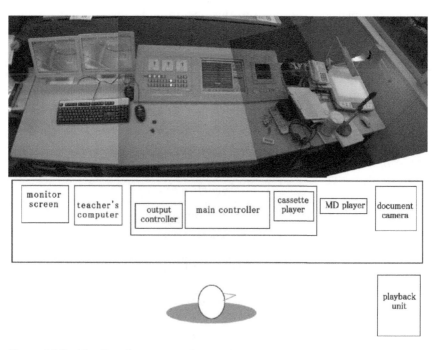

Figure 20.7   The Case 2 system setting.

Table 20.3 A Procedure for the Use of a CALL System during a Lesson

Time	Description of action
0:19:22	Press the button on the main control unit, and select DVD as an input resource and students' PCs as an output channel.
0:19:36	Press the button on the output control unit, and select the room projector and instructor's monitor as an output channel.
0:19:53	Pause the DVD with the remote control.
0:20:47	Press the button on the main control unit, and start recording. Start the DVD with the remote control.
0:21:06	Adjust the audio output level of the DVD with the volume-control slider on the output device unit.

Summary of Classroom Observations

The two cases described here are not exceptional. Creeping featurism, inconsistency of interface design and labeling, and cramped classroom settings were all observed in five universities wherein the classroom observation was conducted. These problems impeded the integration and normalization of technology use within the classroom context.

The two cases also illustrate the current situation that exists in the use of technology in the Japanese EFL context: LL and CALL classrooms were developed to facilitate foreign language teaching, and educational institutions have paid a large amount of funding for that, but what we actually found was that the more the instructors tried to use technology installed in classrooms, the more they faced difficulties in its use. Furthermore, the more the instructors used technology during the lessons, the more they needed to stick to the console unit to push countless buttons, and they thus had extreme difficulty in having face-to-face interaction with their students. In addition, without technical support and teacher training, instructors who would like to move forward in using technology for classes have few opportunities to improve their teaching practice and to become more acquainted with the possibilities of using LL or CALL facilities in language teaching.

DISCUSSION

Through the interviews, three impeditive factors—(a) technology factor, (b) environment factor, and (c) institution factor—became clear, and through the classroom observations, the question of how instructors' use of technology had been impeded in real classroom contexts was clarified.

The author suspects that the instrumental perspective (Warschauer, 1998), which views technology in isolation from the users and their contexts (Kersten, Kersten, & Rakowski, 2004), can be a root cause of the dire situations illustrated in this study. If we base our teaching approach on that perspective, we can easily presume the usefulness of new technology and adopt it without considering the classroom contexts wherein teachers actually use technology in language teaching. Similarly, Bax (2003) criticized the instrumental perspective and called it "'Sole Agent' fallacy" (p. 26), which means that neglecting the factors indispensable for successful CALL implementation discourages its use in teaching.

The author believes these situations can be improved by taking an alternative perspective, an ecological one, into account in designing and implementing technology for language teaching (Bax, 2000, 2003; Chambers & Bax, 2006; Takeuchi, 2007; Tudor, 2002, 2003). According to Tudor (2003), "an ecological perspective involves exploring language teaching and learning within the totality of the lives of the various participants involved, and not as one sub-part of their lives which can be examined in isolation" (p. 4). Therefore, an ecological perspective on the use of technology for foreign language teaching involves exploring language teaching within the totality of the context in which actual language teaching occurs (Warschauer, 1998).

In the light of ecological psychology, Gibson (1966, 1986) stated that the living animal and the environment are interrelated and never to be handled separately. He argues that human action and perception are stimulated and embedded in a situation or a context, and objects or spaces that surround us always give us possibilities for action in a given context, in other words, "affordance." Based on this concept, Norman (1988) used affordance for analyzing the tools that we use in everyday life. From an ecological perspective of second language acquisition, van Lier (2004) proposed ecological linguistics and mentioned that language learning occurs as emerging from the context in which language learners are engaged and wherein they draw on affordance. According to van Lier, affordance for language learning means "a relationship between an organism (a learner, in our case) and the environment that signals an opportunity for or inhibition of action" (2004, p. 4). The common features of the aforementioned studies are to identify actions and perceptions of human beings as a consequence of mutual interaction of person and the environment. In this sense, person and the environment are inseparable in a context (Thorne, 2003; Zukow & Ferko, 1994). Applying this idea to CALL research, it can be said that person (teachers and learners) and technology are interrelated in a classroom context.

Bronfenbrenner (1989) defined human development as "a joint function of person and environment" (p. 188), and formulated the theory based on Lewin (1935) as follows:[7]

D = f(PE)

According to Bronfenbrenner (1989), the "D" term refers to "development," the "P" term refers to "person," and the "E" term refers to "environment." "D" is a function of both personal and environmental factors. In a similar vein, the author believes that the use of technology in foreign language teaching cannot be discussed without the context, and should be integrated into the classroom context. To put into effect an ecological perspective with the foregoing in mind, the author would like to present an extended version of Bronfenbrenner's formula as follows:

U = f(PCT)

In this formula, the "U" term refers to the "use of technology in foreign language learning," the "P" term refers to "person," including teachers and learners, the "C" term refers to "classroom context," and the "T" term refers to "tools." The process of the use of technology in foreign language teaching can be described as a joint function of person, classroom context, and tools. By looking at the use of technology in our field by means of this formula, the author thinks that technology can obtain a "field of meanings" (Wenger, 1990) and can be integrated into the classroom context.

CONCLUSION

The results of this study suggested the three impeditive factors and illustrated how these factors hinder instructors' use of technology in the Japanese EFL context. Furthermore, to ameliorate the dire situations and to achieve integration and normalization of the use of technology in language teaching, the author stressed the ecological perspective. As Garrett (2009) clearly stated, "the full integration of technology into language learning" (p. 719) has come to be one of the central themes of CALL studies. Now CALL is meant to integrate many factors related to foreign language teaching into teaching practices. In the process of designing and implementing teaching practices, the ecological perspective, which involves exploring the use of technology within the totality of the context in which actual language teaching and learning occur, should be taken into account.

NOTES

1. Similarly, Wenger (1990) mentioned that once a tool is used in a local context, it obtains *a field of meaning*. As a result, it becomes invisible among people who use it and achieves cultural transparency.
2. For tools in everyday life, see also Norman (1983, 1988).

3. The junior high school is a private school that has a fully equipped CALL classroom. The level of English language teaching at the school is extremely high. This is because the author included the instructor in the data pool.

4. TOEIC scores ranging from 200 to 600.

5. In the Japanese EFL context, LL or CALL classrooms are usually designed to accommodate about 50 students.

6. Norman (1988) said, "complexity probably increases as the square of the features: double the number of features, quadruple the complexity. Provide ten times as many features, multiply the complexity by one hundred" (p. 174).

7. Bronfenbrenner (1989) also reformulated the formula and redefined it as follows: "Dt = f(t–p)(PE)(t–p)." In this formula, the concept of "a particular point in time" (p. 190) was incorporated, where "t" referred to the time and "t–p" referred to period. By incorporating the dimensions of time, human development shifted from static outcomes to dynamic changes. According to Bronfenbrenner (1989), human development can be defined as follows: "The set of processes through which properties of the person and the environment interact to produce constancy and change in the characteristics of the person over the life course" (p. 191).

REFERENCES

Bax, S. (2000). Putting technology in its place: ICT in modern foreign language teaching. In K. Field (Ed.), *Issues in modern foreign language teaching* (pp. 208–219). New York: RoutledgeFalmer.

Bax, S. (2003). CALL: Past, present and future. *System, 31*, 13–28.

Bronfenbrenner, U. (1989). Ecological systems theory. *Annals of Child Development, 6*, 187–249.

Chambers, A., & Bax, S. (2006). Making CALL work: Towards normalisation. *System, 34*, 465–479.

Corbin, J., & Strauss, A. (2008). *Basics of qualitative research: Techniques and procedures for developing grounded theory* (3rd ed.). London: Sage.

Dörnyei, Z. (2007). *Research methods in applied linguistics: Quantitative, qualitative, and mixed methodologies.* Oxford: Oxford University Press.

Edasawa, Y., Takeuchi, O., & Saeki, N. (1994). Use of language learning laboratory: A questionnaire survey. *LLA Kansai Chapter Monograph Series, 5*, 15–49.

Egbert, J. L., Huff, L., Mcneil, L., Preuss, C., & Sellen, J. (2009). Pedagogy, process, and classroom context: Integrating instructor voice and experience into research on technology-enhanced language learning. *Modern Language Journal, 93*(1), 754–768.

Garrett, N. (2009). Computer-assisted language learning trends and issues revisited: Integrating innovation. *Modern Language Journal, 93*(1), 719–740.

Gibson, J. J. (1966). *The senses considered as perceptual systems.* London: George Allen and Unwin.

Gibson, J. J. (1986). *The ecological approach to visual perception.* Hillsdale, NJ: L. Erlbaum.

Glaser, J., & Strauss, A. (1967). *The discovery of grounded theory.* Chicago: Aldine.

Goodwin, C., & Goodwin, M. H. (1996). Seeing as a situated activity: Formulating planes. In Y. Engeström & D. Middleton (Eds.), *Cognition and communication at work* (pp. 61–95). Cambridge: Cambridge University Press.

Harada, K. (2003). Hitowa donoyouni tashano nayamiwo kikunoka: Gurand-edo seori apurochi ni yoru hatugen kategori no seisei [How do people counsel others in everyday life? Verbal categories developed with a Grounded Theory Approach]. *Journal of Educational Psychology, 51*, 54–64.

Jung, U. O. H. (2005). CALL: Past, present and future—A bibliometric approach. *ReCALL, 17*, 4–17.

Kern, R. (2006). Perspectives on technology in learning and teaching languages. *TESOL Quarterly, 40*, 183–210.

Kersten, G. E., Kersten, M. A., & Rakowski, W. M. (2004). Software and culture: Beyond the internationalization of the interface. In. G. Hunter & F. Tan (Eds.), *Advanced topics in global information management* (Vol. 3) (pp. 56–71). Hershey, PA: Idea Group Publishing.

Kessler, G. (2007). Formal and informal CALL reparation and teacher attitude toward technology. *Computer Assisted Language Learning, 20*, 173–188.

Kuckartz, U. (2007). *MAXQDA 2007*. Berlin: Verbi Software.

Lafford, B. A. (2009). Toward an ecological CALL: Update to Garrett (1991). *Modern Language Journal, 93*(1), 673–696.

Lewin, K. (1935). *A dynamic theory of personality*. New York: McGraw-Hill.

Lewins, A., & Silver, C. (2007). *Using software in qualitative research: A step-by-step guide*. London: Sage.

Norman, D. A. (1983). Some observations on mental models. In D. Gentner & L. Stevens (Eds.), *Mental models* (pp. 7–14). Hillsdale, NJ: L. Erlbaum.

Norman, D. A. (1988). *The psychology of everyday things*. New York: Basic Books.

Potter, W. J. (1996). *An analysis of thinking and research about qualitative methods*. Mahwah, NJ: Lawrence Erlbaum.

Takeuchi, O. (2003). *Yoriyoi gaikokugo gakushuhouhou wo motomete: Gaikokugo gakushu seikousha no kenkyu* [In search of good language learning strategies: Studies on good language learners in the Japanese FL context]. Tokyo: Shohakusha.

Takeuchi, O. (2007). Gakushusha, kyojyusha, media: Gaikokugo kyoiku kenkyu no togoteki wakugumi ni mukete [Learners, teachers, and media: An integrative framework for the foreign language education research]. In O. Takeuchi (Ed.), *Explorations of English language instruction: Papers in honor of Professor Eiji Saito on his retirement from Kansai University* (pp. 90–102). Tokyo: Sanseido.

Thorne, S. L. (2003). Artifacts and cultures-of-use in intercultural communication. *Language Learning & Technology, 7*, 38–67.

Thornton, P., & Sharples, M. (2005). *Patterns of technology use in self-directed Japanese language learning projects and implications for new mobile support tools*. Paper presented at the Proceedings of the 2005 IEEE International Workshop on Wireless and Mobile Technologies in Education. Retrieved from http://ieeexplore.ieee.org/iel5/10547/33360/01579265.pdf

Tudor, I. (2002). Exploring context: Localness and the role of ethnography. *Humanising Language Teaching, 4*. Retrieved from http://www.hltmag.co.uk/mar02/mart1.htm

Tudor, I. (2003). Learning to live with complexity: Towards an ecological perspective on language teaching. *System, 31*, 1–12.

van Lier, L. (2004). *The ecology and semiotics of language learning: A sociocultural perspective*. Boston: Kluwer Academic Publishers.

Warschauer, M. (1998). *CALL vs. electronic literacy: Reconceiving technology in the language classroom*. Paper presented at the CILT Research Forum. Retrieved October 21, 2008, from http://www.cilt.org.uk/research/papers/resfor2/warsum1.htm

Wenger, E. (1990). *Toward a theory of cultural transparency: Elements of a social discourse of the visible and the invisible.* Unpublished doctoral dissertation, University of California, Irvine.

Zapata, G. C. (2004). Second language instructors and CALL: A multidisciplinary research framework. *Computer Assisted Language Learning, 17,* 339–356.

Zukow, P. G., & Ferko, K. R. (1994). An ecological approach to the emergence of the lexicon: Socializing attention. In V. Steiner, C. Panofsky, & L. Smith (Eds.), *Sociocultural approaches to language and literacy: Interactionist perspective* (pp. 170–190). New York: Cambridge University Press.

Contributors

EDITORS

Mike Levy is Professor of Second Language Studies at the University of Queensland, Brisbane, Australia. His research focuses upon Computer-Assisted Language Learning (CALL) and includes studies on the role of technology in *ab initio* language learning, teacher education and learner training, mobile learning for Italian, and distance education for Mandarin Chinese. His publications include *CALL Dimensions* with Glenn Stockwell (Erlbaum, 2006) and *Teacher Education in CALL* with Philip Hubbard (Benjamins, 2006). He is also Chair of the Conference Planning Committee for WorldCALL 2013 (www.worldcall.org).

Françoise Blin is currently Associate Dean for Learning Innovation in the Faculty of Humanities and Social Sciences at Dublin City University, Ireland. She is Vice-President of EUROCALL, co-editor of *ReCALL* (with June Thompson), and deputy editor of *Alsic* (Apprentissage des Langues et Systèmes de Communication). She has been working in CALL since the late eighties and holds a Ph.D. in Educational Technology from the Open University, UK. Her more recent work focuses on the applications of Activity Theory to CALL research, design, and practice.

Claire Bradin Siskin directs the English as a Second Language Writing Online Workshop at Excelsior College in Albany, New York. She has been an enthusiastic practitioner of CALL since 1983. She serves on the editorial boards of both the *Computer Assisted Language Learning Journal* and *CALICO Journal*. She is a past chair of the CALL Interest Section of TESOL as well as the Executive Board of the Computer Assisted Language Instruction Consortium (CALICO). She co-chaired the program for the WorldCALL Conference in Japan in 2008.

Osamu Takeuchi, Ph.D., is Professor of Applied Linguistics in the Faculty of Foreign Language Studies/ Graduate School of Foreign Language Education and Research, Kansai University, Osaka, Japan. Currently, he is Dean of the Faculty and the Graduate School. His work has appeared in such international journals as *System*, *CALICO*, *ReCALL*, *Language Teaching Research*, *Innovation in Language Learning and Teaching*, and *International Journal of Applied Linguistics*. His research interests include language learning strategies, metacognition, motivation, and CALL.

AUTHORS

Professor Carla Barsotti, M.Sc. in Technology, has been teaching English as a Foreign Language (EFL) since 1987. From that time on she has been actively participating in EFL, Education and Technology events. In 2003 she launched the Specialization in Foreign Language Teaching Course at Universidade Tecnológica Federal do Paraná (UTFPR) in Curitiba, Brazil, which she coordinated for 3 years. Carla is currently teaching English as a Foreign Language and Foreign Language Teaching Methodology at UTFPR.

Wai Meng Chan received his M.A. and Ph.D. degrees in German Language and Literature from the German Universities of Würzburg and Kassel respectively. He is an Associate Professor and Director of the Centre for Language Studies at the National University of Singapore. His research currently focuses on learner autonomy, metacognition, new technologies in language learning and learner motivation. He has published a book and several edited books as well as numerous book chapters and journal articles in these fields. He is also Editor of the peer reviewed Electronic Journal of Foreign Language Teaching and a founding member of the NUS Teaching Academy.

Ing Ru Chen received her M.A. in Phonetics from the University of Trier, Germany and has been teaching at the NUS since July 2000. Her research centres on the application of multimedia technologies to foreign language teaching and learning, mother-tongue interference in foreign language acquisition, course design, and materials development.

Deborah (Debbie) Corder is Head of the Department of International and Community Languages at the Auckland University of Technology. She has taught Japanese at secondary and tertiary levels, and more recently developed courses in intercultural competence with colleague Alice U-Mackey. Her research interests are primarily in the interrelated fields of language acquisition, learner autonomy, ICT, and intercultural competence. She is co-author of a series of textbooks for senior school Japanese, and her work has appeared in the series on autonomy in the Authentik Books for language teachers, *CALL-EJ* (with Grant Waller), and *ACM Inroads* (with Alice U-Mackey).

Martin G. Döpel is Lecturer at the Centre for Language Studies of the National University of Singapore, teaching German as a Foreign Language. He received his M.A. from the University of Jena, Germany. His research interests include Web 2.0 applications in foreign language learning and psycholinguistic aspects of foreign language learning with an emphasis on neuropsychological questions.

Ana Gimeno-Sanz, Ph.D. in English Philology, has been a member of the teaching and research staff at the Department of Applied Linguistics, Universidad Politécnica de Valencia (UPV), Spain, since 1985 and is Associate Professor in English language. She has published numerous research papers on language learning and teaching, more specifically in the fields of English for Specific Purposes (ESP) and Computer-Assisted Language Learning (CALL). Dr Gimeno is Head of UPV's CAMILLE Research Group, which is devoted to research in CALL. She has been the Project Manager of several funded multimedia CALL research and development projects which have led to the publication of a number of language courses on CD-ROM: *Español Interactivo* and *Español en marcha* (Barcelona: Difusión, 1998), *Valencià Interactiu* (Valencia: Bromera, 2000), *City Talk* (London: Libra Multimedia, 2000), *¡Bienvenido a bordo!* (London: Unicorn, 2002), *Vida Urbana* (Valencia: SP-UPV, 2004), *Airline Talk* (Valencia: SP-UPV, 2005), and via the internet by means of the *InGenio* authoring tool and delivery environment: *Intermediate Online English* (2004), *Valencià Interactiu—Grau Mitjà* (2004), Czech A1 & A2 (2007), and Slovak A1 and A2 (2007). She is currently President of the European Association for Computer-Assisted Language Learning (EUROCALL).

Yoshiko Goda is Associate Professor at the Research Center for Higher Education and Instructional Systems Program Graduate School of Social and Cultural Sciences at Kumamoto University, Japan. She received her Ph.D. (Science Education) at the Florida Institute of Technology in 2004 with the partial support of a Fulbright scholarship. Her current research interests are self-regulated learning for e-learning, online education program evaluation, Computer-Assisted Language Learning, and innovative communities for global education.

Karin Harbusch is Professor of Computational Linguistics and Artificial Intelligence at the Computer Science Department of the University of Koblenz-Landau since 1995. Her primary interest is in natural-language generation and understanding by computer, in particular based on the formalisms of Tree Adjoining Grammar and Performance Grammar. Applied projects deal with tutorial e-learning systems for first- and second-language teaching, and with computational writing support for severely motor-impaired users. From 1989 till 1995 she held a position as senior researcher at the DFKI (German Research Center for Artificial

Intelligence) in Saarbrücken, where she had received her Ph.D. at Saarland University in 1989. At the DFKI, she participated in several language generation and knowledge representation projects, including the VERBMOBIL research program on spoken language translation.

Philip Hubbard is Senior Lecturer in Linguistics and Director of English for Foreign Students at Stanford University (USA). A professional in Computer-Assisted Language Learning (CALL) for over 25 years, he has published in the areas of software development and evaluation, technology and listening, teacher education, learner training, CALL research, and CALL theory. He is an associate editor of *Computer Assisted Language Learning* and serves on the editorial boards of three other major CALL journals. He recently edited the four-volume series *Computer Assisted Language Learning: Critical Concepts in Linguistics* (Routledge, 2009).

Gerard Kempen (1943) is Emeritus Professor of cognitive psychology at Leiden University and Research Associate of the Max Planck Institute for Psycholinguistics in Nijmegen. From 1976 to 1992 he was Professor of psycholinguistics at the Radboud University in Nijmegen, where he had received his Ph.D. in 1970. His scientific work concerns the grammatical aspects of human sentence production and comprehension. He is studying these topics through a combination of linguistic, experimental-psychological, and computational methods. Since 1980 he has initiated and supervised various theoretical and applied research projects dealing with the computational treatment of Dutch, among other things, for visual-interactive grammar instruction (sentence analysis) in secondary education.

Ferit Kılıçkaya is a research assistant and a doctorate candidate at the Department of Foreign Language Education at the Middle East Technical University, Ankara, Turkey. His main area of interest includes Computer-Assisted Language Learning and testing, educational technology, and language teaching methodology. He has published several articles and reviews in journals such as *CALL-EJ Online, Educational Technology & Society, Teaching English with Technology, Educational Studies* and *The Turkish Online Journal of Educational Technology*. He is currently one of the Editors of *Teaching English with Technology: A Journal for Teachers of English.*

Midori Kimura, Ph.D. in TESOL, is a Professor at the School of Nursing at Tokyo Women's Medical University in Japan. Her research interests include learning strategies, learning styles, and CALL as well as MALL with a special focus on the usage of mobile phones. Her most recent work will be appearing in a book, *Open Source Mobile Learning: Mobile Linux Applications* (now being printed), and other published works are included in *Research Highlights in Technology and Teacher Education*

2009, *The Journal of Medical English Education, The Society of English Studies,* and *JACET Journal.* She is a co-editor of *JACET Journal.*

Teresa Kuwamura is a Lecturer of English in the Faculty of Technology at Osaka Sangyo University, Osaka, Japan. Her work has appeared in the *Bulletin of John Dewey Soceity of Japan,* the *Journal of English and English Education,* and *The Katahira.* She has received a B.A. in China, an M.B.A. in the USA, and a Ph.D. in Japan. Her studies focus on appropriate ways to apply student-centered approaches in English education in Japan taking diversified perspectives, such as comparative and international education, culture, history, pedagogy, philosophy, psychology, and sociology.

Marie-Noëlle Lamy is Professor of Distance Language Learning at the UK Open University. She has 15 years of experience in designing and implementing languages courses for online study, involving extensive use of e-tutorials, text-based as well as voice-based. She has researched extensively in the field of computer-mediated communication for language learning, with a particular interest in real-time conversations in multimodal settings. Her current main foci are investigating methodologies for the description of such conversation, and researching co-construction of cultures by groups of learners in multimodal online environments.

Hsien-Chin Liou is Professor and Department Chair of Foreign Languages and Literature in National Tsing Hua University at Hsinchu, Taiwan, Republic of China. Her work has appeared in *Language Learning and Technology, CALICO Journal, Computer Assisted Language Learning, System,* some books and book chapters. CALL issues she has addressed include the use of concordancers in various contexts for various language skills, the use of Web 2.0 technologies for writing, multimodal literacies, corpora processing and tools for language teaching and learning, and vocabulary learning enhanced by various e-tools.

Suen Caesar Lun is Assistant Professor in linguistics at the Dept. of Chinese, Translation and Linguistics, City University of Hong Kong. He was President of the Linguistic Society of Hong Kong from 2004–2005. Being deeply interested in applying linguistics in real-world applications, he has developed many CALL courseware packages and websites and NLP applications with Langcomp Company Ltd. (http://www.langcomp.com.hk/ <http://www.langcomp.com.hk/>). His idea of CALL can be found in his book *An Integrated Approach to Computer-Assisted Language Learning,* Hong Kong: LangComp Co. Ltd. published in 2006.

Claudia Martins is a Professor of English as a Foreign Language (EFL) and Technology at Universidade Federal do Paraná (UTFPR) in Curitiba,

Brazil. She was also the coordinator of the Modern Foreign Languages Academic Center at UTFPR for three years. She holds an M.Sc. in Production Engineering—Media and Knowledge from Universidade Federal de Santa Catarina (UFSC). Claudia is currently a doctoral student in the Graduate Program in Technology at UTFPR.

Yuri Nishihori is Professor of English in the Faculty of Music at Sapporo Otani University, and Emeritus Professor of Hokkaido University, Sapporo, Japan. Her research interests include applied linguistics, English teaching methodology and educational technology, especially collaborative learning. She has presented her research at several international conferences, including the International Association of Applied Linguistics (AILA), the International Conference on Computers in Education (ICCE) and WorldCALL. She was an executive member of the JACET (Japan Association of College English Teachers) and the president of its Hokkaido Chapter from 2004 to 2010, as well as undertaking the role of counselor for the Japanese Society for Information and Systems in Education (JSiSE) from 2004 to 2009.

Hiroyuki Obari is Professor in the College of Economics at Aoyama Gakuin University in Tokyo. He obtained his M.A. in TESOL from Columbia University and his Ph.D. in Computer Science from University of Tsukuba. He was a visiting research fellow at the University of Oxford from 2007 to 2008. He specializes in CALL, Educational Technology, TESOL, and Speech Recognition. His work has appeared in the AACE papers and CALL related Journals. He has made many presentations at EuroCALL, WorldCALL, e-Learn, ED-MEDIA, GLo-CALL, and ASIA TEFL.

Berit Peltonen, M.A., is a Lecturer in Swedish Business Communication at the Aalto University School of Economics. She is also an author of several textbooks in Swedish Business Communication. Her teaching and research interests include the role and development of guidance and feedback in e-learning courses, the use of audit clips, and student-produced digital videos and podcasts.

Pasi Puranen, M.A., is a Lecturer in Spanish Business Communication at the Aalto University School of Economics where he has developed and taught both online and blended learning courses. His research interests focus on guidance in e-learning and Latin American sociolinguistics. He is also an author of several textbooks in Spanish as a foreign language.

Kenneth Romeo, Ph.D. (http://kenro.web.stanford.edu) is an Academic Technology Specialist for the Language Center and an instructor in English for Foreign Students at Stanford University. He has over 20 years experience teaching English in the US and Japan. He is currently involved in large scale assessment using Stanford's Sakai instance and participated in the publication of the Sakai Teaching and Learning Group's Design Lenses, which will guide future generations of learning management systems.

Dr. Erifili Roubou has been a Director of Studies and English language tutor for the past 10 years. She currently owns and runs an English language school where she carries out various research projects in the field of Computer-Assisted Language Learning (CALL), second language writing, and testing. Her teaching experience involves all levels of proficiency, and age groups from young learners to university students at Aristotle University in Greece. She has presented at many conferences in various countries and has also worked as a reviewer for LangUE 2008 and Essex Graduate Student Papers in Language & Linguistics.

Itesh Sachdev was born and brought up in Kenya, did his primary and early secondary education in Kenya, completed secondary and undergraduate education at the University of Bristol in the UK, and doctoral training in social psychology at McMaster University in Canada. He then taught and conducted research in Applied Linguistics, and was also Head of the School of Languages, Linguistics & Culture at Birkbeck, University of London. Since 2005 he has been at the School of Oriental and African Studies (SOAS, University of London) as Director of the SOAS-UCL Centre for Excellence in Languages of the Wider World, and Professor of Language and Communication in the SOAS Department of Linguistics. He has published widely in the social psychology of language and intergroup relations, having conducted research with various ethnolinguistic groups including those in/from Bolivia, Canada, France, Hong Kong, India, Japan, Taiwan, Thailand, Tunisia and the UK.

Akihiko Sasaki is an English teacher at Kwansei Gakuin Junior High School, Nishinomiya, Japan. He also serves as a member of the working committee of the Japan Association for Language Education and Technology (LET). He received a B.A. in Political Science and an M.A. in Education from Kwansei Gakuin University, and his second M.A. degree in TESOL and the Graduate Certificate in CALL from Monterey Institute of International Studies, USA. His research focus is on the use of CMC, especially e-mail, in English teaching and learning.

Salomi Papadima-Sophocleous is Assistant Professor in Applied Linguistics, specialising in Computer-Assisted Language Learning, and Director of the Language Centre at Cyprus University of Technology. Her work has appeared in *CALICO Journal, Outer Limits: A Reader in Communication & Behavior Across Cultures, The Reading Matrix, Teaching English* with *Technology, Babel, Informatologia, WorldCALL 2009 Proceedings, EuroCALL Review,* and *Educational Novelties for the School of the Future.* She is the author of *Voilà,* printed and digital material for the teaching of French in Australia. She has taught TGreekSL/CALL (RMIT University, Australia) and TEFL/CALL (University of Nicosia, Cyprus) online. She was awarded the Middlesex University prize in 2005 for professional excellence in recognition of her project Development and Implementation of an Online English Placement Test. She has recently received a research grant for the development of digital language teaching and testing materials for languages for specific academic purposes (English, French, Greek, Italian, Spanish, German).

Seijiro Sumi, Ph.D., is a full-time Lecturer in the Faculty of Commerce, University of Marketing and Distribution Sciences, Kobe, Japan. He received an M.A. from Tokyo Metropolitan University and Ph.D. from Kansai University. He also serves as a member of the working committee of the Japan Association for Language Education and Technology (LET). He is currently interested in the integrative application of digital media to language teaching/learning. His work has appeared in *Computers and Education, The Journal of Information and System in Education,* and *Language Education and Technology.*

Akiyoshi Suzuki is Associate Professor of English and American Literature in the Department of English Language and Literature in the Faculty of Letters at Konan Women's University, Kobe, Japan. His work has appeared in the *Journal of English and English Education, Convention of Strategy for College Education and Information, On Effective Utilization of CALL in English of Foreign Language, A Study of University Foreign Language Teaching in the New Era,* and *Journal of Text Study.* He has been developing "E-Job 100", supported by KAKENHI [21520608] and is currently an Executive Director of the Japan Society of Text Studies.

Maija Tammelin, Ph.D., M.A., is a Senior Lecturer in English Business Communication at the Aalto University School of Economics where she also has served as the Director of the Department of Languages and Communication. She has presented widely on CALL issues in international conferences. She is a long-time member of the Academic Advisory Panel of the *ReCALL* journal.

Sylvie Thouësny received a B.A. in German literature and a B.Sc. in computational linguistics. She is currently a Ph.D. student at Dublin City University, Ireland, nearly at the completion stage of her thesis. Her areas of research focus on language learner modeling and dynamic assessment, and include several aspects of computational linguistics such as error analysis, human-computer interaction, and ICALL system design and development. She has presented parts of her work in international and European conferences such as CALICO and EUROCALL, and has articles published and under review. To follow her, do visit http://icall-research.net.

Nathalie Ticheler has taught in a variety of educational settings from primary to higher education, including corporate training for major companies and international organisations. She is an experienced e-learning project manager and author of e-learning materials in French, Italian and Spanish. Nathalie has launched the Flexi-Pack project at the Centre of Excellence for the Teaching and Learning of Languages of the Wider World (School of Oriental and African Studies, University of London). She is now a senior lecturer in French at London Metropolitan University. Nathalie's research focuses on students' experience of Virtual Learning Environments for Modern Foreign Languages in the context of blended learning. Nathalie can be contacted by email (n.ticheler@londonmet.ac.uk) and on Twitter (nvticheler).

Alice U-Mackey is a senior lecturer in the Department of English and Applied Linguistics at the Auckland University of Technology, New Zealand. She has also worked in Burma, Maldives and China and has extensive tertiary teaching experience in the areas of English for academic and specific purposes. Her research interests include academic literacies, group assessments in multicultural classrooms, intercultural communicative competence and ICT. She has presented research papers at international conferences in Canada, Australia, Thailand and Singapore and her work has appeared in the *Journal of Higher Education Research and Development* (with Pat Strauss) and *ACM Inroads* (with Deborah Corder).

Yuxia Wang is a Ph.D. student in applied linguistics at the Department of Chinese, Translation and Linguistics, City University of Hong Kong. Her research focuses on first/second language acquisition, Computer-Assisted Language Learning, and psycholinguistic study.

Index